TREATING SUBSTANCE ABUSE

The Guilford Substance Abuse Series

Howard T. Blane and Thomas R. Kosten, Editors

Treating Substance Abuse

Theory and Technique

SECOND EDITION

Edited by

Frederick Rotgers
Jon Morgenstern
Scott T. Walters

THE GUILFORD PRESS
New York   London

© 2003 The Guilford Press
A Division of Guilford Publications, Inc.
72 Spring Street, New York, NY 10012
www.guilford.com

Printed in the United States of America

This book is printed on acid-free paper.

Last digit is print number: 9 8 7 6 5 4 3 2 1

Library of Congress Cataloging-in-Publication Data

Treating substance abuse : theory and technique / edited by Frederick
  Rotgers, Jon Morgenstern, Scott T. Walters.— 2nd ed., [rev. and
  expanded].
      p.   cm. — (The Guilford substance abuse series)
    Includes bibliographical references and index.
    ISBN 1-57230-897-4 (hardcover)
    1. Substance abuse—Treatment.
      [DNLM: 1. Substance Abuse—therapy. 2. Substance Abuse—
    psychology. 3. Alcoholism—psychology. 4. Alcoholism—therapy.]
    I. Rotgers, Frederick. II. Morgenstern, Jon. III. Walters, Scott T.
    IV. Series.
    RC564.T734 2003
    616.86'06—dc21

                                                    2003012710

About the Editors

Frederick Rotgers, PsyD, ABPP, is Associate Professor and Associate Director of Clinical Training in the Department of Psychology at the Philadelphia College of Osteopathic Medicine. Dr. Rotgers has lectured, taught, and published extensively on a variety of topics related to behavior therapy and addictions. His current research interests include measuring and enhancing motivation to change addictive and other problematic (i.e., criminal) behaviors in underserved populations, and the integration of substance abuse screening and brief intervention into primary care settings.

Jon Morgenstern, PhD, is Vice President and Director of the Division of Health, Treatment Research, and Analysis at the National Center of Addiction and Substance Abuse at Columbia University (CASA). He is also Associate Professor of Psychiatry and Health Policy at the Mount Sinai School of Medicine, where he directs a substance abuse treatment program for disadvantaged mothers. Dr. Morgenstern has expertise in substance abuse treatment and health services research. His areas of interest include cognitive-behavioral treatments, strategies to improve community-based substance abuse programs, and the coordination of treatment across substance abuse, welfare, and child welfare systems. Dr. Morgenstern's research program in substance abuse treatment and health services has been supported by the National Institutes of Health since 1990.

Scott T. Walters, PhD, is Assistant Professor of Behavioral Sciences at the University of Texas School of Public Health, Dallas Regional Campus. His research interests include college student health and substance abuse, brief motivational approaches to treatment, and electronic and mailed interventions. He has authored more than two dozen articles on theoretical and applied aspects of psychology, and two books for children. Dr. Walters has acted as a consultant for several universities, is a frequent speaker to campus, community, and medical groups, and has received national and international awards for his work.

Contributors

Gary R. Birchler, PhD, School of Medicine, University of California, San Diego, and VA Medical Center, San Diego, California

Alan J. Budney, PhD, Department of Psychiatry, University of Vermont, Burlington, Vermont

Kathleen M. Carroll, PhD, Department of Psychiatry, Yale University School of Medicine and VA Connecticut Healthcare System, West Haven, Connecticut

Elizabeth E. Epstein, PhD, Center of, Alcohol Studies, Rutgers—The State University of New Jersey, Piscataway, New Jersey

William Fals-Stewart, PhD, Research Institute on Addictions, University at Buffalo, The State University of New York, Buffalo, New York

Stephen T. Higgins, PhD, Human Behavioral Pharmacology Lab, Department of Psychiatry, University of Vermont, Burlington, Vermont

Daniel S. Keller, PhD (deceased), formerly at the Department of Psychiatry, Division of Alcoholism and Drug Abuse, New York University School of Medicine, New York, New York

Jeremy Leeds, PhD, Director of Counseling and Guidance, Horace Mann School; private practice, New York, New York

Barbara S. McCrady, PhD, Center of Alcohol Studies, Rutgers—The State University of New Jersey, Piscataway, New Jersey

Thomas J. Morgan, PsyD, Center of Alcohol Studies, Rutgers—The State University of New Jersey, Piscataway, New Jersey

Jon Morgenstern, PhD, The National Center on Addiction and Substance Use at Columbia University; School of Psychiatry, Mt. Sinai School of Medicine, New York, New York

Theresa B. Moyers, PhD, Department of Psychology, Center on Alcoholism, Substance Abuse and Addictions, University of New Mexico, Albuquerque, New Mexico

Joseph Nowinski, PhD, Department of Psychology, University of Connecticut, Storrs, Connecticut

Timothy J. O'Farrell, PhD, Department of Psychiatry, Harvard Medical School, VA Boston Healthcare System, Brockton, Massachusetts

Frederick Rotgers, PsyD, ABPP, Department of Psychology, Philadelphia College of Osteopathic Medicine, Philadelphia, Pennsylvania

Edward Rubin, PsyD, Outpatient Behavioral Health Service, Aurora Sinai Medical Center, Milwaukee, Wisconsin

Bill Saunders, PhD, William Montgomery Consulting, Leederville, Australia

Rene D. Sell, MS, Center of Alcohol Studies, Rutgers—The State University of New Jersey, Piscataway, New Jersey

Stacey C. Sigmon, PhD, Behavioral Biology Research Center, Johns Hopkins Bayview Medical Center, Baltimore, Maryland

Tania Towers, MS, Drug and Alcohol Office, Western Australia Department of Health, Mount Lawley, Australia

Jalie A. Tucker, PhD, Department of Health Behavior, School of Public Health, University of Alabama at Birmingham, Birmingham, Alabama

Rudy E. Vuchinich, PhD, Department of Psychology, University of Alabama at Birmingham, Birmingham, Alabama

V. Ann Waldorf, PhD, New Mexico VA Healthcare System, Albuquerque, New Mexico

John Wallace, PhD, Executive Director, The Maxwell Institute of St. Vincent's Hospital Westchester, Tuckahoe, New York

Scott T. Walters, PhD, University of Texas School of Public Health, Dallas Regional Campus, Dallas, Texas

Celia Wilkinson, MS, Drug and Alcohol Office, Western Australia Department of Health, Mount Lawley, Australia

Contents

Introduction

Frederick Rotgers
Jon Morgenstern
Scott T. Walters

This edition of *Treating Substance Abuse: Theory and Technique* (TSA) has been longer in arriving than any of us had hoped. Tragically, soon after we had started to revise the first edition, our colleague and friend Daniel S. Keller died of lung cancer. This new edition is dedicated to his memory.

Shortly after Dan's death, the two remaining editors (Frederick Rotgers and Jon Morgenstern) began a series of positive career changes that were so time consuming that this revision was put on the back burner for many months. After selecting Scott T. Walters as our third editor, we finally got back on track, with the assistance (and gentle but persistent prodding!) of our editor at The Guilford Press, Jim Nageotte. Even then, one of our chapter authors was forced to withdraw due to ill health, and the final manuscript was delayed still further. At long last, however, the process was completed. The volume you hold in your hands represents the outcome of that lengthy process.

In the Introduction to the first edition we stated that the field of substance abuse treatment was a field "in transition." In terms of theory and practice, the field is less in transition now than it was in 1995. Many of the methods and procedures covered in the first edition have begun to be integrated routinely into clinical practice. In particular, motivational and cognitive-behavioral approaches, following the surge of interest in these approaches in research studies, have made great inroads into practice at the grassroots level. Nonetheless, the field remains largely committed to the same traditional philosophies and approaches, mostly grounded in 12-step philosophy, that were dominant at the time of our first edition.

As we said, this field is much less in a state of turbulence than it was at the time of the first edition, perhaps settling into what Thomas Kuhn referred to as "normal science" in which there are active efforts toward solving problems, but within existing theoretical paradigms (Kuhn, 1962). Despite the slowing pace of advances in treatment technologies, the present volume is much revised from the first edition. Since then, a substantial body of research and clinical techniques has emerged that developed mainly from operant behavioral theories focusing on contingency management. Those theories and approaches, to which only a few paragraphs were devoted in the first edition, have now been allocated two chapters of their own.

Most of the chapters in this second edition have been revised, and there are a number of new authors whose work represents emerging theories, techniques, and talents in the field. The decision to provide separate consideration for operant/contingency management approaches led to the need to revise the existing behavioral chapters to reflect that change.

Chapter 13 (Carroll) on pharmacological approaches has been updated to include the latest advances in the pharmacological treatment of substance abuse. Unfortunately, the use of medications specific to the treatment of substance abuse, despite reasonably strong research evidence for their efficacy, has not become widespread in practice. Yet research continues in this area with efforts underway to evaluate combined psychosocial and pharmacological therapies for alcohol dependence (e.g., Project COMBINE; Zweben, 2001) and to develop a "vaccine" against the effects of cocaine (Kantak et al., 2000). Given the outspoken views of representatives from several major government funding agencies (Leshner, 1999), it is not surprising that pharmacological approaches are among the most hotly researched and heavily funded of all approaches to substance abuse treatment.

The last major change in this new edition has been made in response to readers and critics who asked for an integrative, clinically focused chapter that presented information on how clinicians approach clients with substance use disorders in "real life." In Chapter 14 (Rubin), an experienced clinician focuses on how the theoretical and technical knowledge presented in the rest of the book are integrated into actual clinical practice.

OVERVIEW OF THE BOOK

In order to help practitioners better prepare for the significantly increased emphasis on matching clients to treatments (the somewhat middling results of Project MATCH notwithstanding, client–treatment matching continues to have intuitive appeal and research support from smaller scale studies), we have assembled a group of authors who are experts in, and strong proponents of, six major approaches to treatment that are available to nonphysicians: (1) 12-step, (2) psychodynamic, (3) marital/family, (4) cognitive-behavioral, (5) contingency management, and (6) motivational approaches. These approaches were selected for a variety of reasons.

Approaches based on the Alcoholics Anonymous 12-step model are still clearly dominant in the field of substance abuse treatment in the United States, and have continued to dominate despite significant inroads from both motivational and cognitive-behavioral approaches. This influence has no doubt been reinforced by research projects such as Project MATCH (Longabaugh & Wirtz, 2001), which have begun to provide good research evidence for the efficacy of some 12-step-based approaches. Although the theory behind 12-step treatment, as presented in Chapter 1 by John Wallace, has not changed since the first edition of this book was published, the 12-step facilitation approach as presented by Joseph Nowinski in Chapter 2 has been refined and validated as an effective treatment approach for many clients. Nowinski's chapter reflects the recent advances in this approach.

Although psychodynamic theory traditionally has not addressed itself to substance abuse, a number of innovative approaches based in psychodynamic thinking have begun to develop in recent years. These new approaches are particularly attractive because of their potential to enhance the implementation and efficacy of other treatment approaches. In both research and clinical settings, an increased emphasis is being placed on working with clients who have co-occurring psychiatric and substance use disorders (e.g., Rosenthal & Westreich, 1999). Because of this, psychodynamic approaches, though they were not originally developed to treat addictive psychopathology, can provide useful ways of conceptualizing and working with substance users. Jeremy Leeds and Jon Morgenstern have revised their chapter for the present edition (Chapter 3) to reflect ongoing work among psychodynamic theorists of addiction. Daniel S. Keller's chapter (Chapter 4) is still an excellent overview of how to think psychodynamically while using empirically validated approaches to changing substance abuse behavior.

Marital and family approaches to substance abuse treatment have a long and diverse history, and have garnered some of the strongest research evidence for their efficacy. In addition to strong research support, these approaches provide a means of integrating apparently disparate aspects of a client's life into a more coherent treatment and support network that can help produce and maintain changes in substance use. Barbara S. McCrady, Elizabeth E. Epstein, and Rene D. Sell (Chapter 5) provide an updated view of theoretical advances in marital and family approaches. William Fals-Stewart, Timothy J. O'Farrell, and Gary R. Birchler (Chapter 6) present a clinician's overview of the rich variety of marital and family approaches that have been empirically validated and are currently available to therapists.

Cognitive-behavioral approaches, while not widely used clinically, have become more apparent in clinical programs, at least in name. These approaches have amassed the strongest research support for efficacy of any approaches presented in this book (although motivational enhancement and contingency management approaches are rapidly gaining empirical ground!). Cognitive-behavioral approaches are ideally suited to client–treatment matching because they are inherently oriented to the individual, with each client's treatment being potentially different in scope and process depending on the results of thorough pretreatment and ongoing assessments. Frederick Rotgers (Chapter 7) has revised his chapter to reflect ongoing research into the mechanisms of change in cognitive-behavioral treatments. Thomas J. Morgan (Chapter 8) has revised his chapter from the first edition, providing an even more articulated and thorough overview of how cognitive-behavioral approaches are implemented in practice.

Contingency management approaches are behavioral therapies that increasingly have been found to be efficacious since the first edition of this book was assembled. Originating in the theoretical ideas of B. F. Skinner, contingency management approaches share the advantage with marital and family approaches that the client's environment is mobilized in the service of behavior change and maintenance. Strongly supported by research evidence, contingency management treatments can be particularly effective in combination with cognitive-behavioral and 12-step components in a broad-based treatment "package." Rudy E. Vuchinich and Jalie A. Tucker (Chapter 9) present an overview of one theoretical approach that underlies contingency management: behavioral economics. While the behavioral economic approach can be somewhat daunting initially, we believe that it represents an important advance in understanding and treating addictive behavior, and will reward the reader's persistence. Alan J. Budney, Stacey C. Sigmon, and Stephen T. Higgins (Chapter 10) have provided an excellent overview of the diverse ways in which contingency management, and the understandings of human behavior that emerge from theories such as behavioral economics, can be translated into practical interventions for change that have shown both initial success and the ability to produce lasting changes in substance abuse behavior.

Motivational enhancement approaches have continued to garner both research support and clinical popularity. Perhaps the most influential development in the late 20th century substance abuse treatment field, motivational enhancement approaches are now established in the mainstream of substance abuse treatments. Based on research in social psychology and behavior change theories, motivational enhancement approaches attempt to mobilize clients to change maladaptive behavior to more healthful patterns. To some extent these approaches have gained popularity as a reaction against traditional confrontational approaches that focus on aggressively breaking through client "denial." Instead of aggressive confrontation, these motivational approaches take advantage of client ambivalence about the pros and cons of substance use to help produce movement toward change (Miller & Rollnick, 2002). The motivational theory chapter by Bill Saunders, Celia Wilkinson, and Tania Towers (Chapter 11) has been substantially revised by Scott T. Walters and Frederick Rotgers to reflect ongoing theoretical advances in motivational treatments.

Theresa B. Moyers and V. Ann Waldorf (Chapter 12) have provided a useful overview of how to think about and implement motivational approaches in clinical settings.

In addition to the chapters on these six approaches, we have included an updated chapter on psychopharmacological approaches to substance abuse treatment by Kathleen M. Carroll (Chapter 13). Still vastly underutilized considering the strength of the research supporting their efficacy (see, e.g., Miller, Wilbourne, & Hettema, 2002, for a review of effective approaches to alcoholism treatment in which two of the six most empirically validated treatments are pharmacological in focus), particularly in combination with psychosocial treatments, psychopharmacological approaches nonetheless hold great promise as an important component of effective treatment in the future. Resistance to the use of medications still persists in the substance abuse treatment field among more traditionally trained clinicians, who view being "substance free" as the only valid state for a recovering substance abuser to aim for. Nonetheless, with developments in professional practice such as prescription privileges for psychologists, and revisions to the regulations governing the use of opioid substitution treatments (i.e., methadone, buprenorphine), the importance of medications in treatment will likely increase.

Finally, we have included an integrative clinical chapter by Edward Rubin (Chapter 14) that provides a glimpse into the thinking and case formulation of a clinician who uses aspects of many of the approaches presented in this book in real-life clinical practice. While it is relatively easy to think about approaches to treatment in isolation from each other, in the real world clinicians often choose, or need, to incorporate aspects from more than one approach into their work with individual clients. We have added this chapter to assist readers in understanding more clearly how this process occurs in practice.

As with the first edition, this edition is organized into pairs of chapters (with the exception of the chapters on psychopharmacology and clinical integration), composed of a chapter on theory and a chapter on translation of theory into technique. We asked our authors to address a number of questions that we believe are critical to the conduct of treatment. Theory chapter authors were asked to state the assumptions of their approach as clearly as possible, and to address a number of other theory-relevant questions. These questions focused on how the theory under consideration addresses the etiology, maintenance, and change of psychoactive substance use disorders (PSUDs); the role of environmental factors in the etiology, maintenance, and change of PSUDs; the theory's view of the heterogeneity/homogeneity of persons with PSUDs; and the extent to which the theory proposes that different types of clients be treated differently (e.g., depending on drug of choice, demographics, family history, etc.). Finally, we asked authors to address their theory's view of critical tasks necessary for treatment success, and to provide a brief overview of the research support for the theory.

Authors of the technique chapters were specifically asked to translate the theoretical position they have adopted into therapist actions and strategies. Questions were asked about sequencing of treatment activities, how "denial" and "resistance" are addressed, what the role of self-help groups is from the perspective of the treatment under consideration, how treatment termination is decided upon, how treatment modality (e.g., individual, group, family, marital) is selected, and how slips or relapses are addressed. Use of case study material was encouraged.

Our authors are experienced clinicians who are deeply versed in the nuances of the approaches they espouse. As such, we have asked them to write as advocates for their approaches, not simply as reporters of them. Many of our authors are clinical researchers as well, and have been deeply committed to the empirical study of their approaches, as well as to their clinical application. While it is impossible to exclude each author's unique vision completely from his or her chapter, we have attempted to have our authors portray each approach and its derivative techniques in a broad way that is characteristic of how it works in practice.

Several implicit themes emerge as one reads through the chapters. First, and most striking, is the diversity of the approaches presented here. This is particularly surprising given how uniform treatment in the field has been, until very recently. A second theme is the significant extent to which cross-fertilization of ideas and techniques characterizes the various approaches, despite their differing theoretical and technical bases. Finally, it becomes clear that each approach has clear strengths and weaknesses, further reinforcing the conclusion reached by the Institute of Medicine many years ago, that no one approach works with all clients (Institute of Medicine, 1990). This reinforces, for us, the view that some form of client–treatment matching is still the "wave of the future." Our knowledge of how to accomplish effective matching is still primitive, but it seems clear that we must learn to do so if we are to create more effective treatments.

This volume addresses a broad audience. It is suitable for advanced undergraduates, beginning graduate students, and candidates for certification as substance abuse counselors who are learning to do substance abuse treatment for the first time. We also believe experienced substance abuse clinicians, who want to broaden their treatment knowledge without having to wade through a huge scientific literature to do so, will find this book useful in accomplishing that goal. Finally, general psychotherapists and medical practitioners will find this book useful in learning how to approach issues of substance abuse with clients or patients who may be in treatment for other conditions without having to go directly to the scientific literature to do so.

We recognize that this book is not comprehensive, nor do we intend it to be. Rather, it is a focused introduction to what we believe are the most prominent treatment theories, and their derivative techniques. We believe the approaches covered here will form the core of effective substance abuse treatment for the coming decade and beyond.

REFERENCES

Institute of Medicine. (1990). *Broadening the base of treatment for alcohol problems.* Washington, DC: National Academy Press.

Kantak, K. M., Collins, S. L., Lipman, E. G., Bond, J., Giovanoni, K., & Fox, B. S. (2000). Evaluation of anti-cocaine antibodies and a cocaine vaccine in a rat self-administration model. *Psychopharmacology, 148,* 251–262.

Kuhn, T. S. (1962). *The structure of scientific revolutions.* Chicago: University of Chicago Press.

Leshner, A. I. (1999). Science-based views of drug addiction and its treatment. *Journal of the American Medical Association, 282,* 1314–1316.

Longabaugh, R., & Wirtz, P. W. (Eds.). (2001). *Project MATCH hypothesis: Results and causal chain analyses.* (National Institute on Alcohol Abuse and Alcoholism Project MATCH Monograph Series, Vol. 8). Rockville, MD: National Institute on Alcohol Abuse and Alcoholism.

Miller, W. R., Wilbourne, P. L. & Hettema, J. E. (2002). What works? A summary of alcohol treatment outcome research. In R. K. Hester & W. R. Miller (Eds.), *Handbook of alcoholism treatment approaches: Effective alternatives* (3rd ed., pp. 13–63). Boston: Allyn & Bacon.

Miller, W. R., & Rollnick, S. (2002). *Motivational interviewing* (2nd ed.): *Preparing people for change.* New York: Guilford Press.

Rosenthal, R. N., & Westreich, L. (1999). Treatment of persons with dual diagnoses of substance use disorder and other psychological problems. In B. S. McCrady & E. E. Epstein (Eds.), *Addictions: A comprehensive guidebook* (pp. 439–476). New York: Oxford University Press.

Zweben, A. (2001). Integrating pharmacotherapy and psychosocial interventions in the treatment of individuals with alcohol problems. *Journal of Social Work Practice in the Addictions, 1,* 65–80.

1

Theory of 12-Step-Oriented Treatment

John Wallace

Precise definitions of 12-step theory and its derivative, 12-step technique of treatment, are difficult to achieve. The literature of Alcoholics Anonymous (AA), from which all 12-step programs have been derived, does not lend itself to unambiguous interpretation. Moreover, treatment programs that utilize the 12 steps of AA in some manner or another are characterized by considerable heterogeneity. These programs vary in how the steps and concepts of AA are construed and applied and also in the additional theories and techniques they employ. The writings of those theorists who have been categorized as 12-step theorists reveal so many differences in concepts, utilization of particular databases, and emphases that efforts to describe this body of work more often than not result in stereotypes rather than sensitive and accurate descriptions (e.g., Peele, 1985). A further complication is that some authorities sympathetic to both AA and formal treatment approaches would argue that the very term "12-step treatment" is a misnomer or oxymoron because AA is not a treatment program and those treatment programs that do nothing but teach the steps and traditions of AA are not treatment programs either. AA is best thought of as a "fellowship" or, perhaps, a social movement; it does not conduct assessments, arrive at diagnoses, dispense medications, write treatment plans, provide case management, and do group and individual therapy. And treatment programs that do not do at least some of these functions cannot be considered treatment programs either.

Despite these caveats, it is possible to discern some common characteristics among those programs that are sympathetic to AA and make some use of AA concepts while employing other concepts and procedures as well. This chapter focuses on these common characteristics.

Throughout this chapter, then, the term "12-step treatment" refers to certain core concepts, implicit assumptions, informal hypotheses, and explicit ideas that constitute one recognizable approach to addictions treatment and recovery. I make no claim to be a spokesperson for AA or any other 12-step program. The material presented here is best construed as one observer's view on this complex matter and not as a final, definitive statement on what AA is or what 12-step treatment theory is.

CONCEPT OF ADDICTION

The 12-step approach to the origins, maintenance, and modification of addictive behaviors has for some time constituted an informal biopsychosocial-spiritual model of addiction (Wallace, 1989a). Although 12-step talk is the language of laypersons and not that of professional psychologists or other scientists, it is a rich, comprehensive language with many references to the physical, psychological, social, and spiritual aspects of human beings. When, for example, newcomers to AA are told that they have a disease that prevents them from being able to predict and control their drinking in a consistent manner, a biomedical concept has been advocated. But when an AA sponsor tells a newcomer to avoid former drinking companions and drinking situations, the sponsor is making a clear statement about the importance of interpersonal and socioenvironmental factors in recovery. And when members of an AA group share experiences and advice about such psychological matters as depression, anger, loneliness, self-pity, jealousy, resentments, and sexuality, they are obviously involved in a form of folk psychotherapy.

From its inception, AA seemed to offer at least a two-dimensional concept of addiction in its formal literature. William Silkworth (Alcoholics Anonymous, 1976), for example, in the classic work, *Alcoholics Anonymous,* called attention to both biological and psychological factors in alcoholism. For Silkworth, alcoholism was the result of an allergy to alcohol (physical) coupled with an obsession with the substance (psychological). Bill Wilson (1953), the founder of AA, spoke of alcoholism as an "illness" but wrote extensively on the psychodynamic aspects of drinking problems. Within recent years, theorists sympathetic to 12-step programs have contributed formal biopsychosocial models (e.g., Wallace, 1985, 1989c). In short, both the history of AA and modern thinking reveal implicit and explicit concern with multidimensional models of addiction.

DISEASE MODELS

Although both advocates and opponents of biological factors have argued heatedly in favor of or in opposition to a disease concept of alcoholism and other addictions, these arguments have been characterized on both sides by lack of rigorous definitions, misleading generalities, neglect of an abundant body of biological research, and polemic rather than scientific discourse (e.g., Peele, 1988, 1989, 1990). Few of the participants in these proceedings appear to have realized that many disease concepts or models are available and that debate might more profitably center around which of these models more accurately describe addictive phenomena and best fit available data.

In what sense can alcoholism and other drug addictions be considered diseases? Perhaps the simplest answer to this question involves the many biomedical consequences of alcoholism and drug addiction. Alcoholics and addicts are often seriously ill people as a direct result of drug intake. Whether or not one believes in biological etiological factors is simply irrelevant in many practical treatment contexts. Dangerous withdrawal symptoms, overdoses, cardiac conditions, liver disease, pancreatic disease, and so forth must be treated medically despite one's ideology about the origins of these problems. Moreover, the presence of these most serious medical sequelae of alcohol and other drug ingestion clearly indicates that further attempts at drinking or drug taking by the patient must be vigorously opposed by clinicians responsible for the patient's care. In effect, this first and probably least controversial of the disease models can be termed the "medical consequences model."

A considerably more complicated disease model can be termed the "biopsychosocialspiritual consequences/maintenance model." This disease model is multidimensional and hence much richer than the narrow medical consequences model. Interacting biological, psychological, social, and spiritual factors are at issue here rather than medical problems. Furthermore, rather than focusing on the important but extraordinarily complex question of etiology, the biopsychosocialspiritual consequences/maintenance disease model permits both theorists and clinicians to attend to the critical factors involved in changing addictive behaviors by addressing the multiple factors that maintain them once begun. As will be explained shortly, this model asserts that excessive alcohol and other drug use leads to profound biological, psychological, social, and spiritual negative consequences. The distress associated with these multidimensional negative consequences leads to further excessive drug use, which, in turn, leads to more negative consequences and more distress. Hence, a vicious cycle is established that maintains excessive drug and alcohol use. Each of the dimensions of the biopsychosocial model is discussed separately in the following sections.

The Biological Dimension

As a considerable body of research in this century has shown, the brain is an electrochemical information-processing system. Important neuromodulators, neurotransmitters, and neurohormones have been identified and processes involved in presynaptic and postsynaptic neurotransmission of information have been studied extensively. In effect, the human brain is a sea of chemicals. Alcohol and other drugs enter this chemical environment of the brain and produce profound changes. These changes in the chemistry of the brain are associated with important positive and negative cognitive, affective, and behavioral changes. It is probable that the reinforcement value of various drugs lies in their capacities to effect acute changes in brain chemistry. Hence, a drug such as cocaine produces initial feelings of alertness, euphoria, arousal, and energization, probably because of its impact upon dopaminergic, serotonergic, and noradrenergic synapses. But whereas the initial or acute effects of cocaine are to enhance dopaminergic and other neurotransmitter transmission, the drug's longer term or chronic effects are to disrupt such neurotransmission through negative impact upon levels of these important neurochemicals (Dackis & Gold, 1985). As the levels of dopamine and other neurotransmitters fall as a result of continued cocaine use, associated negative changes in mood, affect, cognition, and behavior take place as well. Euphoria gives way to depression; alertness and arousal yield to difficulties in attentional processes and fatigue; feelings of well-being are replaced by irritation and agitation. Cognitive pathology in the form of delusions and hallucinations may suddenly appear and cause the chronic cocaine user further extreme discomfort. But despite these negative outcomes of chronic use, the cocaine addict remains attracted to the chemical in seeming defiance of all that is reasonable and rational. The paradox, however, is readily resolved when we realize that the addict is caught in a vicious cycle: initial positive reinforcement with initial drug use, which leads to abnormal changes in brain chemistry with chronic use, which, in turn, lead to negative mood, affective, and cognitive states. These negative psychological states motivate further drug-seeking behavior because the addict remembers the highly reinforcing, positive psychological states associated with neurotransmitter release and enhancement upon initial use. Similar vicious biopsychological states occur with chronic use of drugs other than cocaine. Alcohol, for example, produces many changes by impacting diffusely upon numerous brain processes and structures. Alcohol in large quantities produces both acute and chronic effects on cell membranes (Goldstein, 1983; Hunt, 1985), neurotransmitter systems (Tarter & Van Thiel, 1985), calcium channels, and brain enzymes (Wallace, 1989b). With regard to the latter, research has shown abnormal adenylate cyclase activity for as long as 4 years after alcohol consumption has ceased (Tabakoff et al., 1988). These many changes in brain structure and processes lead to vicious cycles in which drinking leads to more negative consequences and, in turn, motivates more drug-seeking behavior.

The Psychological Dimension

Chronic excessive use of psychoactive substances may produce important changes in brain chemistry and processes and these changes are linked to further significant alterations in mood and affect. Chronic consumption of large quantities of alcohol may, for example, lead to depression and anxiety. Patients admitted to alcoholism treatment facilities routinely show depressive and anxiety symptoms on admission. By the third to fourth week of treatment, however, these symptoms disappear in the vast majority of patients (Brown, Irwin, & Schuckit, 1991; Brown & Schuckit, 1988). In effect, symptoms of depression and anxiety are often pharmacologically induced in alcoholic patients, who may enter into vicious cycles in which drinking both creates and alleviates (temporarily) these uncomfortable states. Some psychological negative consequences, however, are not linked directly to the pharmacological impact of alcohol and other drugs but are a product of general life happenings of the addicted person. Alcoholics, for example, frequently show serious deficiencies in self-esteem. Although some of these problems in self-regarding attitudes may have preceded active alcoholism, it is probable that negative self-esteem in alcoholics is largely an outcome of such things as shame and embarrassment associated with public drunken comportment, arrests for drunken driving, remorse, guilt or harm done to others while intoxicated, loss of employment, rejection by spouses or lovers, and so forth. Further, many alcoholics show an identity problem. This problem in identity and self-understanding is often the direct outcome of the repeated conflict between the morals and core values of the sober personality at odds with the actions of the intoxicated person. The psychological negative consequences of alcoholism and addiction include low self-esteem; anger; grandiosity; resentments toward others; repressive defenses including denial, rationalization, assimilative projection, minimization of difficulties, avoidance of feelings, and resistance to feedback from others about self; hostility; excessive self-pity and sensitivity; lack of self-confidence; low frustration tolerance; and fears of various kinds. All alcoholics and addicts do not, of course, show every one of these psychological problems, but they do occur with such frequency among addicted populations that clinicians should expect them and plan therapeutic activities that address them. The important point here, however, is not that alcoholics and addicts show a universal set of negative psychological sequelae of chronic drug intake. Rather, it is that psychological negative consequences may also enter into negative cycles that paradoxically maintain the patterns of heavy psychoactive substance use that gave rise to them. In effect, chronic heavy alcohol and other drug consumption is linked to events that eventuate in many psychological problems. The discomfort associated with these psychological problems leads to further drug-seeking behavior and consumption, which in turn leads to an intensification of personal difficulties. And so it goes.

The Social Dimension

Alcoholics and other drug addicts who continue to drink and use drugs must contend with mounting social problems as well as the intense discomfort of the physical and psychological negative outcomes discussed above. Usually the first thing to deteriorate is the complex web of intimate personal relationships that sustain and nurture healthy continued growth and functioning. The marriages of alcoholic and drug-addicted individuals typically become filled with pain, frustration, and anger turning into smoldering resentments, fear, shattered expectations, guilt, sorrow, bitterness, self-pity, depression, and pervasive feelings of hopelessness and helplessness. In the face of this intense emotional stress and discomfort that characterize the majority of addicted relationships, alcoholics and other addicts often feel that they have no other choice but to seek relief by continuing to use the substances that led to their marital problems in the first place. Addicted people as a further consequence of their drinking and drug use do not have well-developed skills for addressing relationship problems, resolving marital conflicts, and nurturing intimate relationships. In effect, they have overlearned the strategy of dealing with the pain of relationship problems by drinking and taking drugs. Moreover, the partners of addicted people also have overlearned maladaptive strategies for coping with relationship problems in marriage. Often obsessed with the need to control an uncontrollable situation, they develop patterns of reacting and responding to their partners' addictive behaviors and actions while intoxicated that usually make matters worse. The wives, husbands, and lovers of addicted people are not the only intimates caught up in the turmoil of addiction. The children of alcoholics and addicts also react to the stress, pain, conflict, and emotional upheaval of the alcoholic and drug-addicted marriage. These children may show many emotional and social problems of their own, including excessive fears, acting out at home and in the community, school and learning difficulties, fighting, delinquency, truancy, early sexual experimentation, lack of self-confidence, and drinking and drug use problems of their own (Wallace, 1987). These problems in parenting and childrearing usher further stress and disorder into a marital system that is already overwhelmed. Unfortunately, additional marital/family stress leads to further drinking and drug use and intensification of family dysfunction and maladaptive problem solution efforts. Obviously, family treatment of some form or another is a necessary part of primary treatment of addiction and occupies a central role in most modern treatment programs that utilize the steps and concepts of AA.

Marital/family difficulties are not the only negative consequences of drinking and drug use that maintain addictive behavior. Alcoholics and addicts show a host of other difficulties that may involve one or more of the following: employment and career troubles, legal and financial problems, disturbed friendships, arrests, incarcerations, community rejection and other forms of social stigma, decline in social status, role identity confusion, role ambiguity and ambivalence, and loss of social position. The pain and stress associated with these unhappy social outcomes usually result in further deterioration of the alcoholic and addict and further drinking and drug use. Obviously, without vigorous intervention and treatment services, this downward spiral into chronic alcoholism and drug addiction is not likely to be reversed. Although some alcoholics and addicts who have gone deeply into addiction have managed to turn their lives around without intervention and treatment, this does not appear to be the case for the majority of those unfortunate persons whose illnesses have become chronic.

The Spiritual Dimension

Spirituality is the fourth and final dimension in the biopsychosocialspiritual consequences/maintenance disease model. More will be said shortly about the focus on spirituality in 12-step theory; however, mention must be made here of the impact of alcoholic drinking and drug addiction upon the spiritual life of a person. For many people, heavy drinking and drug use culminate in intense feelings of alienation, apartness, emptiness, meaninglessness, and lack of purpose in living. Moral values may have been compromised in the erratic acting out of intoxicated behaviors, urges, cognitions, and motivations. Knowledge about self and conviction about personal goals, objectives, and direction appear to become more and more uncertain and confused as addiction deepens. In a sense, alcoholics and addicts of other kinds seem to be ships without rudders cast adrift on turbulent seas. More than one alcoholic has described the terrible sense of inner emptiness and meaninglessness that characterized periods of active alcoholism. Despair is often the outcome of alcoholism and also the stimulus for further drinking. Nothing fills the inner void of alcoholics and addicts like alcohol and drugs do. Never mind that alcohol and drugs ushered in the desperation of spiritual emptiness, alienation, and suffering in the first place. Alcohol and drugs can quickly "fix" these painful states of being. The "fix," of course, is always temporary and usually followed by even greater spiritual distress, but active alcoholics and addicts do not care about delayed punishments. The immediate reinforcement of relief from painful states of being drives addicted people to continue to make choices not in their best interests.

THE PREDISPOSITION DISEASE MODELS

In contrast to the two consequences disease models discussed above, the "predisposition disease model" assumes that alcoholics and other drug-addicted people were set up for addiction by biological differences that preceded the onset of drinking or drug use. From this point of view, genetically transmitted biological risk factors predispose some individuals to addiction once exposure to alcohol and other substances has taken place. In actuality, there are several predisposition models and each of these shows variations.

The first of these types of predisposition models could be called the "genetic determination predisposition model." In this model, environment is considered irrelevant in determining alcoholism and drug addiction. These problems are considered to be determined entirely by genes. All that is required in a genetic determination model is the gene for a specific disorder. Alcoholism, for example, is thought to be the result of an "alcoholism gene." Cocaine dependence is associated with a gene for "cocainism." And heroin addiction is the consequence of a specific gene for this type of addiction. Recent research on genes for alcoholism and cocaine addiction is illustrative of the type of research generated by this model.

A second predisposition disease model is the "genetic influence disease model." This model makes no assumptions about genes for specific disorders and assumes that multiple biological risk factors interacting with psychosocial environmental factors determine addiction. In effect, neither genetics nor environment operating alone is sufficient to produce alcoholism or drug addiction; alcoholism and drug addiction require the joint presence of both biological and psychosocial environmental factors (Tarter & Edwards, 1986).

A third predisposition model is a "mixed genetic determination/influence model." In this model, different types of alcoholism and other types of addiction exist and different etiological theories are necessary to explain each type. Cloninger's (1983) distinction between Type I and Type II alcoholism is an example of this approach. According to Cloninger, Type I alcoholism is explained by a genetic influence disease model as both genetic influence and environmental influence are necessary to produce the illness. Type II alcoholism, however, does not require the presence of environmental risk factors and is considered to be determined entirely by genetic factors operating independently of environment.

Predisposing biological risk factors that have been proposed include the following: defects in one or more neurotransmitter or neuromodulator systems, deficiencies in enzymes involved in neurotransmission, arousal system dysregulation, irregularities in cell membrane processes and structures, and abnormalities concerning various brain condensation products formed when alcohol is consumed (Wallace, 1989b).

THEORETICAL IMPLICATIONS OF DISEASE MODELS FOR TREATMENT

Regardless of the specific disease model chosen, theorists who advocate the importance of biological factors in the origins and maintenance of addictive behaviors appear to show similarities in their approaches to applications in treatment. These similarities are discussed separately in the following sections.

Powerlessness

As the first step of AA asserts, an admission of one's powerlessness over alcohol or some other chemical must take place before progress can be expected. In 12-step theory, the individual need not admit to being an alcoholic or drug addict or to being powerless in general. All that is required is an admission that one's use of psychoactive chemicals is no longer under one's personal control. The person's chemical use has become uncontrolled and/or the person's behavior while using chemicals has become uncontrolled. From this point of view, people who cannot consistently predict and control when, where, and how much they drink and use drugs and/or cannot guarantee their actions once they start to drink or use drugs are perceived as powerless over alcohol or some other chemical. As with other matters, theorists differ in how they approach the issue of loss of control and powerlessness. Some theorists take an all-or-none position and seem to imply that the loss of control is total and that the individual is not only powerless over alcohol or some other chemical but powerless over all aspects of his or her life. Other theorists seem to take a more moderate and balanced position and regard loss of control and powerlessness as matters of degree rather than absolutes. Impaired control and unpredictability of one's behavior once alcohol or drug use has begun are seen as critical. In other words, these more moderate theorists recognize that at various stages in the person's drinking history, considerable control over alcohol may have been evident and may, in fact, still be present. The key here, however, is that the person cannot exercise *consistent control* over chemical use and cannot consistently predict and control his or her behavior once chemical use has begun on any given occasion. Moreover, the reason that the individual has impaired control and cannot consistently control his or her drinking and/or behavior while drinking or using drugs is that the individual is suffering from a disease not unlike other diseases in which choice, will, and moral conviction do not, for the most part, make much difference.

Recognition, Identification, and Acceptance

Before an admission of powerlessness can be made, other changes in the cognitive system must be achieved. Typically, addicted people make tactical use of a variety of defenses that may prevent many of them from seeing even the most devastating negative consequences of alcohol and drug use. Denial, rationalization, minimization, and other forms of repressive defenses make it difficult for the addicted person to see his or her life clearly and to take steps to change. Many of these defenses probably have their roots in shame, guilt, remorse, fear, and strong motivation to continue drinking and drug use. Whatever their origins, these defenses must be overcome and awareness must take the place of the mindlessness and lack of clarity that result from heavy alcohol and other drug consumption. The person must recognize the many negative biopsychosocial consequences that drinking and drug use have caused in his or her life. As treatment progresses, the person is brought to see how many of his or her problems are directly attributable to the disease of alcoholism and/or other drug addiction. In the early stages of treatment and recovery, teaching of a disease concept of some form or another is helpful to the patient in managing otherwise overwhelming feelings of guilt, shame, anger, and remorse that may accompany the uncovering process as defenses fall away. *Identification* with others with similar problems of alcoholism and chemical dependency is useful to the patient and is encouraged. Identification with others also helps to reduce guilt, shame, anger, anxiety, and remorse. Moreover, it eases entry into supportive fellowships such as AA, where the many benefits of community can be made available to recovering people. Emotional support; a sense of belonging; a means to deal with loneliness, alienation, and isolation; shared problem solving; exposure to sober and clean role models; and enhanced motivation to avoid drug and alcohol use are but a few of the many benefits of identification with others who suffer from the same diseases. Finally, *acceptance* of some disease concept and all that it implies for one's future behaviors with regard to alcohol and other drugs is critical. It is not enough simply to know the elements of a disease concept—even a complicated, neurochemical concept—one must also apply the concept to self and accept fully its implications for self. Perhaps the most significant outcome of acceptance of a disease model is the decision to remain abstinent from alcohol and other drugs of addiction.

THE CENTRAL ROLE OF ABSTINENCE

All disease models of alcoholism and other drug addiction stress the central role of abstinence if recovery is to be achieved and maintained. Members of 12-step programs such as AA reject controlled intoxification as a recovery goal for themselves for two simple but important reasons. First, although they personally tried many ways to control their drinking and behavior while drinking, virtually all report eventual failure. Second, virtually none of the members of AA and other 12-step programs report firsthand knowledge of alcoholics and addicts in their home communities who have learned how to be successful at controlled intoxication. What members of 12-step recovery programs see in their own communities are many attempts at controlled intoxication by others and eventual universal failure. Twelve-step theorists report similar observations in both community and clinical contexts. Clinicians who work out of a 12-step orientation report no success at sustained controlled intoxication among those patients they have treated and/or followed. Again, as with general community observations by laypeople, professionally trained clinicians see virtually no sustained, long-term controlled intoxification behaviors among alcoholics and other addicted populations. Moreover, some theorists sympathetic to 12-step theory who have extensive research backgrounds have challenged the optimistic claims by certain controlled drinking researchers and enthusiasts as grossly exaggerated and incapable of standing up to rigorous scientific analyses (e.g., Wallace, 1990, 1993). Also, attempts to replicate or substantiate previous optimistic findings on controlled drinking have failed (Pendery, Maltzman, & West, 1982; Rychtarik, Foy, Scott, Lokey, & Prue, 1987), whereas new research on alcoholics has demonstrated stable moderate drinking to be a rare outcome among treated alcoholics (Helzer et al., 1985).

Despite the absence of lay ethnographic observations on successful sustained controlled intoxication by alcoholics and other addicts and despite the absence of a scientifically acceptable body of evidence in favor of controlled intoxication, some critics of 12-step theory have continued to dismiss the insistence on abstinence and to urge instead the widespread adoption of controlled intoxication treatment goals (Peele, 1983; Searles, 1993). The position of these critics, who, for the most part, are psychologists, is difficult to comprehend because psychology as a rigorous scientific discipline insists on conclusions drawn from carefully conducted and methodologically sound studies. Furthermore, the issue of controlled intoxication treatment goals for alcoholics and addicts is not a trivial one. Because alcoholics who continue to drink are at sharply increased risk for many biopsychosocial consequences including death; disease; traumatic injury; legal, financial, marital, and employment difficulties; and psychological/psychiatric problems, advocacy of controlled intoxication treatment goals for alcoholics and addicts raises many professional and ethical questions, and especially so in the absence of a convincing body of scientific evidence in favor of such goals.

From a 12-step theory perspective, little progress can be expected in treatment and recovery if alcoholics and addicts continue to attempt to drink alcohol and use unauthorized drugs. There are several reasons why this is the case. First, the pharmacological actions of drugs such as alcohol and cocaine increase the likelihood of compulsive use rather than decrease such use in addicted people. Changes in brain chemistry with continued use probably serve as important internal cues for compulsive use. Also, alcoholics and other addicts often appear to possess poor impulse control, low frustration tolerance, weakly controlled anger, impatience, and various cognitive impairments (Tarter, Alterman, & Edwards, 1987). Because alcohol and certain other drugs appear to exacerbate these difficulties, it seems most appropriate for alcoholics and addicts to avoid these chemicals altogether. In order to stay clean and sober, addicts and alcoholics need all their wits about them, not less. Second, the continued use of psychoactive substances keeps addicted people caught in the mind-set of solving problems with chemicals rather than through searching for personal, emotional, cognitive, interpersonal, and spiritual growth and development. And as alcohol and other drugs trigger urges and cognitions about continued use, alcoholics and addicts who attempt to drink and use drugs with control seem to end up even more obsessed with the substances. In many cases, even those small numbers of alcoholics who managed through incredible effort to achieve some controlled drinking gave it up in favor of abstinence because of the reported misery and unhappiness of being continually obsessed with the "next drink" and the enormous amount of work required in holding their drinking down to a set quota of a few drinks a day.

Not only do attempts to drink and use drugs keep alcoholics and addicts caught up in chemical solutions to problems of living, they separate addicted people from clean and sober friends and 12-step fellowship programs. It is difficult to feel a part of AA if your brain is thoroughly soaked in marijuana and you are sitting in a roomful of clean and sober people rejoicing in their sobriety. In contrast to 12-step fellowship programs, there has been no enduring support group devoted to the pursuit of moderate intoxication for alcoholics, moderate cocaine use for cocaine addicts, moderate cigarette smoking for nicotine addicts, and so forth. Although there have been attempts to establish some of these, none has yet been proven to stand the test of time as have AA, Narcotics Anonymous, and other abstinence-oriented programs.

SPIRITUALITY AND THE PROBLEM OF POWERLESSNESS

Once addicted people have admitted their powerlessness over alcohol and/or other drugs, they find themselves faced with a new dilemma. If they cannot personally control their behavior with regard to these chemicals, who will do it for them? The 12-step answer to this dilemma is at first blush disarmingly simple, but it is far more complicated on further analysis. According to the second and third steps of AA, addicted people are urged to believe in and turn their will and their lives over to a power greater than themselves. This emphasis on spirituality has been a boon to many and a stumbling block to others. Some critics have seized upon the similarities between AA and religion and have rejected the AA claim that it is a spiritual program and not a religious one. This emphasis by critics on similarities, however, ignores the many differences between AA and organized religions. An orange is round and so is the world, but an orange is not the world. Similarities do not prove identities. Of course, the literature of AA and the talk of some of its members contain double messages and ambiguities that encourage misperception. But, in the final analysis, despite similarities and double messages, AA and its offspring 12-step theory cannot be considered to constitute religions. The steps of AA, for example, are not requirements but suggestions for recovery and, as such, cannot constitute dogma. Although it does have a founder in the person of Bill Wilson, AA has no central religious figure or leader who is worshipped and adored, as do Christianity, Buddhism, Hinduism, and Judaism.

In approaching the distinction between religion and spirituality, the thoughts of the transpersonal psychologist Ken Wilber (1993) may prove helpful. Wilber draws a distinction between what he terms "exoteric" religions and a form of spirituality he terms "esoteric." In Wilber's words:

> Exoteric or "outer" religion is mythic religion, religion that is terribly concrete and literal, that really believes, for example, that Moses parted the Red Sea, that Christ was born from a virgin, that the world was created in six days, that manna once literally rained down from heaven, and so on. Exoteric religions the world over consist of those type of beliefs. The Hindus believe that the earth, since it needs to be supported, is sitting on an elephant which since it needs to be supported, is sitting on a tortoise which in turn is sitting on a serpent. . . . Lao Tzu was nine hundred years old when he was born, Krishna made love to four thousand cow maidens, Brahma was born from a crack in a cosmic egg, and so on. That's exoteric religion, a series of belief structures that attempt to explain the mysteries of the world in mythic terms rather than direct experiential or evidential terms. . . . Esoteric spirituality, on the other hand, is "inner or hidden." The reason that esoteric . . . is hidden is not that it is secret or anything, but that it is a matter of direct experience and personal awareness. Esoteric (spirituality) asks that you believe nothing on faith, or obediently swallow any dogma. Rather, esoteric (spirituality) is a set of personal experiments that you conduct scientifically in the laboratory of your own awareness. Like all good science, it is based on direct experience, not mere belief or wish, and it is publicly checked or validated by a peer group of those who have also performed the experiment. (p. 176)

In a very real sense, 12-step theory embraces a point of view that closely approximates Wilber's esoteric mysticism. Members of AA perform an experiment (in this case, the experiment is to try to follow the suggested 12 steps of the program) and then observe over time through direct experience the consequences of having done so. But what of this notion of a power greater than self in which one may believe and to whom one gives one's will and one's life? How may the concept of a higher power be approached without resorting to conventional religiosity? Twelve-step fellowship programs neatly dodge thorny problems here simply by defining the AA group as a power greater than self. There is a certain cunning in this position because the problem is not that addicted people need to find a conventional god but that they need to give another approach a try. In AA terms, they need to "get out of the driver's seat." Left to their own devices, many addicted people fail again and again but still keep returning to the belief in their own willpower as the means to conquer their addictions. By turning over their will and their lives to others at the beginning of their recoveries, addicted people become open to new cognitions, alternative behavioral strategies for dealing with their problems, and fresh approaches to dealing with their chemical addictions.

While the group as a power greater than self can serve many addicted people well in the beginning stages of recovery, it is also useful in 12-step theory to introduce patients to other ways of construing a "God of their own understanding." Some people, of course, do enter recovery programs with well-developed religious convictions and prefer to continue with these. Others, however, have virtually no understanding of how to proceed in these matters or are openly hostile to anything that even remotely resembles religiosity. Resistance to spirituality may constitute a reasoned intellectual position or may flow directly from highly negative childhood experiences with organized religions. In either case, addicted people may benefit from consideration of alternative ways of construing these matters. As the theologian Paul Tillich (1952) asserted, God is a person's ultimate concern in life. From this perspective, almost anything can become a god or higher power. People have made gods of money, sexuality, fame, prestige, social position, and so forth. In the case of addicted people, alcohol and drugs often achieve this power of ultimate concerns and, as such, take precedence over all other aspects of the addict's life. Marriage, family, friendships, jobs, careers, health, and well-being often take a backseat to the addict's drive to seek out his or her drug of choice and "get high." In effect, drugs and alcohol become powers greater than self, directing forces that drive all aspects of the addict's feelings, cognitions, and behaviors. In a real sense, the addict's problem is not to find a higher power, because he or she already has one. The trick is for the addict to switch from a destructive higher power to a constructive and beneficial one. As sobriety lengthens, the person may consider nondeistic directing forces for his or her life other than the recovery group. Examples of these higher powers are love, knowledge, creativity, and justice. Ordering one's life and seeking direction in terms of abstract principles rather than concrete religious figures is one way to develop a nondeistic spirituality for oneself. This is not without historical precedent. Many great men and women in history found comfort, strength, and direction in principles rather than in the mythic structures of exoteric religions. And for many alcoholics and addicts, a strong, even passionate, commitment to some power or principle greater than self seems necessary if the powerful allure of psychoactive chemicals and the addict lifestyle is to be overcome.

In the final analysis, the 12-step theory emphasis on turning one's will and life over to the care of a power greater than self is an attempt to deal with the grandiosity, extreme self-centeredness, egotistical concerns, inability to delay gratification, faulty decision-making processes, and urgent needs of many active alcoholics and addicts. "Do it my way," "Me first!," "I'm right and you're wrong," "Look at it from my point of view," and "I want it and I want it right now!" could very well be the theme songs of many active alcoholics and addicts. Spiritual growth and development as defined above are means to overcome extreme self-centeredness and to achieve significant and necessary changes in the structure of the self and in one's way of being in the world.

AWARENESS, SELF-EXAMINATION, AND SELF-CRITICISM

Because of the alcoholic's and addict's use of repressive defenses and general mindlessness when drinking and using drugs, 12-step theory emphasizes the importance of achieving and utilizing knowledge about self. In 12-step fellowship programs, the writing of a personal inventory and then sharing this inventory with at least one other person is one means through which personal shortcomings as well as strengths can be realized. In 12-step treatment programs, the strong emphasis on group therapy and individual counseling is devoted to the same end. Although 12-step-oriented therapists differ in counseling techniques and theoretical orientations, most seem to work toward increasing the patient's awareness of his or her motivations; typical ways of dealing with stress, anger, rejection, and fears; and the consequences of an active alcoholic or addict lifestyle. Awareness of one's feelings and the need to share these feelings in a safe, supportive, and caring interpersonal context are stressed.

Twelve-step therapists also stress awareness of emotional states, attitudes, and actions that may signal the beginning of an active relapse process. According to many 12-step theorists, the alcoholic or addict is never completely "fixed." Individuals are encouraged to think of themselves as always in recovery and never as recovered. Some theorists, however, reject this point of view and argue that addicted people can recover completely from addictive disease, as do persons with illnesses of other types. Whatever the theorist's position on this issue of "recovering" versus "recovered," virtually all theorists and clinicians stress the importance of continued self-scrutiny and self-examination in avoiding relapse.

Along with continued self-scrutiny, individuals are encouraged to engage in self-criticism as well. Several steps of the AA fellowship program speak directly to these matters. It is suggested to members that they make a list of all the people they harmed during their period of active addiction and wherever possible, make amends to them. Making amends is thought to have several desirable outcomes. First, making amends for past wrongdoing toward others enables the alcoholic or addict to deal with excessive guilt, remorse, and continued fear over past actions. Second, it often results in mending relationships that were once broken by active alcoholism and drug addiction. In many cases, these mended relationships are ones critically important to the alcoholic's and addict's sense of community and self-esteem. Third, making amends permits the addicted person to see his or her past alcoholic and addicted behaviors clearly and for what they were by reducing the need for continued use of repressive defenses such as denial, minimization, and rationalization. In addition to the amends steps, persons in the AA fellowship program are urged to continue to take their personal inventories on a daily basis and when wrong to promptly admit it and take the necessary actions to correct the situation. This approach encourages the addicted person to own his or her actions and to take responsibility. Openness to self-criticism on a daily basis also reduces the addict's need to continue to use repressive defenses with regard to his or her behavior.

In a very real sense, the Buddhist concept of mindfulness characterizes the necessary passage of addicted people from states of blind acting out, lack of insight, and poor self-knowledge to the states of heightened awareness and joyful consciousness that are considered the hallmarks of ideal recoveries. Buddhists and others committed to spiritual growth and development utilize the tools of meditation, prayer, and other rituals to achieve mindfulness. In the fellowship of AA and in some formal 12-step treatment programs, these tools are encouraged as well.

PERSONAL RESPONSIBILITY, POWERLESSNESS, AND HELPLESSNESS

It is sometimes argued that encouraging people to view their addictions as diseases takes away their sense of personal responsibility. From this point of view, alcoholics and addicts will simply continue to drink and use drugs while claiming that they have a disease and cannot help themselves. Twelve-step theory neither endorses shirking of personal responsibility for one's addiction nor sees such shirking of responsibility as a necessary outcome of the teaching of disease models of addiction. The usual position taken on this matter by 12-step theorists and clinicians is that because of genetic and other biological etiological factors, addicted people are not responsible for having developed an addictive disease, but they most certainly are responsible for dealing with the illness once they know they have it. Indeed, rather than encouraging addicted people to disclaim responsibility, 12-step theory advocates a thoroughgoing sense of responsibility, not only for addictive behaviors but for all aspects of one's conduct in the world. In 12-step approaches, people are held responsible generally for their actions and are not permitted to "cop out" by blaming their illness or, for that matter, anything else. Part of the misperception here stems from confusion of the concepts of powerlessness and helplessness. In 12-step theory, addicted people are indeed encouraged to view themselves as powerless over their drug of choice, but they are not encouraged to perceive themselves as powerless in general. Because addicted people are powerless over a chemical does not mean that they are helpless. If one is an addicted person, many actions can be taken to help oneself. The addicted person may not be able to choose when to stop using cocaine in the middle of a cocaine run, but he or she is certainly able to choose to attend a treatment program or a Cocaine Anonymous group when not in the middle of a run. Addicted people can choose to become actively involved in their therapy groups if in treatment, or actively involved in their 12-step fellowship groups if in one of these programs. Once clean and sober, addicted people can exercise choices about all aspects of their life, including jobs, relationships, marriages, parenting, investing, and so forth. In early stages of recovery, however, such choices are better made in consultation with professionals and, when appropriate, with sponsors in fellowship programs. As recovery progresses, the ideal outcome is a self-governing person with the ability to make choices that are in his or her best interests.

MENTAL ILLNESS AND 12-STEP THEORY

There is no conflict between psychiatric and 12-step theories with regard to so-called dual diagnoses. It is well recognized and accepted by the majority of 12-step theorists that some alcoholics and addicts may suffer from certain mental and emotional illnesses. These illnesses must be diagnosed and treated accordingly. In many cases, treatment will of necessity include use of antipsychotic and/or antidepressant medications. Twelve-step theorists, however, do object to the overprescribing of psychoactive medications that can accompany poorly informed psychiatric treatment of alcoholics and addicts in early stages of recovery. As research has shown (e.g., Brown et al., 1991; Brown & Schuckit, 1988), most of the psychiatric symptoms seen in the first days and weeks of primary treatment are the outcome of alcohol and other drug use and do not constitute the bases for formal diagnoses of primary psychiatric disorders. Symptoms of depression and anxiety commonly seen in many alcoholics in the beginning of treatment usually resolve without psychoactive medication within 3 weeks of primary treatment in a supportive and caring environment.

On the other hand, 12-step theorists stress the need for routine psychological assessments, psychiatric screenings, and intensive workups in individual cases when symptoms do not resolve and primary psychiatric disorders are suspected. Failure to treat an accompanying depressive disorder in an alcoholic is as serious a blunder as treating with antidepressant medications in the absence of a primary affective disorder.

In the past, 12-step theorists were often in conflict with poorly informed and improperly trained psychiatrists who perceived alcoholism and drug addiction as symptoms of underlying psychiatric illness and who often produced secondary addictions by treating alcoholics inappropriately with benzodiazepines and other antianxiety agents with addiction potential. These conflicts, however, have been reduced considerably as more and better training in the addictions has been made available to psychiatrists and other medical personnel and as accurate information about addictive disease has become more widely available.

PRIORITY SETTING AND TIME BINDING

Most 12-step theorists agree that the therapeutic change process should be an orderly one and should consist of clear priority-setting activities. Newcomers to AA, for example, are often advised to deal with "first things first." This phrase is usually taken to mean that in the early stages of recovery, attempts to deal with issues other than those directly involved with drinking or drug use should be delayed until a stable base of sobriety has been achieved. It is not that 12-step theorists and clinicians believe that other issues are unimportant and should be avoided permanently. It is more a question of *when* certain things get addressed and not a question of whether to address them at all. In the absence of sobriety, the problems of the vast majority of chemically dependent people do not improve despite attempts at problem solving. As we have already noted, drinking and drug use have important multiple impacts upon individuals, including negative effects on the brain and cognitive processes involved with reasoning, judgment, problem solving, and decision making. As these cognitive deficits have been shown to improve as sobriety lengthens, it makes very good sense to delay addressing complex problems for a time. Of course, with regard to some problems, delay may not be possible and issues other than drinking and drug use must be dealt with from the outset of treatment. A primary affective disorder, for example, must be dealt with early in recovery. Family issues also must be dealt with early in recovery. However, in treating families, the same concern with priority setting applies. Clinicians working from a 12-step perspective generally endorse more structured family therapy approaches with more modest initial recovery goals and objectives in the beginning of treatment.

Throughout recovery, then, the phrase "First things first" serves as a reminder that problem solving should proceed in an orderly fashion moving from primary concerns to more secondary matters as treatment proceeds. In a sense, this approach to problem solving encourages the person to go at his or her problems in manageable units rather than flying off in all directions at once. The phrase "Easy does it" is intended to accomplish the same goal by slowing down the tempo of problem-solving attempts, and hence restricting the numbers of personal problems that can be addressed at any one time. "Easy does it" also cautions the alcoholic and addict to avoid a high-intensity, emotionally charged approach in which problems must be solved and solved now. Because most problems in the real world often require considerable amounts of time to solve and usually involve frustration and delay of gratification, problem-solving styles characterized by impatience, impulsiveness, and inability to delay gratification are not optimal for addicted people and are probably associated with relapse.

Perhaps one of the more ingenious ideas to come out of 12-step theory is the simple but important concept of *time binding*. Newcomers to AA and 12-step-oriented treatment programs are constantly urged to take life "24 hours at a time" because alcoholics and addicts seem to have more difficulty than others in maintaining a here-and-now perspective. Many chemically dependent people make themselves miserable by living in the past or projecting into the future. A focus on the past can keep the alcoholic stuck in the painful stuff of regret, guilt, and remorse over actions and events that occurred while drinking. On the other hand, an obsessive preoccupation with the future stirs anxiety, fear, and dread over events that may or may not take place. By placing one's consciousness in the reality of each day as it unfolds, addicted people can learn to avoid the painful emotional triggers that are often associated with relapse. In effect, addicted people need to learn how to learn from their histories and not wallow in events they can no longer do anything about. And they need to learn how to plan for the future without projecting themselves into a future that may or may not unfold. In both cases, they need to learn to live in the reality of the here-and-now. Time binding is an important theoretical idea in helping them to do so.

CHANGE, ACCEPTANCE, AND GRATITUDE

The Serenity Prayer so popular in the fellowship of AA asks God to grant "the serenity to accept the things I cannot change, the courage to change the things I can, and the wisdom to know the difference." Curiously, most of the discussion in AA, however, seems to center around the need for acceptance and seldom on the courage to change. Perhaps this is because alcoholics and addicts perceive themselves and each other as having had major difficulties with acceptance in the past and now need to concentrate on that aspect of their development. In 12-step theory, however, change is viewed as at least as important as acceptance for a stable, enduring, and fulfilling recovery. In many cases, alcoholics or addicts may make themselves miserable by persisting in attempts to accept some situations or problems that are, in fact, not in their best interests or even completely unacceptable. Difficult and destructive marriages and other intimate relationships that should be changed but are "accepted" are prime examples of situations that alcoholics and addicts in recovery often seem to be willing to put up with rather than address directly. Demeaning, unfulfilling, and boring jobs performed under the direction of impossible bosses in sick organizations are another situation in which recovering alcoholics and addicts find themselves stuck and miserable. Unfortunately, many alcoholics and addicts will choose relapse as a way of getting out of these difficult situations. By getting thrown out for being intoxicated, they allow alcohol and other drugs to make the decisions for them. Clearly, much more work needs to be done in 12-step-oriented contexts on how addicted people can develop the attitudes and skills necessary for bringing about necessary and beneficial changes in their lives.

In general, however, change is an important ingredient of 12-step theory and clinical practice. Treatment from this perspective is all about change—change in cognitions about self and others, change in the way problems are construed and solved, change in the way emotions are experienced and dealt with, and change in troublesome, difficult situations that reduce the quality of life in recovery or even increase the likelihood of relapse. If a person completes primary treatment and has changed nothing other than some verbal behavior concerning his or her intentions with regard to drinking or drug use, a continued stable and enduring recovery is not likely.

But despite all that has been said about the importance of change, acceptance is also critical. While actively drinking and using drugs, addicted people as a rule did not learn how to accept things very well. Disappointments were drowned in alcohol. Loss of a promotion or a job meant time to get drunk or high. Illness, death of a loved one, divorce, financial losses, or other major life reversals were not accepted but used as excuses for becoming intoxicated. Even the petty irritations of everyday life led to drinking and/or drug use. Hence, while 12-step theory does stress the importance of changing those things that can and must be changed, it also emphasizes the need for addicted people to learn the skills and attitudes that comprise acceptance. As the saying in AA goes, sometimes alcoholics need to learn how to "sit still and hurt." That is, sit still and hurt without drinking or resorting to drug use.

Perhaps the single most crucial attitude that addicted people can learn is an "attitude of gratitude." The pessimism, cynicism, and chronic dissatisfaction that characterize active alcoholics and drug addicts and appear to drive the continuance of their addictions must yield to a degree of optimism, trust, and sense of fulfillment. By helping recovering alcoholics and addicts to see and appreciate the value of what they do have rather than complaining bitterly about what they do not have, 12-step-oriented clinicians can encourage the development of cognitive structures in their patients that support decisions to remain abstinent and seek fulfillment in activities that do not involve the use of alcohol and drugs.

REFERENCES

Alcoholics Anonymous. (1976). *Alcoholics Anonymous.* New York: Alcoholics Anonymous World Services.

Brown, S. A., Irwin, M., & Schuckit, M. A. (1991). Changes in anxiety among abstinent male alcoholics. *Journal of Studies on Alcohol, 52,* 55–61.

Brown, S. A., & Schuckit, M. A. (1988). Changes in depression among abstinent alcoholics. *Journal of Studies on Alcohol, 49,* 412–417.

Cloninger, C. R. (1983). Genetic and environmental factors in the development of alcoholism. *Journal of Psychiatric Treatment and Evaluation, 5,* 487–496.

Dackis, C. A., & Gold, M. S. (1985). Bromocriptine as a treatment of cocaine abuse. *Lancet, 1,* 1151–1152.

Goldstein, D. B. (1983). *Pharmacology of alcohol.* New York: Oxford University Press.

Helzer, J. E., Robins, L. N., Taylor, J. R., Carey, K., Miller, R. H., Combs-Orme, T., & Farmer, A. (1985). The extent of long-term moderate drinking among alcoholics discharged from medical and psychiatric treatment facilities. *New England Journal of Medicine, 312,* 1678–1682.

Hunt, W. A. (1985). *Alcohol and biological membranes.* New York: Guilford Press.

Peele, S. (1983, April). Through a glass darkly: Can some alcoholics learn to drink in moderation? *Psychology Today,* pp. 38–42.

Peele, S. (1985, January–February). Change without pain. *American Health,* pp. 36–39.

Peele, S. (1988). Can alcoholism and other drug addiction problems be treated away or is the current treatment binge doing more harm than good? *Journal of Psychoactive Drugs, 20,* 375–383.

Peele, S. (1989). *Diseasing of America—Addiction treatment out of control.* Lexington, MA: Lexington Books.

Peele, S. (1990). Why and by whom the American alcoholism treatment industry is under siege. *Journal of Psychoactive Drugs, 22,* 1–13.

Pendery, M. L., Maltzman, I. M., & West, L. J. (1982). Controlled drinking by alcoholics?: New findings and a reevaluation of a major affirmative study. *Science, 217,* 169–175.

Rychtarik, R. G., Foy, D. W., Scott, T., Lokey, L., & Prue, D. M. (1987). Five- to six-year follow-up of broad-spectrum behavioral treatment for alcoholism: Effects of training controlled drinking skills. *Journal of Consulting and Clinical Psychology, 55,* 106–108.

Searles, J. S. (1993). Science and fascism: Confronting unpopular ideas. *Addictive Behaviors, 18,* 5–8.

Tabakoff, B., Hoffman, P. L., Lee, J. M., Saito, T., Willard, B., & Deleon-Jones, F. (1988). Differences in platelet enzyme activity between alcoholics and nonalcoholics. *New England Journal of Medicine, 313,* 134–139.

Tarter, R. E., Alterman, A. I., & Edwards, K. L. (1987). Neurobehavioral theory of alcoholism etiology. In C. Chaudron & D. Wilkinson (Eds.), *Theories of alcoholism* (pp. 73–102). Toronto: Addiction Research Foundation.

Tarter, R. E., & Edwards, K. L. (1986). Antecedents to alcoholism: Implications for prevention and treatment. *Behavior Therapy, 17,* 346–361.

Tarter, R. E., & Van Thiel, D. H. (Eds.). (1985). *Alcohol and the brain: Chronic effects.* New York: Plenum Press.

Tillich, P. (1952). *The courage to be.* New Haven, CT: Yale University Press.

Wallace, J. (1985). Predicting the onset of compulsive drinking in alcoholics: A biopsychosocial model. *Alcohol: An International Biomedical Journal, 2,* 589–595.

Wallace, J. (1987). Children of alcoholics: A population at risk. *Alcoholism Treatment Quarterly, 43,* 13–30.

Wallace, J. (1989a). Ideology, belief, and behavior: Alcoholics Anonymous as a social movement. In *Writings: The alcoholism papers of John Wallace* (pp. 335–352). Newport, RI: Edgehill.

Wallace, J. (1989b). The relevance to clinical care of recent research in neurobiology. In *Writings: The alcoholism papers of John Wallace* (pp. 85–207). Newport, RI: Edgehill.

Wallace, J. (1989c). A biopsychosocial model of alcoholism. *Social Casework: The Journal of Contemporary Social Work,* 325–332.

Wallace, J. (1990). Controlled drinking, treatment effectiveness, and the disease model of addiction: A commentary on the ideological wishes of Stanton Peele. *Journal of Psychoactive Drugs, 22,* 261–280.

Wallace, J. (1993). Fascism and the eye of the beholder: A reply to J. S. Searles on the controlled intoxication issue. *Addictive Behaviors, 18,* 239–251.

Wilber, K. (1993). *Grace and grit: Spirituality and healing in the life and death of Treya Killam Wilber.* Boston: Shambhala Press.

Wilson, B. (1953). *Twelve steps and twelve traditions.* New York: Alcoholics Anonymous World Services.

2

Facilitating 12-Step Recovery from Substance Abuse and Addiction

Joseph Nowinski

This chapter presents a model for facilitating recovery from alcohol or drug abuse or addiction. The model is intended for use by practitioners who do not necessarily have extensive knowledge of or experience with 12-step fellowships such as Alcoholics Anonymous (AA) or Narcotics Anonymous (NA) but who wish to actively facilitate their patients' use of such programs as a means of not drinking or not using drugs. Patients need not be dependent either on alcohol or drugs in order to benefit from the model presented here; rather, they need merely to meet the primary criterion for becoming members of AA (or NA), namely, having "a desire to stop drinking" (Alcoholics Anonymous, 1952, p. 139) or to stop using drugs. However, the reader should be aware that these fellowships have as their overall goal abstinence from (as opposed to controlled use of) alcohol or drugs. By definition, these fellowships were founded and exist for the benefit of those who have failed to control their use of alcohol and/or drugs (Alcoholics Anonymous, 1976, pp. 21, 24, 30–31).

GOALS AND OVERVIEW

Twelve-Step Facilitation (TSF; Nowinski & Baker, 2003; Nowinski, Baker, & Carroll, 1992) includes a range of interventions that are organized into a "core," or basic, program; an "elective," or advanced, program; and a conjoint program. Interventions in the core program are most appropriate for what could be termed the "early" or initial stage of recovery from alcohol or drug dependence. By "early recovery," we generally mean that stage of change in which an individual takes his or her initial steps from active substance abuse toward abstinence. The interventions included in the TSF core program could also be said to be directed primarily at the first four stages of change as described by the transtheoretical model of change (Prochaska, DiClemente, & Norcross, 1992; Saunders, Wilkinson, & Towers, 1996). These include *precontemplation*, referring to a relative unawareness of any need to change one's behavior at all; *contemplation*, meaning the process of coming to a decision to change; *preparation*, or marshaling resources for change; and *action*. This entire stage of the change process is typically marked by ambivalence, or what is commonly referred to as *denial* in the recovery field. The primary focus of this chapter will be on the TSF core program.

TSF also includes a set of interventions that can be brought to bear when working with patients who have moved to the *maintenance* stage of change (Prochaska et al., 1992, p. 1101). In recovery terms, these are men and women who have shown some sustained sobriety as well as some evidence of having bonded to a 12-step fellowship. Some of the topics included in the advanced program of TSF may also be useful with patients who have relapsed after some period of sobriety.

The conjoint program, which is the third component of TSF, may be used with patients at any stage of change. It is intended to enlist the help of significant others in the change process by teaching them the Al-Anon concepts of *enabling* and *caring detachment* (Al-Anon Family Group Headquarters, 1986a).

Finally, TSF includes a structured termination session. The goals of this session are to assess progress to date and to develop a posttreatment follow-up plan of action.

TSF was intended to be utilized as a time-limited (12- to 15-session) intervention. Initially developed as an individual treatment, it has been adapted for use with groups (Maude-Griffin et al., 1998; Seraganian, Brown, Tremblay, & Annies, 1998). In either format TSF is a highly structured intervention whose sessions follow a prescribed format. Each begins with a review of the patient's *recovery week*, including any 12-step meetings attended and reactions to them, episodes of drinking or drug use versus sober days, urges to drink or use drugs, reactions to any readings completed, and any journaling that the patient has done.

The second part of each session consists of presenting new material, consisting of material drawn from the core, elective, or conjoint programs. Each session ends with a wrapup that includes the assigning of *recovery tasks*: readings, meetings to be attended, and other pro-recovery behavioral work that the patient agrees to undertake between sessions.

The various TSF interventions are grouped as follows:

Core (basic) program

- Introduction and assessment
- Acceptance

- People, places, and routines
- Surrender
- Getting active

Elective (advanced) program

- Genograms
- Enabling
- Emotions
- Moral inventories
- Relationships

Conjoint program

- Enabling
- Detaching

Early Recovery

Broadly speaking, early recovery can be broken down into two phases: *acceptance* and *surrender*. "Acceptance" refers to the process in which the individual overcomes denial. "Denial" refers to the personal belief that one either does not have a substance abuse problem, and/or that one can effectively and reliably control one's drinking or drug use. In motivational terms, acceptance represents a vital insight: that the patient has in fact lost the ability to effectively control his or her use. Acceptance is marked by a realization that the patient's life has become progressively more unmanageable as a consequence of his or her alcohol or drug use, and furthermore that individual willpower alone is an insufficient force for creating sustained sobriety and restoring manageability to one's life. Given that realization, the only sane alternative to continued chaos and personal failure is to admit defeat (of one's efforts to control use), and to accept the need for abstinence as an alternative to controlled use.

As important as insight is, insight alone is not sufficient for recovery. That is where the concept of *surrender* comes in. "Surrender" basically means a willingness to take action, and specifically to embrace the 12 steps as a guide for recovery and spiritual renewal. AA and NA are programs of action as much as they are programs of insight and personal growth. Surrender follows acceptance and represents the individual's commitment to making whatever changes in lifestyle are necessary in order to sustain recovery. Surrender requires action, including frequent attendance at AA and/or NA meetings, becoming active in meetings, reading AA/NA literature, getting a sponsor, making AA/NA friends, and giving up people, places, and routines that have become associated with substance abuse and which therefore represent a threat to recovery. In TSF the action and commitment that are the hallmarks of surrender are guided to some extent by the facilitator; but they are also heavily influenced by the individuals whom the patient encounters and begins to form relationships with within 12-step fellowships. One especially significant relationship that TSF actively advocates for in early recovery is that of the *sponsor.*

Involvement in 12-step fellowships will inevitably expose both the patient and the therapist to a number of key 12-step traditions and concepts, such as the concept of a *higher power* (Alcoholics Anonymous, 1976, p. 50), the advocacy of fellowship over professionalism (Alcoholics Anonymous, 1952, p. 166), and the concepts of *group conscience* and *spiritual awakening* (Alcoholics Anonymous, 1952, pp. 106, 132). Because these concepts and traditions are so central to 12-step fellowships and their philosophy of recovery, the practitioner must not only be familiar with them but must be prepared to discuss them and their implications for action. Effective assignment of recovery tasks does not require that the therapist be in recovery, but it does demand familiarity with the culture and traditions of 12-step fellowships. For this reason therapists who have no personal knowledge of 12-step fellowships are encouraged to familiarize themselves with the basic AA texts, such as *Alcoholics Anonymous* (Alcoholics Anonymous, 1976), *Twelve Steps and Twelve Traditions* (Alcoholics Anonymous, 1952), and *Living Sober* (Alcoholics Anonymous, 1975). When working with drug abusers the basic NA text (Narcotics Anonymous, 1982) is very useful. Finally, therapists who are naive concerning 12-step fellowships are encouraged to attend several open AA, NA, and/or Al-Anon meetings prior to implementing TSF.

PRINCIPLES OF TWELVE-STEP FACILITATION

TSF, as a model of intervention, seeks to be both philosophically and pragmatically compatible with the 12 steps of AA. Accordingly, TSF is based on certain principles that follow from the 12 traditions of AA, and that should be understood if the intervention is to achieve this desired compatibility. Potential facilitators might do well to reflect on these principles and to "work through" any reactions they may have to them prior to embarking on an intervention.

Locus of Change

TSF considers the primary locus of change with respect to patients' drinking or using behavior to lie less in the hands of the therapist and more in the hands of 12-step fellowships such as AA and NA. In other words, our goal is the patient's active participation and involvement in 12-step fellowships, for we rely on that involvement to support the patient's recovery. That is the main reason why we prefer the word "facilitation" to words such as "therapy" or "treatment." The facilitator is obviously a highly skilled professional who must possess not only good psychotherapy skills but also a working knowledge of 12-

step fellowships. However, the therapist must also be able to resist becoming a patient's recovery program, as opposed to AA and/or NA becoming that program. In order to accomplish this, the facilitator must develop considerable skill in knowing when to provide advice and support personally versus when to encourage the patient to seek these things through AA or NA. As skilled as the facilitator may be, he or she must accept the idea that the patient's recovery is not dependent solely on the skills he or she acquires through therapy or on the support of the therapist; rather, therapists who employ TSF believe that sustained recovery relies heavily on skills the patient acquires through active fellowship with other recovering persons and on their ongoing support. Such a therapeutic stance places the responsibility for recovery squarely on the shoulders of the patient and defines the therapist–patient role as one of collaboration to achieve the goal of involvement in AA and/or NA.

Motivation

From its inception AA has characterized itself as a fellowship that is "based on attraction rather than promotion" (Alcoholics Anonymous, 1952, p. 180). Through this statement AA established a tradition of not seeking to attract members through overt advertising or promotion, much less through coercive techniques of any kind. AA's historic rate of growth is such that it has been likened to a "social movement" (Room, 1993). This growth, in turn, has relied in great part on the notion of identification and attraction, and also on the 12-step, which states: *"Having had a spiritual awakening as the result of these steps, we tried to carry this message to alcoholics, and to practice these principles in all our affairs"* (Alcoholics Anonymous, 1952, p. 106).

AA assumed from the outset that if an alcoholic attended meetings, listened to the stories of other alcoholics, and identified with them, then sooner or later he or she would naturally be motivated to try the program laid out in the 12 steps. The 12th step, meanwhile, supported the institution of sponsorship, in which individuals who have succeeded in sustaining recovery through AA or NA over a period of years, and who have remained active in it, will take newcomers under their wing for a period of time. They do so in order to support the newcomer and to teach him or her the traditions, etiquette, and other "rules of the road" that have evolved over the years in 12-step fellowships.

The AA/NA philosophy of attraction has implications for the therapist who wishes to use TSF. TSF eschews a heavily confrontational approach in favor of what could be called "carefrontation." This latter approach is more similar to what a newcomer to AA or NA will likely encounter at meetings. Typically, newcomers are greeted heartily; but there is no "hard sell," but instead a low-key approach that is welcoming and emphasizes "giving it a try" and "keeping an open mind."

The effectiveness of more coercive approaches at achieving sustained

sobriety has not been thoroughly tested. Although some have argued co-
gently that most people who seek help are pressured to do so in some way
or another (Anderson, 1991), it remains our conviction that involvement in
AA or NA is most effectively accomplished through a shaping approach,
emphasizing positive reinforcement of any and all progress made—in other
words, through an approach that is compatible with the traditions of these
fellowships.

Spirituality

One aspect of 12-step recovery that clearly separates it from other models of
intervention lies in its active promotion of spirituality. The guiding books of
AA—*Alcoholics Anonymous* (1976) and *Twelve Steps and Twelve Traditions*
(1952)—are replete with references to the importance of spirituality to recovery, and the 12th step, already cited here, asserts that following the program of
personal growth as outlined in the 12 steps will lead in the end to a spiritual
"awakening."

Here are some examples of the way that 12-step fellowships speak of spirituality:

> We have learned that whatever the human frailties of various faiths, those faiths
> have given purpose and direction to millions. People of faith have a logical idea of
> what life is all about. Actually, we used to have no reasonable conception what-
> ever. (Alcoholics Anonymous, 1976, p. 49).

> On one proposition, however, these men and women [alcoholics] are strikingly
> agreed. Every one of them has gained access to, and believes in, a Power greater
> than himself. (Alcoholics Anonymous, 1976, p. 50)

> . . . as a result of practicing all the Steps, we have each found something called a
> spiritual awakening. (Alcoholics Anonymous, 1976, p. 106)

Twelve-step fellowships regard spirituality as a force that provides direction and meaning to one's life, and they equate spiritual awakening with a re-
alignment of personal goals, specifically, with a movement away from radical
individualism and the pursuit of the material toward community and the pursuit of serenity as core values.

When conducting TSF, the clinician should be prepared to discuss the issue of spirituality. At several different points in treatment (Nowinski & Baker,
2003, pp. 73–81; Nowinski et al., 1992, pp. 2, 4, 47–48) the facilitator is asked
to engage the patient in a specific discussion of his or her spiritual beliefs.
Guidelines are provided for these discussions, which generally focus around
the issues of willpower, powerlessness, and faith, as well as on the issues of personal values and goals.

Pragmatism

Interestingly, although many people think of AA and its sister fellowships as primarily spiritual programs (and sometimes confuse them with religions), historically pragmatism has been as central to AA as spirituality. One official AA publication, *Living Sober* (Alcoholics Anonymous, 1975), is subtitled *Some Methods AA Members Have Used for Not Drinking.* This book contains a wealth of practical advice—much of it very compatible with cognitive-behavioral therapies—for avoiding "taking the first drink." Consider the following sampling from its Table of Contents:

- Using the 24-hour plan
- Changing old routines
- Making use of "telephone therapy"
- Getting plenty of rest
- Fending off loneliness
- Letting go of old ideas

In TSF the facilitator attempts to educate the patient with respect to some practical methods for staying sober. The facilitator consistently admonishes the patient to focus on "one day at a time" (another very pragmatic approach), and encourages the patient to solicit and follow practical advice from fellow AA members and his or her sponsor on issues ranging from the best ways to deal with difficult situations, to how to cope with cravings, to what to do after a slip, and so on. Of course the most basic advice given to all alcoholics and addicts is simple: don't drink (or use) and always go to meetings. In TSF each facilitation session ends with the facilitator assigning one or more *recovery tasks*, which are specific and pragmatic suggestions for action, including meetings, readings, journaling, and the like. In this way TSF mirrors the pragmatism of AA itself.

A Collaborative Approach

In setting a tone for the intervention, the 12-step facilitator takes an approach that is best described as "collaborative." He or she consistently strives to engage the patient in a constructive collaboration with the goal of achieving sobriety. The facilitator relies on the third tradition of AA as a foundation for this collaboration: *the only requirement for AA membership is a desire to stop drinking* (Alcoholics Anonymous, 1952, p. 139). This tradition is deliberate in its wording. It means that it is not essential for the patient to embrace each and every tenet of AA, or to adopt a particular spiritual philosophy. This attitude is supported by the following statement: "Alcoholics Anonymous does not demand that you believe anything. All of its Twelve Steps are but suggestions" (Alcoholics Anonymous, 1952, p. 26).

Following on the above, TSF encourages therapists to be flexible within the broad guideline of establishing a collaborative relationship with the patient toward the end of helping him or her stopping drinking or using. Confrontation in TSF is common, but it never takes the form of threat. For example, the 12-step facilitator will never terminate treatment because a patient drinks between sessions (or even shows up intoxicated).[1] On the other hand, the facilitator will consistently confront the patient about drinking or drug use and its connection to denial, and will consistently attempt to move the patient through the process of acceptance and surrender. The facilitator, committed to the idea that "90 meetings in 90 days" is the best strategy for the person in early recovery, will continue to ask for and encourage frequent attendance at meetings, but she or he will never make compliance with this suggestion a condition of treatment. Similarly, the 12-step facilitator will identify and point out denial to the patient, and will talk frankly with the patient about any "slips" that he or she has. But the facilitator always accepts addiction as a "cunning and clever" illness, and therefore expects both denial and relapse (at least in early recovery) as natural parts of the overall recovery process. Again, the 12-step facilitator seeks to be a shaper of behavior, relying heavily on rapport and reinforcement.

Focus

The focus of TSF is on helping the patient *begin* the process of recovery. The primary goal of TSF is to help the patient begin the process of bonding to a 12-step fellowship by understanding its key concepts and learning how to utilize its resources for support and advice.

Although collateral issues may (and frequently are) raised by patients in the course of treatment, facilitators are advised to avoid "drift," that is, a loss of focus on drinking or drug use and on becoming active in AA or NA, in favor of some other issue. Facilitators make every effort to validate patients' legitimate concerns—for example, about work, marriage, or family issues. But they also should be alert to patients' use of collateral issues as a means of avoiding either the subject of alcohol or drug use or the facilitator's expectations concerning them. While concurrent therapies may be necessary at times (e.g., for the acutely depressed patient, or for the patient with a co-occurring chronic

---

[1] TSF has specific guidelines for therapists to follow in the event that patients show up for meetings intoxicated, if they binge, or if their overall mental status deteriorates. The general guideline is that sessions are terminated if the patient is intoxicated although the therapist's first task is to ensure the patient's safety and make suggestions regarding contacting the AA. Hotline, getting to a meeting, or the like. TSF may be temporarily suspended if a patient requires detoxification.

mental illness), in general the TSF model advocates prioritizing problems, with early recovery from alcohol or drug abuse at the top of the list. At the very least, treatment of substance abuse should be coequal with treatment of mental illness in any comprehensive treatment plan, since a failure to address it independently (e.g., to assume that it may spontaneously remit once another problem is addressed) is always a serious mistake.

OBJECTIVES

The primary goals of early recovery, namely, acceptance and surrender, are achieved not only through dialogue with the facilitator but also through action on the part of the patient. Toward this end TSF seeks to achieve a number of specific objectives that can be broken down broadly into two related categories: (1) active involvement and (2) identification and bonding.

Active Involvement

To be sure, active involvement in 12-step fellowships such as AA and NA means going to meetings. But merely attending meetings does not qualify as *active* involvement. Very often practitioners who are unfamiliar with the 12-step model may stop their intervention at this point, or even short of it. "I suggested that my patient go to an AA meeting," a clinician might say, "but she told me that she tried that once and didn't like it."

Much as any psychotherapy involves helping patients work through resistances to change, facilitating active involvement means helping the patient to examine and work through resistances to active involvement in AA and/or NA. Working within a 12-step frame of reference, one is apt to encounter the word "denial" used instead of "resistance," though the two are in fact conceptually equivalent.

"Getting active" begins with going to meetings. For the individual who is just beginning to give up alcohol or drugs, 12-step fellowships have traditionally advocated attending 90 meetings in 90 days (i.e., a meeting a day, if not more, as a minimum goal). The exact origins of this common wisdom are vague, as are the origins of much of the "culture" of AA and the advice that is commonly offered to newcomers. However, such advice squares well with research on relapse (Marlatt & Gordon, 1985), which shows consistently, across addictions, that the majority of relapses occur within 90 days of initial abstinence.

AA and NA meetings vary a great deal with respect to membership, tone, and format. Because AA is by tradition deliberately decentralized (Alcoholics Anonymous, 1952, pp. 160, 172), no two meetings will be exactly alike. The result is a fellowship that is eclectic in form and open to continual change. The

facilitator should understand that there are not only discernable regional differences in the overall tone of meetings, say between those held in Connecticut and those held in California, but that there is a growing trend toward various "specialty" meetings. It is common, for example, to find men's, women's,
Latino, and gay AA/NA meetings listed, not to mention nonsmoking meetings. In larger communities, one can typically also locate meetings for professionals, for clergy, and so on. The San Francisco Bay Area lists special AA
meetings for atheists, for agnostics, and for meditators. Not all meetings, moreover, will be officially registered with AA's central office. Many are started by
AA and NA members and grow by word of mouth.

Though AA as an organization purposefully exerts no effort to assure that
meetings are organized or run in a prescribed way, there are a number of AA
and NA traditions, as well as discernable types of meetings. Traditions include,
of course, anonymity. They also include a rule against *cross-talk*, meaning interrupting a speaker to question him or her. So-called *service work*, such as making
coffee, setting up and taking down chairs, and passing the hat for voluntary
contributions to pay for any costs associated with supporting the meeting are
other traditions likely to be seen across groups. Finally, most groups will establish a series of rituals and rites, such as ways of starting and ending meetings;
ways of recognizing the achievement of certain landmarks, such as one, two,
five, and 10 years of sobriety; and so on.

There are also, by tradition, several different types of meetings, starting
with *speaker meetings*, in which an individual tells his or her story of addiction
and recovery, generally following this format: "How it was then, what happened, and how it is now." Invariably the theme of these stories is that of the
phoenix: the capacity of the human spirit to rise from the ashes of defeat. The
key to this dramatic change in each case is the individual's courage to admit
that alcohol or drugs has made life unmanageable (acceptance), and to replace
individual willpower with fellowship and the 12 steps as a pathway to recovery
and spiritual renewal (surrender).

Another type of meeting is the *open discussion* meeting. Here a designated
member or members raises an issue (e.g., resentment, loneliness, spirituality)
that members respond to in turn, sharing their thoughts or experiences relative
to the subject.

A third type of meeting is called a *step meeting*. Usually a group will focus
on one of the 12 steps for a month at a time. At the beginning of the meeting
the step is read aloud. Members then respond to the step, explaining how they
are "working" it in their daily lives. Some groups go through the entire 12
steps in this way; other groups may limit themselves to certain steps only—for
example, the first three—and cycle through them repeatedly.

Some AA and NA meetings are *open*, meaning that one need not necessarily admit to having a problem with alcohol or drugs in order to attend. Such
meetings are good to recommend to patients who are not yet sure that they

have a problem, or who want to stop drinking or using. They are also useful for therapists who want to learn more about 12-step fellowships before implementing TSF in their practices. Other meetings are *closed*. These meetings should be attended only by persons who are ready to admit to alcoholism or addiction, and who say they want to stop.

In facilitating early recovery, the facilitator should monitor not only *how many* meetings a patient attends, but also *what kinds* of meetings he or she attends. This can be done conveniently by asking patients to maintain a personal "recovery journal" in which they record meetings attended, what type they are, and their own reactions to them. By exploring these entries at the outset of each session (the review of the patient's "recovery week"), the therapist can help to create momentum in treatment and greatly enhance the overall facilitation effort.

Facilitators should make an effort to encourage patients to try out several different types of meetings, including open discussion, step, and speaker meetings. They should also encourage patients to attend one or two specialized meetings (e.g., a men's or a women's meeting). After the patient has attended a number of different meetings, she or he can be encouraged to begin thinking about making one of them his or her *home group*. This means making a commitment to attending that meeting regularly and to accepting some service work responsibility at the meeting. The secretary of the meeting is the individual who generally assigns service work responsibilities, which are typically rotated after a period of time.

Choosing a home group and accepting some responsibility for service to it moves the newly recovering patient to a deeper level of active involvement. Another level is achieved as the patient begins to utilize *telephone therapy*. This is another long-standing AA/NA tradition, attributed to one of AA's founders, Bill Wilson, who is reported to have once decided to call someone instead of taking a drink.

Giving and getting phone numbers is another normal part of the AA/NA culture, and patients should be prepared for it. Of course, they should feel free to decline to give out their phone number initially, if this idea makes them feel uncomfortable. However, the therapist should normalize this tradition and explain its purpose, which is to build a support network of fellow AA/NA members who are sympathetic to the goal of not drinking or using drugs, and who can be called on in times of need. In this regard it is important to explain to patients who are not experiencing any immediate urges to drink or use (and who may therefore be inclined to see no immediate need for such contacts) that it is important to establish a network of AA friends *before* one needs them.

On another level, getting and using phone numbers, like becoming more active in meetings, serves to gradually reconstruct the patient's social circle. Over time it can lead to less contact with old, drinking or using friends and more contact with new, sober friends. Since research suggests that social support is a significant factor in recovery (Sobell, Cunningham, Sobell, & Toneatto, 1993), this process of progressively establishing a new social network can be thought of as a core objective of TSF.

The last objective with regard to facilitating active involvement in AA or NA concerns *sponsorship.* A sponsor is by tradition a sort of mentor: an individual who has traveled the road before you and who can serve as your guide. AA succinctly describes the role and significance of the sponsor in early recovery in this way: "Not every A.A. member has a sponsor. But thousands of us say we would not be alive were it not for the special friendship of one recovering alcoholic in the first months and years of our sobriety" (Alcoholics Anonymous, 1975, p. 26).

Sponsors by tradition are of the same sex as the newcomers, for the obvious reason of minimizing the possibility of dual agendas. For gay and lesbian patients, the same caveat applies: a sponsor ought not to be someone with whom a romantic attraction is likely to become established.

The sponsor–sponsee relationship is usually a close one. For newcomers especially, sponsors will often establish a pattern of daily telephone (and sometimes face-to-face) contact. They may meet the newcomer at meetings and facilitate his or her meeting new people. The sponsor may suggest meetings that would be particularly good for the newcomer to attend. Sponsors may also introduce newcomers to AA social events and may try to the best of their ability to answer questions about the 12 steps or the fellowship itself. Because of the need to maintain clear boundaries, the facilitator (even if she or he is personally in recovery) cannot become a patient's sponsor. Nevertheless, the facilitator needs to take a proactive role in helping the patient to find a sponsor very early in the recovery process. Often this issue will be brought up directly in meetings: the meeting chairperson will ask, first, if there are any newcomers present, and second, if there is anyone in need of a sponsor. Alternatively, the patient can be coached in how to ask for a sponsor at that point in a meeting when it is open to requests.

Taken together, the above set of objectives serve to establish a broad basis of social support for sobriety while simultaneously breaking the patient away from people, places, and routines that have long been associated with alcohol or drug use. Along with identification, it is a core aspect of the TSF program. Obviously it is an active therapeutic process, and one that goes well beyond the simple (and passive) suggestion that a patient "try going to AA."

Identification and Bonding

It is axiomatic within AA that it is the similarities among alcoholics, not the differences, that are important. What is being referred to, of course, is the "similarity" of not being able to control drinking. Bill Wilson expressed it this way:

We are average Americans.[2] All sections of this country and many of its occupations are represented, as well as many political, economic, social, and religious backgrounds. We are people who normally would not mix. But there exists among us a fellowship, a friendliness, and an understanding which is indescribably wonderful. (Alcoholics Anonymous, 1952, p. 17)

It is common, indeed natural, for the newcomer to AA and NA to experience discomfort. After all, alcoholism and addiction still carry with them a significant social stigma. In addition, people who have little or no direct knowledge of 12-step fellowships are apt to hold many stereotyped attitudes and beliefs. For example, they may have the idea that AA and NA are religions or that their members are obsessed with God. Many worry that they will be asked to commit themselves to a cult, or that they will find themselves surrounded by skid-row bums. In all of these ways and more, patients' anxieties may cause them to persist in seeing themselves as different, while ignoring the essential similarity between their own experiences with substance abuse and those of everyone else in the room.

The first thing the facilitator needs to do is to normalize and empathize with patient's initial reticence to identify with those attending a meeting, or even to walk into a meeting. Reading the above quote can initiate a productive discussion of this issue, as can having the patient share entries that were written in his or her recovery journal after going to a meeting. The facilitator needs to remain alert for resistance to identification and to help the patient work it through. The first strategy for doing so is education. Solicit and discuss any stereotypes the patient has about AA/NA, their members, or what happens at meetings. Then ask the patient to go to some open speaker and discussion meetings and to simply listen. Ask the patient to recount what she or he heard, being vigilant for stereotypes versus realities.

The facilitator should routinely ask the patient who is new to AA or NA if there was a person, or a particular part of a story or discussion, that she or he could relate to (i.e., *identify with*). Building on this foundation, the facilitator can gradually promote the patient's capacity for identification. Naturally this calls for no small amount of judgment and skill—for example, in knowing just how much identification to press for. Sometimes identification is simply too threatening to the patient to be accepted in whole.

Others methods for facilitating identification are keeping a journal (already mentioned) or reading AA and NA material. Especially useful for purposes of promoting identification are the many personal stories of addiction

---

[2] AA has grown considerably since these words were written. According to the AA General Services Office, as of December 31, 1998, there were 101,000 AA groups spread out over 145 countries. Total membership at that time exceeded 4 million.

and recovery that appear in *Alcoholics Anonymous* (1976) and *Narcotics Anonymous* (1982). For patients with a great deal of social anxiety, attempting to identify through reading at home may be easier at first than identifying through listening at meetings.

However identification is achieved, it is a highly desirable outcome of 12-step facilitation for it has the effect of *bonding* the patient to the fellowship. Often, in the very early stages of recovery, it is getting active per se that is most crucial. In order to sustain involvement and ensure sobriety over the long run, though, a deeper sense of identification and connection—of bonding—may be crucial. Furthermore, in general, it is in the context of this bonding that many AA members begin to pursue more advanced work such as creating moral inventories (Steps 4 and 5) and to experience firsthand some of the spiritual renewal that has long been associated with AA. Indeed, it may be impossible for an individual to experience the "spiritual awakening" that the 12th step speaks of in the absence of this bonding process.

Taken together, active involvement and identification form a solid basis for recovery. The more effective the facilitator, in collaboration with the patient, is in establishing these dimensions of recovery, the more likely, we think, it is that the patient will sustain his or her sobriety.

Assessment

Facilitating recovery using a 12-step model begins much as any good treatment for substance abuse should begin: with a thorough assessment. The specific approach to assessment employed in TSF has been described in detail elsewhere (Nowinski & Baker, 2003; Nowinski et al., 1992) and for reasons of space will be described only briefly here.

Assessment is important for two reasons. The first and most obvious reason is that we want to determine if the prospective patient is indeed addicted to alcohol or drugs. In reality, however, research has established that "problem drinkers" just as much as true alcoholics can benefit from TSF (Project MATCH Research Group, 1997). Therefore, the use of TSF need not be limited to "severe" or "end-stage" alcoholics or addicts.

A second and perhaps less obvious objective underlying assessment has to do with the issue of motivation. Part of the purpose of taking a thorough alcohol and drug history, as well as a careful inventory of consequences, is to establish a collaborative therapeutic relationship with the patient and, ideally, to reach a *consensus* regarding diagnosis and treatment. This may require the facilitator to refer back frequently in subsequent sessions to data collected during the assessment. Therefore, it is important that the clinician keep good records of information he or she has gathered. Toward this end, it is recommended that the patient be given a copy of the assessment and be asked to review it as one of his or her first *recovery tasks* between sessions.

An alcohol–drug history is a graphical representation of chronological changes in the type and amount of mood-altering substances used by the patient, along with correlated events and effects. Creating an alcohol–drug history is best done using a chart such like that shown in Table 2.1.

In this hypothetical example, the patient reported first use of alcohol at age 11. At that time he sipped from his father's supply of beer, primarily on weekends. Drinking made him feel "silly," but sometimes it made him feel sick. He reported that his mother and father fought often at about the same time. By age 13 his use of alcohol had increased to two or three beers, two or three times a week. This made him feel "high," suggesting that he was experiencing some pleasurable affect as a consequence of his drinking, and was using alcohol primarily for its euphoric effects. At about this same time, his father left the home.

By the time he was 14 our hypothetical patient was drinking beer as well as smoking marijuana three to four times a week. He reports that this made him feel "mellow," which suggests that he was at that point using substances to control his mood and to create a sense of relaxation and calm. He also reports getting into trouble at school and having much conflict at home at this point in time.

Although Table 2.1 is necessarily brief for purposes of illustration, the clinician should take care to fill in a similar chart as completely as possible, adding as much detail as the patient will offer. Again, the objective is to engage the patient in a collaborative effort in the creation of this autobiography, most especially to document the *progression* of substance use over time and all significant events correlated with it. If this takes more than a single session, so be it.

After the alcohol–drug history is completed, the patient should be given a copy and asked to study it between sessions. At the next session the facilitator should review it again with the patient, filling in any additional details that the patient recalled as a result of this recovery task.

TABLE 2.1. Alcohol–Drug History

Substance/age	Type/amount		Frequency	Effects	Significant events
Alcohol/11	Beer: sips from Dad's supply		Weekends	"Silly" "Sick"	Mom and Dad fighting.
Alcohol/13	Beer: 2–3	×	2–3/wk	"High"	Dad left.
Alcohol	Beer: 2–3	×	3–4/wk	"Mellow"	Doing poorly in school/ fighting at home.
Marijuana/14	1–2 joints	×	3–4/wk		

The second major part of the assessment is an inventory of *consequences* of alcohol and drug use. Again, both for purposes of clarity and to enhance motivation, this is best done chronologically. The facilitator can introduce this part of the assessment with an opening statement similar to the following:

> "Let's take some time to examine some of the issues, conflicts, and problems that you've experienced over your life, and let's see if any of them are connected in any way to your use of alcohol or drugs."

Negative consequences of alcohol or drug use should be explored both chronologically and categorically. Be sure not to leave out (or allow the patient to avoid) examining each of the following areas.

Physical Consequences

Included here (especially for older patients) are the physical consequences of long-term substance abuse, including
hypertension, gastrointestinal problems, sleep disorders, weight loss, alcohol- or drug-related injuries and accidents, emergency room visits, blackouts, heart problems, liver disease, and kidney disease. Keep in mind that it is estimated that approximately 50% of all general hospital beds in the United States are occupied by patients whose medical illnesses are alcohol- or drug-related (National Institute on Alcohol Abuse and Alcoholism, 1990).

Legal Consequences

Alcohol and drug use often lead to legal troubles such as DWI (driving while intoxicated) arrests, arrests for possession or sale of illegal substances, arrests for disorderly conduct, and the like. Also include alcohol- or drug-related illegal activities (e.g., sale, theft, prostitution) that the patient was either not arrested or convicted for.

Social Consequences

Social consequences of alcohol or drug use include relationship, family, or job conflicts. Substance abusers often alienate their partners, perform progressively more poorly at work, and are dysfunctional as parents. They may destroy their marriages, lose their jobs, and alienate their friends. It is important to do a thorough inventory of such losses, in chronological order, and to connect them to the patient's alcohol–drug history as appropriate.

Psychological Consequences

Habitual use of alcohol and drugs, even in the absence of clear dependency, typically leads to negative psychological consequences such as anxiety and depression. Other consequences include poor anger control, sleep and eating disorders, irritability, amotivational syndrome, and confused thinking. As habitual use gives way to dependency, and as negative consequences accrue, suicidal thinking and suicide attempts are not uncommon.

Sexual Consequences

Not only is alcohol and other substance abuse associated with sexual dysfunction in both males and females (Powell, 1984), but alcohol and drug use and dependency are often correlated with sexual victimization and exploitation. The facilitator should explore the patient's sexual history to determine if sexual dysfunction, victimization, or exploitation are present, and if so whether they are correlated with substance abuse. Frank discussion of sexuality is often omitted from assessment even though it is often a potential motivator for recovery. Guidelines for conducting substance-abuse-related sexual histories have been published elsewhere (Nowinski & Baker, 2003).

Financial Consequences

It is a good idea to have the patient estimate how much money she or he has spent on alcohol or drugs in the 2 years prior to the assessment. Expenses should include both the cost of the substances themselves and the costs of any consequences. The latter include such costs as traffic tickets, legal defense or representation, and lost income. For example, a cocaine addict may have spent $50,000 on cocaine over 2 years; but may also have lost a job worth $40,000 per year; had to hire one lawyer to represent him in court, and another to represent him in divorce action; and had a bank foreclose on his house. These financial consequences are all justifiably included as costs of addiction.

*   *   *

Once both the alcohol–drug history and the inventory of consequences have been completed, the assessment itself ends with the facilitator sharing a diagnosis and treatment plan. Obviously, this should come as no surprise to the patient if the assessment process has truly been a collaborative venture. Still, the patient and the clinician may disagree, especially if the clinician thinks the patient is addicted, but the patient still does not believe that he or she is addicted. What is important for the clinician to note is that it is not essential for the pa-

tient to acknowledge alcoholism or addiction in order to proceed with TSF.
The sole criteria for making use of AA, and therefore using TSF, is a *desire to
stop drinking.* Addiction is not a prerequisite.

TREATMENT

It is to be hoped that a successful assessment has not only confirmed a clinical diagnosis for both the clinician and the patient, but has also motivated the patient to
want to stop drinking or using drugs. In some cases this motivation will mean
that the patient will be willing to follow the therapist's advice—for example, to
begin attending meetings, doing some reading, keeping a journal, and so on.

Many patients may acknowledge that drugs and/or alcohol have indeed
caused serious consequences, and may even express a desire to stop drinking;
nonetheless, their behavior may reveal a resistance to taking any of the actions
that recovery requires. Others may produce a history replete with consequences, and appear to be leading an unmanageable life, yet still deny addiction. In each of these situations successful treatment demands that the therapist
be able to establish a collaborative relationship with the patient. Within AA
and other 12-step fellowships the transition from outright denial, to passive acknowledgment of a problem, to active participation in a 12-step fellowship as a
means of achieving recovery is known as "working the steps." This is also the
crux of early recovery. It is a process wherein the patient could be said to move
from *denial,* to *acceptance,* to *surrender.*

Acceptance

The first step of AA and NA as it appears in their respective "Big Books" read
as follows:

> We admitted we were powerless over alcohol—that our lives had become un-
> manageable. (Alcoholics Anonymous, 1976, p. 59)

> We admitted we were powerless over our addiction—that our lives had become
> unmanageable. (Narcotics Anonymous, 1982, p. 8)

Although many individuals take issue with the word "powerless" in these
statements, it is important for clinicians who wish to use TSF to understand
exactly how that concept is used within the fellowships of AA and NA, which
is *contextual.* In other words, 12-step fellowships speak of powerlessness only in
the context of alcohol or drug use. Step 1 refers specifically to *powerlessness over
alcohol or drug use*; it does not imply any kind of generalized powerlessness.

The powerlessness that is spoken of in Step 1 does have to do with acknowledging the limitations of individual willpower. Twelve-step fellowships were and are built on acceptance of a simple yet profound recognition: that individual willpower can be overwhelmed by the addiction process. Once addicted, efforts to control use will only lead to failure and frustration, and eventually to hopelessness. Furthermore, once addicted, individuals are not as likely to sustain sobriety alone as they are through mutual support. In order to stay sober, AA admonishes the alcoholic to "quit playing God" (Alcoholics Anonymous, 1976, p. 62), and to accept the notion that "any life run on self-will can hardly be a success" (Alcoholics Anonymous, 1976, p. 60).

In essence, then, the first step represents a statement of humility. It reflects an acceptance of personal limitation: that life has become *unmanageable*, that this unmanageability is the result of substance abuse, and that willpower alone has not been enough to change that. Philosophically, the first step (and AA itself) has been characterized as a challenge to the radical individualism that has long been a core theme in U.S. culture (Room, 1993).

In discussing Step 1 with patients, the therapist will find it extremely useful to have the alcohol–drug history and the chronology of consequences at hand. The focus of therapist–patient dialogue should be on the *progressive pattern of unmanageability in the patient's life and the limitations of personal willpower.* If the patient's history and chronology do not make a case for total loss of control, it should at least show a pattern of growing unmanageability that can be pointed out—repeatedly, if necessary—to the patient. The patient can also be encouraged to describe some of the methods that she or he has used in the past in order to limit or stop her or his use of alcohol or drugs. In this regard the facilitator would do well to share the following excerpt with the patient:

> Here are some of the methods we have tried: Drinking beer only, limiting the number of drinks, never drinking alone, never drinking in the morning, drinking only at home, never having it in the house, never drinking during business hours, drinking only at parties, switching from scotch to brandy, drinking only natural wines, agreeing to resign if ever drunk on the job, swearing off forever (with or without a solemn oath), taking more physical exercise, reading inspirational books, going to health farms and sanitariums, accepting voluntary commitment to asylums—we could increase the list ad infinitum. (Alcoholics Anonymous, 1976, p. 31)

In the face of evidence of growing unmangeability and failure to control use, the patient who continues to resist suggestions that she or he needs to admit defeat (of willpower) and therefore needs to give up alcohol or drugs altogether could be said to be in *denial.*

Any discussion of Step 1 should proceed toward acceptance of the need for abstinence in a series of steps, as follows:

1. The patient acknowledges that he or she has a "problem" with
    alcohol or drugs—that life has become, or is becoming, progressively
    more unmanageable.
2. The patient acknowledges that individual efforts to limit or stop
    drinking or using have failed (i.e., accepting powerlessness in the con-
    text of substance use).
3. The patient acknowledges the need to give up alcohol and/or drugs
    as opposed to trying to limit or their control use.

As simple and straightforward as the above sounds, clinicians find that
moving a patient from denial to acceptance usually is more of a *process* than an
event—and a painful one at that. For many individuals with alcohol or drug
problems, acceptance represents an insight that is achieved gradually and only
reluctantly. It is also an awareness that is frequently accompanied by intense
emotional reactions (to acceptance of personal limitation and the loss of alcohol or the drug of choice as a "friend" and coping mechanism), such as anger,
that the facilitator must be able to empathize with. As a rule, acceptance without emotion is suspect. More typically, patients will experience most or all of
the emotional stages associated with grief and loss as they move through the
stages of acceptance. The clinician does well to raise this issue of emotional responses to Step 1, to normalize it, and then to explore it with the patient.

People, Places, and Routines

From acceptance, which roughly corresponds to the *contemplation* stage of
change (Prochaska et al., 1992), TSF moves on to help the patient *prepare* for
change. The vehicle for this preparation is the Lifestyle Contract, an example
of which is shown in Table 2.2.

The Lifestyle Contract is based on the notion that addiction evolves into
a virtual lifestyle that is supported by a range of "people, places, and routines."
In order to support his or her recovery, once the decision has been made to
pursue abstinence as a long-term goal, the substance abuser must be prepared
to make changes in each of these areas. The Lifestyle Contract, which is devel-

TABLE 2.2. Lifestyle Contract

	Dangerous to recovery	Supportive of recovery
People	Drinking friends	AA members Nondrinking friends
Places	Bars, casinos	AA meetings Nondrinking friends' homes
Routines	Drinks after work	Meeting AA friends Exercise

oped collaboratively by the patient and the therapist, becomes a blueprint for this life change.

The Lifestyle Contract also assumes that simply "giving things up" will not be a successful strategy for change in the long run. To truly support recovery, people, places, and routines that are supportive of recovery must be substituted for those that pose a threat to recovery. Viewed another way, the Lifestyle Contract is an inventory of the lifestyle that supports drinking or drug use versus an alternative lifestyle that supports sobriety.

It is recommended that the therapist work with the patient to develop a Lifestyle Contract early in treatment, but only after the patient has achieved at least some degree of acceptance of the need to give up alcohol or drugs.

Surrender

Surrender follows acceptance and the development of the Lifestyle Contract. It represents the patient's decision to seek outside help and abandon personal willpower as a means of controlling or stopping use of alcohol or drugs. Like acceptance, surrender is more typically a process than an event. Again, it is a process that evokes intense emotion. It is reflected in Steps 2 and 3 of Alcoholics Anonymous:

> We came to believe that a Power greater than ourselves could restore us to sanity. We made a decision to turn our will and our lives over to the care of God *as we understood Him.* (Alcoholics Anonymous, 1976, p. 59)

The italics at the end of the third step appear in the original text and are emphasized in order to point out that the AA view of God or a higher power is a pluralistic one. There is neither an organized priesthood nor a specific dogma within AA or NA; rather, these are deliberately decentralized fellowships. The closest thing to a dogma are the 12 steps themselves, which are framed not as dogma but as suggestions.

AA does have a long spiritual tradition, to the extent that the 12 steps challenge us to believe in a center of power that is greater than our individual wills. Substituting faith in the group (or some other higher power) for faith in personal willpower has been construed as a form of spiritual conversion or awakening:

> Faith is a dynamic process of construal and commitment in which persons find and give meaning to their lives through trust in and loyalty to shared centers of value, images and realities of power, and core stories. Conversion in AA perspective begins when one reaches and acknowledges a state of helpless desperation in the effort to maintain the false self and the illusion that one can manage one's drinking. Gradually it comes to mean making a commitment to enter into the 12

steps and become part of the 12 traditions of Alcoholics Anonymous. (Fowler, 1993)

If Step 1 involves *accepting the problem* (i.e., alcoholism or drug addiction), then Steps 2 and 3 can be thought of as *accepting the solution*, which requires the addict to reach out. Within 12-step fellowships this is commonly referred to as "turning it over"—that is, moving away from self-centeredness and an excessive belief in the power of individual willpower toward a willingness to reach out to and accept the strength of fellowship. This is more than an abstract notion: it will be directly reflected in patients' *hope for recovery*, in their *willingness to become active in the fellowship*, and in their *openness to receiving advice*. When an individual begins to "surrender" in this fashion, she or he begins to appreciate that accepting powerlessness over alcohol or drugs does not in any way imply helplessness over addiction.

AA and NA are fellowships that were established by and for the "hopeless," in other words, by and for people whose personal struggles to control addiction had led to personal defeat and desperation. Individuals whose problems with alcohol and drugs are less severe than that may have a harder time identifying with some of the shared images, values, and stories that form the spiritual foundation of these fellowships. Nevertheless, so long as life has become increasingly unmanageable as a result of drinking or drug use, the individual may become motivated to give it up. Furthermore, as stated earlier, even "problem drinkers" (as opposed to true alcoholics) have benefited from TSF.

The clinician should engage the patient in a specific and ongoing dialogue about willpower, faith, and surrender. It is suggested that at least one entire session be devoted to reading Steps 2 and 3 and discussing the patient's reactions to them. Questions like the following can be used as a guideline for this discussion:

- "As a youth, who were your heroes, and who are they now?"
- "What are your most cherished values? In other words, what personal qualities in others do you admire most?"
- "How do you feel about people who ask others for help when they feel stuck, and why?"
- "Are you open to the idea that people struggling with similar problems can help each other more than each of those people can help themselves?"
- "Whose advice are you most likely to follow?"
- "Do you ever pray? When, and why?"
- "Are you open to the idea that there are some personal problems that a person can solve only by reaching out for help and support from others?"

- "Do you believe that others could help you stay clean or sober?"
- "What is your idea of God?"
- "Who in the world do you trust the most, and why?"
- "Are you willing to do what someone else who has overcome alcoholism or drug addiction tells you to do? When would you, and when wouldn't you, follow his or her advice?"
- "How do you feel about using the support of people in AA or NA to help you stay clean and sober?"

This sort of dialogue is more than an intellectual adventure. It is central to introducing the patient to the spiritual foundation of 12-step fellowships. Not all therapists will be comfortable engaging patients in this sort of dialogue. All therapists would be wise to ponder such questions themselves before entering into this kind of dialogue. In the end it can be very productive to venture down this road, since it represents a highly effective route to working through patients' resistances to becoming active in AA or NA and making full use of their social and spiritual resources. An all-too-common alternative to this kind of dialogue is for the therapist to merely accuse the patient of being in denial, which only encourages further resistance. Rather than pursuing that course, it is generally more productive to explore issues related to letting go of the illusion of personal omnipotence and to overcoming reluctance to reach out to others.

Getting Active

The fifth and final component of early treatment centers around facilitating the patient's active participation in AA and/or NA. "Getting active," in 12-step parlance, means "working the steps." AA puts it this way: "Just stopping drinking is not enough. Just not drinking is a negative, sterile thing. That is clearly demonstrated by our experience. To stay stopped, we've found we need to put in place of the drinking a positive program of action" (Alcoholics Anonymous, 1975).

A popular meditation book expresses similar sentiments in this way: "Work and prayer are the two forces which are gradually making a better world. We must work for the betterment of ourselves and other people. Faith without works is dead" (Anonymous, 1975, p. 83).

The message here is clear: recovery requires faith, but it also requires action. Steps 1 and 2 in particular can be thought of as necessary but not sufficient conditions for staying clean or sober. To facilitate recovery, the clinician must be prepared to continually work with the patient toward the goal of his or her active involvement in a 12-step fellowship, namely, going to meetings frequently and listening well, getting phone numbers and building a support network, seeking a home group and taking on a responsibility, seeking out a sponsor, and reading AA/NA material.

Two useful vehicles for pursuing the goal of getting active are keeping a *recovery journal* (described earlier) and doing *recovery tasks.* The latter are not unlike "homework" that is often employed in cognitive-behavioral therapies which, like TSF, also involve patient–therapist collaboration and active work on the part of the patient. It is recommended that the clinician end each session with a series of specific recovery tasks, and begin each session with a review of the patient's "recovery week," including progress made on recovery tasks.

Recovery tasks and the subsequent review should cover each of the following areas:

- Readings from AA and/or NA literature.
- Suggestions about specific meetings to attend.
- Progress made on the use of telephone therapy, selecting a home group, taking on responsibility, and getting a sponsor.

Clinicians may wish to employ techniques like role playing in order to facilitate reaching specific objectives (e.g., using the telephone, speaking up at meetings) that are difficult for patients suffering from high social anxiety. Therapists must also be prepared to shape behavior—in this case, active participation—through positive reinforcement of the patient's efforts. It is not uncommon, for example, for patients to make several false starts when first "testing the waters" of AA or NA. They may get as far as the door of a meeting, for example, only to turn around at the last second. They may come to a meeting late and leave early. Or they may attend only one meeting after promising to attend three.

Obviously, to be able to shape behavior, the facilitator must first know about it. A blaming or unreceptive attitude on the part of the facilitator is likely to cloud communication when what is needed is openness. The patient should be made to feel safe disclosing what he or she actually did between sessions. This is not inconsistent with his or her also knowing what the clinician would *like* him or her to have done. Rather than scolding or punishing the patient in any way, the therapist should recognize and reinforce all the patient's positive efforts to change, and then work collaboratively with the patient to identify the causes of any resistance. If the cause is something like social anxiety, then techniques like role playing may help. If the cause is linked to resistance to ideas like powerlessness, as discussed earlier, then a different approach may be in order.

READINGS

Here are some suggestions for readings that might be assigned relative to the subjects of acceptance, the Lifestyle Contract, surrender, and getting active:

Acceptance

Twelve Steps and Twelve Traditions: pp. 21–24.

Alcoholics Anonymous: "The Doctor's Opinion," "Bill's Story," "More About Alcoholism."

Narcotics Anonymous: "Who Is An Addict," "Why Are We Here?" "How It Works."

Living Sober: pp. 7–10.

Surrender

Alcoholics Anonymous: "There Is a Solution,"
"More About Alcoholism," "How It Works."
Narcotics Anonymous, pp. 22–26.
Twelve Steps and Twelve Traditions, pp. 25–41.
Living Sober, pp. 77–87.

Lifestyle Contract/Getting Active

Alcoholics Anonymous: Personal stories (to be selected by facilitator).
Living Sober: Chapters 3, 6, 8, 10, 11, 13, 14, 15, 18, 22, 26, 27, 29.

Therapists should be familiar with any readings assigned and be prepared to discuss them during the review period at the outset of each TSF session. Consideration should be given to the patient's reading level and available time when making reading assignments. For patients who cannot read, audiotapes of AA publications are available through Alcoholics Anonymous World Services, PO Box 1980, New York, NY, 10163-1980. Similarly, most AA and NA texts are available in various translations.

Readings should not be limited to the above. Rather, these are offered as appropriate suggestions. With experience, the facilitator will develop personal preferences as well as a sense for "what fits who" with respect to readings.

MEETINGS

In order to make meaningful recommendations about which meetings to suggest to a patient, the facilitator must obtain current official AA and NA meeting schedules. These are available through regional AA or NA offices. Local numbers for AA and NA groups are listed in the white pages of many telephone books. They may also be obtained at AA and NA meetings. This brings up an important point: clinicians wishing to utilize TSF are strongly encouraged to occasionally attend open AA, NA, and/or Al-Anon meetings, to maintain current meeting schedules, and, if possible, to develop their own small network of AA and NA contacts who may be useful resources for getting shy newcomers to meetings, explaining the AA/NA "rules of the road," and so on.

Many recovering persons express a great deal of gratitude to those first "friendly faces" encountered at meetings. The facilitator should not assume this responsibility personally; instead, she or he is better off developing relationships with recovering men and women who are at a point in their own recovery process where they are ready to do this sort of "12th step" work. Therapists should not hesitate to reach out for such help, since it is an integral part of the AA culture to help those who need help.

Conjoint Program

It is not uncommon for interventions based on a 12-step model to include a family and/or marital component. Such an inclusion recognizes the reality that substance abuse effects not only the abuser but also his or her significant others. A detailed intervention for significant others of substance abusers has been described elsewhere (Nowinski, 1998).

TSF incorporates an abbreviated conjoint program into its model. The TSF conjoint program is consistent with the philosophy of Al-Anon, which is a 12-step fellowship for significant others of substance abusers (Al-Anon Family Group Headquarters, 1986a).

The objectives of the TSF conjoint program, which generally spans no more than two or three sessions, is to provide a spouse or significant other with an overview of the facilitation program that the patient is undergoing, to do an initial assessment of possible partner substance abuse, and to introduce the significant other to Al-Anon and two of its key concepts: enabling and detaching.

TSF recognizes that relationships, including marriages and parent–child relationships, are often rendered deeply dysfunctional and wounded as a result of addiction. It recognizes also that marital and/or family therapy are often much needed by alcoholics and addicts in recovery. At the same time, TSF is based on the idea that *early* recovery is best served by focusing on acceptance, surrender, and getting active. In a similar vein, TSF seeks to help significant others get a *start* on recovering from the effects of addiction, and believes that programs like Al-Anon offer the best resources for that start. Accordingly, before a patient who is just beginning recovery and his or her partner or family are referred for marital or family therapy, TSF attempts to engage them in fellowships that can offer understanding, support, and advice.

Partner Substance Abuse

The issue of partner substance abuse cannot be ignored by the practitioner working with persons on early recovery for the obvious reason that it represents a threat to the early recovery of the primary patient. But TSF does not insist on total abstinence from partners who are merely social drinkers. However, basic questions such as those listed below should be asked in order to determine whether a partner is best referred for treatment as well:

- "Do you drink or use drugs at all? If so, what do you drink [use] and how often?"
- "Have you ever felt [or has anyone else ever suggested] that you have a problem with alcohol or drugs?"
- "Have you ever suffered any consequences of any kind related to alcohol or drug use?"
- "Has drinking or drug use ever interfered with your day-to-day life or made it 'unmanageable' in any way?"

Based on a simple and brief inquiry such as this, along with any information that the clinician has gathered from the patient, a decision can be made about whether it should be suggested to a partner that he or she should also seek further help. At the same time the facilitator will know whether partner substance abuse should be taken into account when constructing the primary patient's Lifestyle Contract.

Introducing Al-Anon and/or Nar-Anon

Al-Anon and Nar-Anon are fellowships that parallel AA and NA. However, these fellowships were formed not to support recovering addicts or alcoholics, but rather to support those who are in relationships with alcoholics or addicts. As do AA and NA, both Al-Anon and Nar-Anon begin with statements of "powerlessness." In this case, however, it is the behavior of the alcoholic or addict that the individual is powerless over. Coming to terms with this personal limitation (Step 1 of Al-Anon) is a process that parallels the alcoholic's or addict's coming to terms with his or her powerlessness over alcohol or drugs. Many of the same psychodynamics (e.g., denial) must be acknowledged and worked through. Similarly, the decision to reach out to others (Al-Anon) for support and guidance has its parallels in Steps 2 and 3 of AA.

Learning to stop doing things that either purposefully or inadvertently allow the alcoholic or the addict to continue drinking or using (*enabling*), and to let go of any illusion of being able to control the alcoholic or addict (*detaching*), are central to Al-Anon and Nar-Anon. It is only through learning detachment, it is believed, that partners and family members can begin to recover their own mental health. Al-Anon and Nar-Anon provide both the social and the spiritual support for this process. Al-Anon expresses the overall goal this way:

"Detach!" we are told in Al-Anon. This does not mean detaching ourselves, and our love and compassion, from the alcoholic. Detachment, in the Al-Anon sense, means to realize we are individuals. We are not bound morally to shoulder the alcoholic's responsibilities. (Al-Anon Family Group Headquarters, 1986, p. 54)

After giving partners an overview of TSF and inquiring into their own use of alcohol or drugs, the facilitator devotes the bulk of the conjoint program to discussing the issues of enabling and detaching and encouraging the partner to get active in Al-Anon or Nar-Anon. In this way the conjoint program, however brief, parallels the facilitation program itself. *Enabling* is defined as any behavior that has the effect of allowing the alcoholic or addict to ignore facing the reality that drinking or drug use is making his or her life unmanageable. Examples are given, such as those listed below:

- Making excuses to cover up for the patient when she or he would otherwise get into trouble as a consequence of alcohol or drug use.
- Providing money or other support for acquiring alcohol or drugs.
- Justifying (rationalizing) inappropriate or illegal behavior while under the influence of alcohol or drugs.

The significant other is asked to give specific examples of how she or he has enabled the patient to continue to drink or use. The motivations behind these actions are also explored. Typically, it is concern for the well-being of the patient, or fear of the consequences (e.g., to the family) of not enabling, that motivates enabling. For example, a spouse might fear the loss of income if she refused to call in "sick" for a drunk spouse. Others might fear physical abuse if they say no to a demand for money that they know will be spent on alcohol or drugs. Less often, enabling is motivated by a desire to avoid facing one's own alcohol or drug problem.

Detaching can be thought of as a process of learning not to enable, but it also can be conceptualized more positively as learning what to do *instead of* enabling. The facilitator engages the partner in some discussion of this change, using examples of enabling as a springboard. To follow on the above example, instead of calling in "sick" for the alcoholic who in fact is hungover, the partner could sympathize with the drinker's dilemma but still refuse to make the call for him or her.

Learning to detach takes courage. It can be supported by the therapist, to be sure, but it is through the fellowships of Al-Anon and Nar-Anon that partners will find the greatest amount of support and comfort for their task. Toward this end the facilitator should suggest several specific Al-Anon or Nar-Anon meetings that the partner could attend, and follow up on these suggestions at the outset of subsequent sessions.

Termination

If TSF has been successful, then termination essentially consists of "turning over" the patient to the care of a 12-step fellowship. The more successfully the patient and the therapist have collaborated toward this end, the more likely it is that the patient will continue his or her progress toward lasting sobriety. This prediction is based in part on AA member surveys, which show that the best predictor of future sobriety is current active participation in AA (Alcoholics Anonymous General Services Office, 1999). In addition, the contribution of AA/NA meeting attendance to maintaining abstinence has received empirical support (Fiorentine, 1999).

Because the overarching goal of TSF is involvement in AA and/or NA, termination should in part consist of an honest appraisal of how much progress has been made toward that end. Questions such as the following are in order:

- "How many meetings per month, on average, do you now attend? What kinds of meetings are they?"
- "Do you have a home group?"
- "On average, how many AA/NA friends do you call by phone each week? How many AA/NA people call you?"
- "Do you have a sponsor?"
- "Have you taken on any responsibility at a meeting—for example, making coffee, setting up, or cleaning up?"

Besides monitoring AA/NA activity, the facilitator should check to see whether the patient has absorbed key 12-step concepts, and whether his or her attitudes about addiction and recovery have changed at all as a result of participation in TSF. Questions such as the following can be useful for this purpose:

- "To what extent do you think that alcohol or drug use made your life unmanageable prior to coming to the program?"
- "Do you believe now that alcoholics and addicts can 'control' their drinking or drug use?"
- "Do you think that willpower is enough to achieve sobriety, or do addicts need to reach out to others?"
- "What do the following concepts mean to you: *denial, enabling, higher power?*"
- "What role, if any, has AA or NA played so far in your effort to stay clean and sober?"
- "What are your plans relative to AA (or NA) now that this program is coming to an end?"

Finally, the facilitator should take a moment (preferably prior to the actual termination session) to reflect on the issue of the relative responsibilities of patient and therapist in this model. In this regard, the concept of detaching is as relevant to the facilitator as it is to any significant other in the patient's life. Clinical experience suggests that the best the facilitator can hope to do is to introduce key concepts in ways that the patient can understand them, actively encourage the patient to give 12-step fellowship a try, confront the patient constructively with the role that alcohol or some drug has played in making the patient's life unmanageable, and answer questions about AA or NA to the best of his or her ability. How many sober days the patient has had, and how active she or he has become in AA or NA, is not within the control of the facilitator. In the final analysis, the facilitator must be able to "turn over" the patient and his or her future to the care of whatever higher power the facilitator happens to believe in.

Advanced Work

This chapter has focused on a structured, time-limited intervention for what has been called "early" recovery. It is unlikely that any more ground than what has been described here could reasonably be covered in brief therapy. Indeed, the goals of TSF are ambitious. I do not recommend attempting to do more advanced work with patients until they have a minimum of 6 months of uninterrupted sobriety and have satisfied all goals of the core program.

TSF does include an advanced or "elective" program (Nowinski & Baker, 2003, pp. 95–154; Nowinski et al., 1992, pp. 59–96) that provides therapist guidelines for covering the following topics: genograms, enabling, emotions, moral inventories, and relationships. A discussion of this material is beyond the scope of this chapter; however, parts of the elective program may be considered for patients who have consolidated their early recovery and are ready to work, for example, on Steps 4 and 5 (the so-called moral inventory), or who are ready to begin the process of healing wounded relationships.

Case Study

The following is offered as an illustration of how the TSF model of intervention described in this chapter may be applied.

Bob and Kathy, married for 20 years, came to see the author ostensibly for help with long-standing marital difficulties that had reached crisis proportions since their youngest child had left home for college. Though it was initially obscured by discussions and arguments about money and sex, it became apparent after a while that Bob had a drinking problem that needed to be evaluated.

He was asked to come in individually for two sessions to talk about this problem.

The assessment sessions revealed that Bob had several signs of alcohol dependency. He had a powerful tolerance, drank daily, and had experienced a number of drinking-related consequences, not the least of which was a seriously strained marriage. In addition, it was discovered that he was in trouble at work as a consequence of his drinking, a problem he'd kept secret from his wife.

Bob at first was reticent to change the focus of therapy from his troubled marriage to his drinking. He was assured that his concerns about the marriage were legitimate and would be dealt with. But he was told that first he needed to examine his drinking and either take action about it or risk losing his job and/or his marriage.

The story of Bob's private struggle for control over alcohol was a testament to stubborn determination as much as it was a classic story of the power of addiction. Having started out sipping beers stolen from the refrigerator as a youth barely 12 years old, Bob had been drinking for nearly 30 years. Things didn't get "really bad," though, according to him, until after he was married and the kids were born. Two things happened then. First, he felt obligated to stay in a job that paid well but that he had intended to leave. Second, his relationship with Kathy, in his words, became "diluted" as a consequence of the demands of family life—meaning that sex between them became a very occasional thing, and that she paid much less attention to him in general than she did when they were a couple.

It was around this time that Bob developed the habit of having "a cocktail or two" every night after work and before dinner. For a long time Kathy went along with this, though she did notice that "a cocktail or two" eventually became three, four, or more. She didn't much care for alcohol herself, and she had little personal experience with it in her own family. Out of naivete she took Bob's ability to "drink others under the table"—in other words, his tolerance—to be a good thing. Ironically, she believed that this ability to "hold his liquor" was actually a sign that Bob could *not* become addicted.

As time went on, the process of addiction gradually set in. Instead of eating lunch with his colleagues in the company cafeteria, Bob started going out alone for lunch two or three times a week to a local bar where he'd grab a sandwich and a couple of cocktails. By the time he got home he was anxious to "relax"—his euphemism for having more cocktails. Kathy and the kids soon found that anything that stood between Bob and his cocktails made him irritable. He didn't want to be bothered with problems until he was "relaxed." Of course, by that time he was also intoxicated, emotionally unstable, and prone to losing his temper. In time the family learned to avoid him. Kathy took to solving most of the household problems by herself, or else she let them go. The kids, meanwhile, led their own lives and had minimal communication with their father.

Though he was very hesitant to admit it for a long time, privately Bob had struggled long (and ultimately unsuccessfully) to control his drinking. He hadn't wanted to be like his own father: a "quiet drunk" who was less flamboyant than Bob in his drinking, but who had "liked his liquor" no less, and who had also been a social isolate and a "nonfactor" (as Bob described both himself and his father) within the family.

The story of Bob's private efforts to control his drinking sounded like something right out of the AA Big Book: drinking only wine, drinking only beer (no cocktails) at lunch, drinking from a smaller glass, adding more ice cubes to his cocktails, and so on. While he was conscious on some level of gradually losing control, he continued to tell himself that he was really alright. It was not until his boss smelled liquor on his breath that the shell of self-deceit that Bob had built was finally and abruptly shattered. He was called onto the carpet and told that a second such incident would result in disciplinary action. It also affected, he felt sure, his subsequent performance evaluation, which was lukewarm to say the least.

By the time he and Kathy came for "marriage counseling," Bob had managed to fall 2 years behind on his tax returns and owed the government several thousand dollars. According to Kathy, the house they lived in was falling apart faster and faster on account of maintenance projects that Bob refused to hire someone to do but kept putting off doing himself. Their son, who had just turned 18, was failing half of his courses in his freshman year in college; meanwhile their daughter "hated" Bob and alternately fought with and ridiculed him. On top of all this, Kathy had been sexually turned off to Bob for some time, which left him feeling frustrated and filled with self-pity.

The assessment process involved carefully chronicling first the progression of Bob's drinking, from cocktails on weekends to cocktails at lunch, how he had built a tolerance, and how drinking affected him (i.e., making him irritable and withdrawn). We then proceeded to talk at length about the methods that Bob had used to "control" his drinking, followed by discussion of all the ways in which his life had become increasingly unmanageable. At the end of this process Bob was willing to admit that he had a drinking problem and "probably" needed to stop drinking altogether. At that point, however, he was not willing to entertain the idea of using AA as a resource for helping him implement his desire to stop drinking. On the other hand, he was willing to defer marriage counseling while he met with the author to work on his drinking problem.

In subsequent sessions Bob reported that he was drinking less than before, but had not gone more than 1 day without a drink. At that point the author moved ahead to a discussion of Step 1, reading it aloud and then talking with Bob about it at length, making sure he covered the following points:

- "What does this statements mean to you? What is your initial reaction to it . . .
  - *Emotionally*: How does it make you feel?
  - *Intellectually*: What thoughts do you have in response to it?"
- "How do you relate to the concept of *powerlessness*? What kinds of things can people be powerless over in their lives?"
- "Can you see how some people might be 'powerless' over alcohol or drugs?"
- "Have you ever felt powerless over something in your life? What have you felt powerless over?"
- "At this point do you believe that you can still control your use of alcohol? What makes you believe this?"
- "In what ways has your life become more *unmanageable* over the past several years? Where are the areas of conflict? In what ways are things not going well for you?"

The *recovery tasks* discussed at this time focused on getting Bob to begin reading some of the material in the Big Book, especially "Bill's Story" and "We Agnostics." This material was particularly relevant to Bob, who was personally alienated from organized religion and who stereotyped AA as a religion. In addition he was a strong believer in self-determination, to the point where it was all but impossible for him to find the humility necessary to admit that he'd been ultimately unsuccessful, on his own, in controlling his drinking.

Reluctantly, and only after a frank discussion of humility combined with an appeal to be more open-minded, Bob agreed to attend a few different AA meetings as an observer. He agreed to a recovery task that involved going to meetings, listening to the stories being told, and trying to focus on *identifying* as much as possible with the theme of progressive loss of control, acceptance, and surrender. He was not asked to speak or to participate in any other way. On the other hand, he was advised to avoid focusing his attention on how he was different from other people at these meetings—for example, in terms of background, education, or financial circumstances.

One frequent problem of alcoholics who resist giving AA a try is their internalized stigma about alcoholism. Bob was no exception to this. He held very negative stereotypes about alcoholics, and fully expected to discover himself in the company of derelicts and criminals when he went to AA. Of course, he discovered just the opposite, which made it easier to encourage him to continue. In fact, he made a friend at one of the very first meetings he went to, and this person eventually became his first sponsor.

The next focus of treatment was denial. Bob had attempted to avoid coming to terms with his loss of control over drinking as fiercely as any alcoholic. His first line of defense had always been to get angry whenever the subject was brought up by his wife. After blowing up, he'd usually change the subject, either launching into an attack on Kathy, or else complaining long and loudly about some other problem, like finances, his in-laws, or their sex life. In response to the ever-growing list of household chores that went undone, he pleaded fatigue—after all, he said, he worked hard all week and needed the weekends to "unwind."

Not surprisingly, Bob's denial extended outwardly to his behavior, and even inwardly to his own thought processes. For example, he went out of his way to associate with men who drank as much or even more than he did, and then comforted himself by drawing the comparison between his own use and theirs. Of course, he concluded that he was merely "average" (and therefore "normal") among his peers. At times when he felt guilty pouring that fifth or sixth martini, he'd tell himself that he "deserved" it—for example, because of the stress of having to endure an unsatisfying job. His trouble at work he tried writing off to a combination of bad luck and a vindictive boss; his increasing tendency toward sexual impotence he attributed to his wife's rejection of him and her preoccupation with their children.

As is often the case, once Bob was able to admit to someone else (i.e., to me) the ways in which he'd denied his drinking problem, the more open he became to accepting it. At this point he was even willing to admit it to Kathy and did so in a conjoint session. He continued to express reservations about whether he was a "true alcoholic," as he put it, but he was willing to keep going to AA on the premise that he did have the requisite desire to stop drinking.

As brief as this case example is, I hope it gives the reader a flavor for TSF as a mode of intervention. With respect to process, it incorporates elements of education, confrontation, interpretation, and suggestion. It is based on the 12-step model of addiction and recovery, and it clearly relies upon sophisticated clinical skills for its successful implementation.

REFERENCES

Al-Anon Family Group Headquarters. (1986a). *Al-Anon faces alcoholism* (2nd ed.). New York: Author.

Al-Anon Family Group Headquarters. (1986b). *One day at a time in Al-Anon*. New York: Author.

Alcoholics Anonymous. (1952). *Twelve steps and twelve traditions*. New York: Alcoholics Anonymous World Services.

Alcoholics Anonymous. (1975). *Living sober: Some methods A.A. members have used for not drinking*. New York: Alcoholics Anonymous World Services.

Alcoholics Anonymous. (1976). *Alcoholics Anonymous: The story of how many thousands of men and women have recovered from alcoholism* (3rd ed.). New York: Alcoholics Anonymous World Services.

Alcoholics Anonymous General Services Office. (1999). *Alcoholics Anonymous 1998 membership survey.* New York: Author.

Anderson, D. J. (1991). *Perspectives on treatment: The Minnesota experience.* Center City, MN: Hazelden.

Anonymous. (1975, December 29). *Twenty-four hours a day.* Center City, MN: Hazelden.

Fiorentine, R. (1999). After drug treatment: Are 12-step programs effective in maintaining abstinence? *American Journal of Drug and Alcohol Abuse, 25*(1), 93–116.

Fowler, J. W. (1993). Alcoholics Anonymous and faith development. In B. S. McCrady & W. R. Miller (Eds.), *Research on Alcoholics Anonymous: Opportunities and alternatives* (pp. 113–135). New Brunswick, NJ: Rutgers Center of Alcohol Studies.

Marlatt, G. A., & Gordon, J. R. (Eds.). (1985). *Relapse prevention: Maintenance strategies in the treatment of addictive behaviors.* New York: Guilford Press.

Maude-Griffin, P. M., Hohenstein, J. M., Humfleet, G. L., Reilly, P. M., Tusel, D. J., & Hall, S. M. (1998). Superior efficacy of cognitive-behavioral therapy for urban crack cocaine users: Main and matching effects. *Journal of Consulting and Clinical Psychology, 66*(5), 832–837.

Narcotics Anonymous. (1982). *Narcotics Anonymous* (4th ed.). Van Nuys, CA: Narcotics Anonymous World Services.

National Institute on Alcohol Abuse and Alcoholism. (1990). *Alcohol and health.* Washington, DC: Author.

Nowinski, J. (1998). *Family recovery and substance abuse.* Thousand Oaks, CA: Sage.

Nowinski, J., & Baker, S. (1992). *The twelve-step facilitation handbook: A systematic approach to early recovery from alcoholism and addiction.* New York: Lexington Books.

Nowinski, J., & Baker, S. (2003). *The twelve-step facilitation handbook: A systematic approach to recovery from alcoholism and addiction.* Center City, MN: Hazelden.

Nowinski, J., Baker, S., & Carroll, K. (1992). *Twelve-step facilitation therapy manual: A clinical research guide for therapists treating individuals with alcohol abuse and dependence* (DHHS Publication No. ADM 92-1893, Project MATCH Monograph Series, Vol. 1). Rockville, MD: National Institute on Alcohol Abuse and Alcoholism.

Powell, D. (Ed.). (1984). *Alcoholism and sexual dysfunction: Issues in clinical management.* New York: Haworth Press.

Prochaska, J. O., DiClemente, C. C., & Norcross, J. C. (1992). In search of how people change: Applications to addictive behaviors. *American Psychologist, 47,* 1102–1114.

Project MATCH Research Group. (1997). Matching alcoholism treatments to client heterogeneity: Project MATCH posttreatment drinking outcomes. *Journal of Studies on Alcohol, 58,* 7–29.

Room, R. (1993). Alcoholics Anonymous as a social movement. In B. S. McCrady

& W. R. Miller (Eds.), *Research on Alcoholics Anonymous: Opportunities and alternatives* (pp. 167–187). New Brunswick, NJ: Rutgers Center of Alcohol Studies.

Saunders, B., Wilkinson, C., & Towers, T. (1996). Motivation and addictive behaviors: Theoretical perspectives. In F. Rotgers, D. S. Keller, & J. Morgenstern (Eds.), *Treating substance abuse: Theory and technique* (pp. 241–265). New York: Guilford Press.

Seraganian, P., Brown, T. G., Tremblay, J., & Annies, H. M. (1998). *Experimental manipulation of treatment aftercare regimes for the substance abuser.* (National Health Research and Development Program [Canada] Project No. 6605-4392-404). Unpublished paper, Concordia University, Montreal, Canada.

Sobell, L., Cunningham, J. A., Sobell, M., & Toneatto, T. (1993). A life-span perspective on natural recovery (self-change) from alcohol problems. In J. S. Baer, G. A. Marlatt, & R. J. McMahon (Eds.), *Addictive behaviors across the life span: Prevention, treatment, and policy issues* (pp. 93–113). Newbury Park, CA: Sage.

3

Psychoanalytic Theories of Substance Abuse

Jeremy Leeds
Jon Morgenstern

PSYCHOANALYSIS AND PSYCHOANALYTIC PSYCHOTHERAPY

Although it is probably the best known system and theory of psychotherapy, psychoanalysis is difficult to define. Controversy and innovation have been the rule since the theory's inception and have continued unabated through the present. Pine (1990), in trying to summarize and integrate various strains of psychoanalytic theorizing, speaks of the "central place of conflict and of the multiple functions of behavior" (p. 5). Gabbard (1992) characterizes psychoanalytic psychiatry as a "*way of thinking* about both patient and clinician that includes unconscious conflict, deficits and distortions of intrapsychic structures, and internal object relations" (p. 991). Other authors focus on how diffuse the concept of psychoanalysis is. Eagle (1984) notes the ferment within psychoanalytic theory. He points to the wide range of criticisms and innovations, some of which call into question the basic Freudian tenets. He ends his work by calling for "recapturing" the early psychoanalytic and even prepsychoanalytic emphasis on the disclaimed versus the claimed, the impersonal "it" versus the personal "I," the dissociated versus the integrated (p. 212). Greenberg and Mitchell (1983) categorize the "current diversity of psychoanalytic schools of thought" in two basic groups: those like Freud, who build around a concept of drives and their vicissitudes; and those like Sullivan and Fairbairn, who give primary importance to "relations with others" (p. 3).

In this chapter, we use the broadest of these definitions of psychoanalysis. We use "psychoanalysis and psychoanalytic psychotherapy" to mean a theory and practice with a focus on making the unconscious conscious, in which the range of unconscious material and its sources can be said to extend from the biological to representations of relations with others. Our purpose is to describe how theorists and clinicians from various points on the psychoanalytic spectrum have understood substance abuse and its treatment.

Psychoanalytic theories are theories of *motivation*—of why, for example, a person initiates or maintains a dependence on a substance or substances. "Motivation" can encompass both needs a person has and an absence of awareness of these needs and of their significance. Such "needs" often conflict with each other, with social norms, and with those of others. They then might come into awareness and behavior first in the form of "symptoms."

Originally, for Freud, "symptom" was the form in which a repressed idea or memory comes to consciousness. It does so in an unrecognizable form because it is distorted by psychological defense. Thus a symptom is a *compromise*. It is the product of *conflict* between the repressed idea and the defense against it (Laplanche & Pontalis, 1973, p. 76).

Whether or not one maintains the original Freudian conception of drive and defense, the concept of symptom—the outward expression of an internal conflict, or of the conflict between an internal need and some external limitation—is one of the enduring ideas of psychoanalysis. Bringing to consciousness the underlying conflict that has resulted in symptoms is a psychoanalytic therapy. It is usually assumed that "making the unconscious conscious" is a major contributor to the alleviation of the symptom, though the distance between insight and cure is often a wide and troubling one.

Substance abuse has generally been categorized within this psychoanalytic concept of symptom. However the underlying difficulties and conflicts are conceptualized, it is generally assumed in psychoanalytic theory that substance abuse is a response to such conflict. A history of psychoanalytic concepts of substance abuse is therefore by and large a history of the kind of symptom psychoanalysts have conceptualized substance abuse as being.

It is a seemingly logical next step, after identifying what substance abuse is symptomatic of, to say that understanding the "underlying cause" of the symptom is the key to its removal. This is perhaps logical but not necessary or, in fact, always valid. Often, psychoanalytic *understanding* has been confused with psychoanalytic *cure,* to the detriment of both. Whether psychoanalytic understandings of substance abuse are veridical is one major question; whether and how they are helpful in treatment are two conceptually separate questions.

History and Concepts

As the range of ideas and techniques in psychoanalysis as a whole is wide, with a long and involved history, so it has been for psychoanalytic treatment of substance abuse. In part, the evolution of the theory of substance abuse treatment mirrors changes in psychoanalysis as a whole. Blatt, McDonald, Sugarman, and

Wilber (1984), in an important paper on psychodynamic theories of opiate addiction, note that early psychoanalysts failed to distinguish between types of addiction, viewing all addiction as "oral phenomena" with similar unconscious meanings (p. 161). This was at a time when the field was generally concerned with "id" issues: the study of the internally based drives and how they played out in the patient's world.

Beginning with Rado (1926), analysts looked to formulate different typologies of addiction, based on the substance used and the internal state of the user. These early typologies were developed through the prism of the psychoanalytic paradigm known as "ego psychology." Historically subsequent to the above focus on "id" concerns, ego psychology is broadly a perspective reflecting a movement within mainstream (Freudian) psychoanalysis toward interest in how people developed their own adaptations to the world.

As we will see, other and often more recent psychoanalytic conceptions have mirrored the shift in the field to the concern, noted by Greenberg and Mitchell (1983) above, with relations with other people.

In the Blatt et al. (1984) schema, psychoanalytic theories of motivation for opiate addiction fall into three categories. The first is the "establishment of a need-gratifying, symbiotic state"; the second is "a defense against critical, harsh and dysphoric self-judgment (e.g., guilt and shame)"; and the third is a "defense against potential psychotic disintegration" (p. 163). The authors developed these categories by "integrating the traditional emphasis of drives and defensive functions with object relations theory" (p. 163). This article was an important attempt to move psychoanalytic understanding of substance abuse toward the more current understandings of psychological functioning. We see our work as an attempt to continue this process.

CURRENT STATUS

In a recent article, we (Morgenstern & Leeds, 1993) surveyed and discussed the current status of psychoanalytic theories of substance abuse. Readers with an interest in pursuing the topic in greater depth are encouraged to read this article. Based on that discussion, we will summarize the range of current psychoanalytic thinking (necessarily leaving out important points from our larger discussion) and briefly discuss its strengths and limitations.

In contrast to its contributions to a wide range of other disorders, psychoanalysis has made rather meager recent contributions to the understanding of substance abuse. There are many possible explanations for this lack of theory. One is the perception that drug abuse renders one unsuitable for psychoanalytic treatment. Because abusers resort to altering their internal states rather than to try to understand them, insight is precluded. Hence the widespread refusal to treat these patients and the tendency to refer them to 12-step programs. A related explanation is that a history of poor outcome in attempts at treatment (Brickman, 1988) created a sense that psychoanalysis was not a treatment of choice for these disorders. Nonetheless, several psychoanalytic thinkers have made important contributions to the understanding of substance abuse. We have chosen to focus on four current authors who are of particular interest and significance: Leon Wurmser, Edward Khantzian, Henry Krystal, and Joyce McDougall.

All four thinkers view substance abuse as a particular instance of a more general kind of disorder or pathology which is familiar to students of psychoanalysis. As such, the four theorists span a wide range of current psychoanalytic theorizing in general: drive theory (Wurmser), object relations theory (Krystal), self psychology theory (Khantzian), and McDougall's theory of psychosomatic disturbance. We have organized the thinkers in a chart (Table 3.1), based on what each considers to be wrong with the substance abuser and what effect each thinks an abuser seeks from a drug.

While all four of these thinkers are aware and make note of the physiological aspects of substance abuse and addiction, their main focus is on the psychological aspects of the process.

Wurmser

Wurmser sees himself in a traditional psychoanalytic drive-theory context. While he favors a "deeply grounded combination treatment," involving self-help groups, pharmacological treatment, education, and family counseling (1985, p. 95), he reserves a primary place for traditional psychoanalysis in the treatment of substance abuse disorders. It is his theory that substance abusers suffer from overly harsh and destructive superegos, which threaten to overwhelm the person with rage and fear. Substance abuse is an attempt to flee from such dangerous affects. These emotions are the result of traditional *conflicts* between psychic agencies, specifically, the harshness of the superego.

Wurmser thinks actual, overwhelming, early traumas are the origins of

TABLE 3.1. Contemporary Psychoanalytic Theories of Drug Dependence

Theorist	Prototypical pathology	Vulnerability	Wished-for effect
Wurmser	Neurotic conflict	Condemned self	Liberation
Khantzian	Self-deficit	Damaged self	Repair/regulation
Krystal	Impaired object relations	Borderline self	Merger/ecstasy
McDougall	Psychosomatic disturbance	Externalizing self	Avoidance/escape

Note. From Morgenstern and Leeds (1993, p. 196). Copyright 1993 by the American Psychological Association. Reprinted by permission.

this state of being (1984, p. 230). He speaks of "unusually severe *real* exposure to violence, sexual seduction, and brutal abandonment, and/or of *real* unreliability, mendacity, betrayal, and abandonment, and/or of *real* parental intrusiveness or secretiveness" (p. 253). Such events lead to hostility to authority, rebelliousness, and defiance. They also lead to a harshness of internal authority and doubts about one's basic worth. One of his patients speaks of "a shadowy feeling of massive guilt, almost of mythical proportions" (1985, p. 90).

Drugs serve at least temporarily to disable the threatening internal authority and to neutralize the feelings of doubt and anxiety that appear so overwhelming. However, in disabling the superego, drugs do not affect only the specific unwanted feelings and thoughts; they severely limit other superego functions as well. These include internal stability of mood and affect, the "ego ideal," self-observation, understanding of the boundaries of outer reality, and self-care (1984, p. 232). This accounts for the way substance abusers present to the therapist. They are often grandiose, avoidant, and manipulative; they are unaware of the dangers of their behavior. All this fits within Wurmser's notion of the use of drugs as an "archaic, global" way to avoid the feelings and impulses of pain, anxiety, and shame that so threaten the substance abuser.

Given this understanding, Wurmser's main focus in psychoanalytic treatment is the analysis of the superego. He believes that a moralistic stand toward addicts' behavior is counterproductive in that the problem is not too little superego but too much. Thus the therapist needs to offer a "strong emotional presence" and "an attitude of warmth, kindness and flexibility" (1985, p. 94).

Khantzian

Khantzian has developed a widely known group psychotherapeutic treatment for substance abusers. His work is based on the conception that *deficits,* not conflicts, underlie the problems of substance abusers. That is, weaknesses and inadequacies in the "ego" or "self," rather than conflicts between psychic agencies, are at the root of the problem.

For Khantzian, holes in the organization of the self—how a person protects, regulates, cares for, and thinks of him- or herself—lead a person to seek the particular effect of some drug that will counteract the deficit. Khantzian is the only one of the four here surveyed who gives this degree of importance to the specific" drug of choice" for the abuser. For example, opiate addicts seek the drug's antiaggressive effect:

> Our experience suggests that the problems with aggression in such individuals are in part a function of an excess reservoir of this intense affect—partly constitutional and partly environmental in origin—interacting with psychological (ego) structures which are underdeveloped or deficient and thus fail to contain such affect. (1980, p. 35)

On close examination, we have been impressed repeatedly that the so-called "high" or euphoria produced by opiates is more correctly a relief of dysphoria associated with unmitigated aggression. (1980, p. 32)

Cocaine addicts, on the other hand, exhibit a different range of predisposing factors:

1. Pre-existent chronic depression (dysthymic disorder)
2. Cocaine abstinence depression
3. Hyperactive/restless/emotional lability syndrome or attention-deficit disorder
4. Cyclothymic or bipolar illness (Khantzian & Khantzian, 1984, p. 758)

Although difficulties in affect regulation and tolerance are common in all drug addictions, the specific affects and the level of disturbance vary widely in Khantzian's schema. He does not consider abusers to be necessarily as psychologically disturbed as Wurmser or indeed the next two theorists do.

Khantzian and his colleagues have developed a modified dynamic group therapy (MDGT; Khantzian, Halliday, & McAuliffe, 1990) to address the characterological underpinnings of substance abuse. The four foci of the groups are "1) affect tolerance, 2) the building of self-esteem, 3) the discussion and improvement of interpersonal relationships, and 4) the development of appropriate self-care strategies among the substance abusers" (McLellan, Woody, Luborsky, & O'Brien, 1990, pp. ix–xii).

Krystal

Krystal offers two theories of why individuals abuse substances. It is not clear if and how the two relate, but each makes an important contribution. Both presuppose severe disturbance in early development.

One theory is based on an object relations understanding of pathology. The drug is experienced by the abuser symbolically as a primary maternal object. That is, the drug stands in for the functions usually attributed to an actual maternal figure. The addict relates to the drug based on the disturbed pattern of relationship to such maternal figures as he or she has experienced developmentally. As Krystal says, "The drug dependent patient craves to be united with his ideal object, but at the same time dreads it" (1977, p. 243). This is a variant of borderline pathology.

Krystal, like several other analysts (Kernberg, 1975; Rinsley, 1988), conceptualizes substance abuse in this light. The abuser's relation to the drug of abuse is an acting out in adulthood of primitive, infantile fantasies. Thus, the usual intense, unstable personal relations, rageful behavior, problems with self-care, and compulsive substance abuse are all part of an ongoing destructive drama. Krystal (1978) sees this as the "basic dilemma" of the substance abuser.

The second theory Krystal employs centers on the abuser's disturbed affective functions. This theory is known as "alexithymia."

Krystal believes that addicts differ from others in that they do not recognize the cognitive aspects of feeling states. That is, instead of experiencing differentiated feelings as "sad," "angry," "happy," and so forth, alexithymics experience global physiological states and tensions. This makes it difficult to use emotions as guides to self-understanding and eliminates or at least severely limits an important source of information and feedback. It means one cannot read the significance of specific arousal states; arousal itself becomes a source of anxiety. Therefore, one attempts to eliminate it by sedation or discharge. Substance abuse is one means of doing so.

Krystal believes that severe disturbance in object relations is at the base of substance abuse. This is in contrast to the "conflict" or "deficit" models above. He is also more pessimistic about the treatment of substance abusers, as one would be with any such severe borderline pathology. He advocates treatment in a program setting, with several therapists, to dilute transference, which would otherwise become too intense and possibly unmanageable. Although, like Khantzian, he recommends a focus on self-care and the tolerance of affects, he sees this as a first step in treatment, which must be accompanied by an analysis of the ambivalence and aggression being acted out by the patient through substance abuse.

McDougall

McDougall sees substance abuse as one of a variety of addictive behaviors, including eating disorders, compulsive sexual behavior, and addictive relationships. She sees all these as psychosomatic disorders. They are ways of dealing with distress that involve externalizing and physicalizing what are initially psychic disturbances. Psychosomatic phenomena are

> all cases of physical damage or ill health in which psychological factors play an important role. These include: accident-proneness or the lowering of the immunological shield when under stress so that one more readily falls victim to infectious disease, as well as the problems of addiction, which are a "psychosomatic" attempt to deal with distressful conflict by temporarily blurring the awareness of their existence. (1989, p. 19)

Psychosomatic phenomena are a "discharge in action" rather than thought. Instead of elaborating feeling states internally, a psychosomatic solution is an externalization of the experience. Although everyone uses such defenses on occasion, substance abusers and others with psychosomatic disorders do so habitually. One outcome is that those feelings and experiences that would be painful or dangerous if actually experienced and felt internally are instead seen as unremarkable.

The psychosomatic–addictive solution is a defensive maneuver against unconscious emotions and fears. McDougall sees these as of a basic, akin to psychotic, nature: "deep uncertainty about one's right to exist and one's right to a separate identity . . . fear of losing one's body limits, one's feeling of identity or the control over one's acts" (1982, p. 382). Addiction is a way to avoid the internal feeling of deadness and emptiness that threatens the substance abuser. The use of drugs is part of the "false self" the person creates to ward off these painful and dangerous feelings.

While McDougall is more optimistic than many other analysts about the possible success of treatment with these patients, the extensive defenses against internal life make it a difficult and lengthy process. She advocates that attention be paid to the development of an internal life and, at the same time, to the patient's level of suffering and fear that increasing internal awareness may evoke.

CRITIQUE OF THEORY

Blatt et al. (1984) point out several difficulties with psychoanalytic studies of addiction from a rigorous methodological standpoint: "1) conclusions drawn from either single case studies or clinical reports based on only a few addicts, 2) a frequent failure to distinguish among different types of addiction or the level of severity of the addiction, 3) attempts to understand predispositional factors from data gathered after the addiction has taken place, and 4) difficulties establishing adequate control or comparison groups" (p. 161). These criticisms are similar to those often directed against psychoanalysis as a whole. They are, however, more telling in the case of addictions for two reasons. First, there is little evidence that psychoanalytic treatment is effective when provided to substance abusers. This is widely acknowledged even within the psychoanalytic community (Brickman, 1988; Gerald, 1992).

Second, significant advances have been made in understanding addictive behaviors during the last 20 years. Even contemporary analytic theories have largely ignored this important knowledge base. As a result, analytic theories and treatment techniques are out of step with an increasingly well-validated paradigm that views addictive disorders from an integrative biopsychosocial perspective. In looking at the current status of psychoanalytic theories and treatment, we must first summarize the new paradigms and their divergence from analytic models.

The analytic theories we have surveyed by and large share a common set of assumptions about substance abuse. First, they conceive of substance use as a symptom of an underlying disorder. They differ concerning the nature of that disorder. Second, they tend to view the current psychological problems of the substance abuser as having existed prior to and causing the substance abuse. Third, they tend to conceive of substance use disorders as homogeneous, descriptively as well as etiologically. Although little attention is paid to definitions, all theories imply that compulsive use is categorically present or absent and degrees or dimensions of severity are not important. Similarly, each theorist views his or her theory as explaining all cases of substance use disorder and does not suggest that there may be different forms or subtypes of the disorder with different etiologies and psychodynamics. This is less the case with a theorist such as Khantzian, who posits different varieties of self-medication; however, he still puts all problems within this self-medication, drug-of-choice context. Fourth, most theories would consider the presence of substance use disorder in a patient as generally indicative of severe underlying pathology. As a result, most tend to be relatively pessimistic regarding the outcome of analytic treatment.

These assumptions diverge significantly from emerging knowledge about addictive disorders derived from empirical studies. The divergence of the psychoanalytic paradigm from empirically derived theories can be described succinctly as centering around three issues: (1) the homogeneity versus the heterogeneity of substance abusers, (2) the impact of prolonged use on the personality and symptom picture of the substance abuser, and (3) the degree to which the pathogenesis of substance abuse can adequately be explained solely by psychogenic factors. We next briefly summarize these points of divergence.

Homogeneity versus Heterogeneity

Studies from diverse areas, such as psychiatric epidemiology (Regier et al., 1990), genetic epidemiology (Cloninger, 1987), clinical psychopathology (Babor, 1992), and treatment outcome (Kadden, Cooney, Getter, & Litt, 1989) indicate that substance abusers are a heterogeneous group differing in patterns of onset, course, symptom picture, family history, and comorbid psychopathology. Of particular relevance are findings from the Epidemiologic Catchment Area study (Robins & Regier, 1991) indicating that substance abuse co-occurs with a wide variety of other disorders, including personality disorders, bipolar disorders, schizophrenia, and anxiety disorders, as well as alone without evidence of other psychopathology. This and other evidence (Meyer, 1986; Nathan, 1988) has led experts to reject the position that any one set of characterological features predisposes or is always involved in the pathogenesis of an addictive problem. This has indeed been acknowledged by analysts such as Krystal (1984), but the consequent expected reformulation of analytic positions has not yet been made.

In addition, empirically based paradigms consider specific patterns of substance use important in understanding and treating substance use problems. These paradigms reject the notion that substance use problems are either categorically present or categorically absent. Instead, they view substance use problems as existing on a continuum of severity and attempt to provide clear operational criteria to establish whether use is normative or pathological. Such distinctions are important in determining appropriate treatment selection and goals.

Psychoanalytic approaches have not paid adequate attention to this dimension and instead have focused on characterological and general psychodynamic issues. A significant limitation of analytic approaches is their failure to differentiate between patterns and severity of substance use. As a result, the analytic approach reinforces the homogeneity position by lumping together individuals with varying levels of problem severity.

The Impact of Substance Use on Presenting Psychopathology

Psychoanalysts have generally assumed that the presenting psychological problems of substance-abusing patients were stable manifestations of underlying character and therefore etiologically significant. However, current empirically based paradigms examining data from a variety of sources suggest that the presenting psychological problems of substance abusers may be transient and may be the consequence rather than the cause of substance abuse. In particular, many have argued that the pharmacological effects (e.g., on mood and anxiety) of substances and the loss of important social reinforcers that occurs during prolonged use are often responsible for the significant level of psychopathology found in substance abusers presenting for treatment. When considering the issue of additional psychopathology, empirical paradigms would classify substance users into a minimum of three types: (1) those with no additional problems, (2) those whose psychological problems are secondary to substance abuse, and (3) those whose psychopathology predates their substance use. Implications for the treatment of these groups would differ. Those with secondary psychopathology may not require additional treatment because their symptoms may remit after a period of abstinence, whereas those with primary psychopathology would require additional treatment. This can be contrasted to the analytic position that all substance abusers suffer from primary characterological problems and all require extensive treatment to address these problems.

Zinberg (1970), from within the psychoanalytic camp, addressed these concerns relatively early on. He advocated attention to the cumulative importance of drug, set, and setting in the development of addictive disorders. "Drug" is the pharmacological effect of the substance, "set" is the frame of mind of the user, and "setting" is the social and environmental context in which the user finds him- or herself (p. 5). He presents a critique of psychoanalytic thinking conceptually similar to that presented here, stressing the inadvisability of reading backward from substance abuse to "underlying" characterological issues.

The Pathogenesis of Substance Use Disorders

There is increasing empirical support for the dependence syndrome concept as a model to describe pathogenic processes in substance use disorders (Ziedonis & Kosten, 1993; Morgenstern, Langenbucher, & Labouvie, 1994). Overall, current consensus holds that most addictive behaviors are multiply determined by cultural, psychological, behavioral, and biological forces. In addition, a variety of clinical and laboratory studies offer strong evidence that more severe substance use is driven by biobehavioral forces and that cultural and psychological factors are of secondary importance (Babor, 1992).

Figure 3.1 illustrates this notion in a somewhat simplified manner. On the left, the dependence syndrome model is used to portray a transition from socially sanctioned drug use to mild, moderate, and severe forms of dependence. On the right are the dominant underlying mechanisms that control use at the various stages of the transition. Normal use is largely controlled by cultural and social factors. For instance, social modeling influences beliefs concerning the positive effects of alcohol and drugs. However, certain select individuals develop personal idiosyncratic beliefs in the power of alcohol or drugs to provide escape from painful affects or to escape from social responsibilities. For these individuals, substance use becomes driven by a need to regulate internal states and consumption of drugs deviates from normal to pathological use. Either because of internal conflicts or deficits or because of severe and/or prolonged stressors, these individuals are particularly vulnerable to the immediate positively reinforcing quality of drugs (i.e., their ability to alter mood quickly and effectively). At this level of mild dependence, motives and structures described by analytic theories may be the dominant underlying mechanisms that determine use.

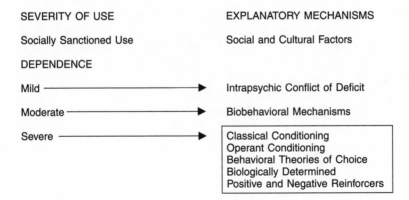

FIGURE 3.1. The relationship between dependence severity and pathogenesis.

However, if at this point drinking or drug use increases, an entirely different set of forces related to learning theory and biologically mediated reinforcement comes into play to determine use. Some of these biobehavioral mechanisms are listed in the figure. While it is beyond the scope of this chapter to describe these mechanisms, of particular importance is the notion that environmental stimuli—people, places, and things—become paired with biologically determined positive and negative reinforcers. With increasing use, concentrated cycles of reciprocal reinforcement occur, and these stimuli function as powerful reinforcers that elicit overwhelming cravings. In addition, new studies indicate that alcohol and drugs act directly on pleasure and pain centers in the brain and thus are uniquely powerful reinforcers (Wise, 1988).

In sum, empirically based theories postulate that the biobehavioral mechanisms operative in moderate and severe dependence offer the most adequate explanation for the power, tenacity, and seemingly irrational character of drug addiction. In support of this position, such theories note that all widely used and effective treatments, whether drawn from behavioral or self-help traditions, use techniques designed to counter these biobehavioral mechanisms. Analysts have usually attributed the poor efficacy of insight-oriented techniques to the severe psychopathology of the addict. A more parsimonious explanation may be that insight does not work at moderate or severe levels of dependence because the dominant nature of the mechanisms driving addiction are not primarily psychological in nature.

Tolstoy famously wrote, "All happy families are alike; each unhappy family is unhappy in its own way" (1877/2001, p. 1). Psychoanalysis is one unhappy family in the substance abuse/dependence field; but it must be said in all fairness that there is plenty of unhappiness to go around. There has been quite little in terms of successful treatment of substance abuse, and what there has been has not correlated with any particular theoretical approach (see Project MATCH; Project MATCH Research Group, 1997). One then begins to wonder if perhaps all of these unhappy families are indeed alike: the severe limitations of all psychotherapy (including, incidentally, self-help approaches) in treating substance abuse are not particular to any theoretical approach. The scope and nature of the problem may call for different kinds of solutions, at least in combination with talk and insight.

CONCLUSION

What is the future of psychoanalytic substance abuse treatment? Based on the above, it is not hard to see why there is currently a crisis of confidence from within psychoanalysis in the efficacy of psychoanalytic understanding and treatment of substance abuse. Brickman (1988), in a representative view, states that traditional psychoanalytic approaches to the treatment of addictions have been lacking in effectiveness. He questions the psychoanalytic presupposition that substance abuse patterns can be influenced by insight (p. 360). Several recent contributions to the literature advocate the use of 12-step programs such as Alcoholics Anonymous as adjuncts to psychoanalytic psychotherapy (e.g., Brickman, 1988; Gerald, 1992). These approaches divide the treatment of the abuser into two parts: the substance use is addressed in 12-step programs, broader psychological issues are addressed in psychoanalysis. Others would suggest that psychodynamic treatment not even begin until the resolution of the substance abuse problem and an extended period of abstinence (Kaufman, 1994). At the same time, there is an increasing interest in integrating various perspectives within the substance abuse field, and psychodynamic theorists and practitioners have been a part of this. One of the many examples is the Second Annette Overby Memorial Symposium, a meeting held in 1992, sponsored by the National Psychological Association for Psychoanalysis (1992), entitled "Working with Alcoholics and Substance Abusers in Private Practice."

It is clear that the field is in a period of flux, with the challenge of a new integration looming. Much of the recent focus on stages of change (Prochaska & DiClemente, 1983) and motivational interviewing, both potentially promising innovations in substance abuse treatment, is at least compatible with a psychoanalytic approach. Both focus on the ambivalence toward change that the dependent person experiences and acts on, a topic well-suited for psychodynamic exploration.

Along with a growing contribution of research in understanding substance abuse patterns, psychoanalytic perspectives in understanding and treating addictive disorders have an important contribution to make. It seems clear that substance abusers are a heterogeneous group, and not all suffer from any one form of character pathology or other psychological difficulty. Nevertheless, studies show that a significant portion do have character problems (Morgenstern, Langenbucher, Labouvie, & Miller, 1994). To date, there are no professional psychological treatments, with the exception of Khantzian's MDGT, that specifically target character problems within the context of substance abuse treatment. Whatever the empirical evidence shows about the overall psychoanalytic conceptions, it is imperative that clinicians make an attempt to understand the person who suffers, and not just "the substance abuser" in the abstract. This unified person, with thoughts, fears, needs, and anxieties that may or may not be related to substance abuse, is too often ignored in the design of treatments and the conceptualization of "who" a substance abuser is. Psychoanalytic theories will be crucial in addressing these concerns and in the creation of a new synthesis of empirical and clinical insight in the understanding and treatment of substance abuse.

REFERENCES

Babor, T. F. (1992). Nosological considerations in the diagnosis of substance use disorders. In M. Glantz & R. Pickens (Eds.), *Vulnerability to drug abuse.* Washington, DC: American Psychological Association Press.

Blatt, S., McDonald, C., Sugarman, A., & Wuber, C. (1984). Psychodynamic theories of opiate addiction: New directions for research. *Clinical Psychology Review, 4,* 1–34.

Brickman, B. (1988). Psychoanalysis and substance abuse: Toward a more effective approach. *Journal of the American Academy of Psychoanalysis, 16*(3), 359–379.

Cloninger, C. R. (1987). Neurogenetic adaptive mechanisms in alcoholism. *Science, 236,* 410–416.

Eagle, M. (1984). *Recent developments in psychoanalysis.* New York: McGraw-Hill.

Gabbard, G. O. (1992). Psychodynamic psychiatry in the "Decade of the Brain." *American Journal of Psychiatry, 149*(8), 991–997.

Gerald, M. (1992). Working with alcoholics and drug abusers in private practice: A psychoanalytic–chemical dependency model. *Psychology of Addictive Behaviors, 6*(1), 5–13.

Greenberg, J. R., & Mitchell, S. A. (1983). *Object relations in psychoanalytic theory.* Cambridge, MA: Harvard University Press.

Kadden, R. M., Cooney, N. L., Getter, H., & Litt, M. D. (1989). Matching alcoholics to coping skills or interactional therapies: Posttreatment results. *Journal of Consulting and Clinical Psychology, 57,* 698–704.

Kaufman, E. (1994). *Psychotherapy of addicted persons.* New York: Guilford Press.

Kernberg, O. (1975). *Borderline conditions and pathological narcissism.* New York: Aronson.

Khantzian, E. J. (1980). An ego-self theory of substance dependence. In D. J. Lettieri, M. Sayers, & H. W. Pearson (Eds.), *Theories of addiction* (NIDA Research Monograph No. 30, DHHS Publication No. ADM 80-967). Washington, DC: U.S. Government Printing Office.

Khantzian, E. J., Halliday, K. S., & McAuliffe, W. E. (1990). *Addiction and the vulnerable self: Modified dynamic group therapy for substance abusers.* New York: Guilford Press.

Khantzian, E. J., & Khantzian, N. J. (1984). Cocaine addiction: Is there a psychological predisposition? *Psychiatric Annals, 14*(10), 753–759.

Krystal, H. (1977). Aspects of affect theory. *Bulletin of the Menninger Clinic, 41,* 1–26.

Krystal, H. (1978). Self-representation and the capacity for self-care. *Annual Psychoanalysis, 6,* 209–246.

Krystal, H. (1984). Character disorders: Characterological specificity and the alcoholic. In E. M. Pattison & E. Kaufman (Eds.), *Encyclopedic handbook of alcoholism.* New York: Gardner Press.

Laplanche, J., & Pontalis, J. B. (1973). *The language of psychoanalysis.* New York: Norton.

McDougall, J. (1982). *Theaters of the mind: Illusion and truth on the psychoanalytic stage.* New York: Basic Books.

McDougall, J. (1989). *Theaters of the body.* New York: Norton.

McLellan, A. T., Woody, G. E., Luborsky, L., & O'Brien, C. P. (1990). Foreword. In E. J. Khantzian, K. S. Halliday, & W. E. McAuliffe, *Addiction and the vulnerable self: Modified dynamic group therapy for substance abusers* (pp. ix–xii). New York: Guilford Press.

Meyer, R. E. (1986). How to understand the relationship between psychopathology and addictive disorders: Another example of the chicken and egg. In R. E. Meyer (Ed.), *Psychopathology and addictive disorders* (pp. 3–16). New York: Guilford Press.

Morgenstern, J., Langenbucher, J., & Labouvie, L. (1994). The generalizability of the dependence syndrome across substances: An examination of some properties of the proposed DSM-IV dependence criteria. *Addiction, 89,* 1105–1113.

Morgenstern, J., Langenbucher, J., Labouvie, L., & Miller, K. (1994, August). *The comorbidity of alcoholism and Axis II disorders in a clinical population.* Paper presented at the annual meeting of the American Psychological Association, Los Angeles.

Morgenstern, J., & Leeds, J. (1993). Contemporary psychoanalytic theories of substance abuse: A disorder in search of a paradigm. *Psychotherapy, 30,* 194–206.

Nathan, P. (1988). The addictive personality is the behavior of the addict. *Journal of Consulting and Clinical Psychology, 56,* 183–188.

National Psychological Association for Psychoanalysis. (1992). *Working with alcoholics and substance abusers in private practice.* Second Annette Overby Memorial Symposium, New York.

Pine, F. (1990). *Drive, ego, object and self.* New York: Basic Books.

Prochaska, J. O., & DiClemente, C. C. (1983). Stages and processes of self-change of smoking: Toward an integrative model. *Journal of Consulting and Clinical Psychology, 51,* 390–395.

Project MATCH Research Group. (1997). Matching alcoholism treatments to client heterogeneity: Project MATCH posttreatment drinking outcomes. *Journal of Studies on Alcohol, 58*(1), 7–29.

Rado, S. (1926). The psychic effects of intoxicants: An attempt to evolve a psychoanalytical theory of morbid cravings. *Internal Journal of Psychoanalysis, 7,* 396–413.

Regier, D. A., Farmer, M. E., Rae, D. S., Locke, B. Z., Keith, S. J., Judd, L. L., & Goodwin, F. K. (1990). Comorbidity of mental disorders with alcohol and other drug use. *Journal of the American Medical Association, 264,* 2511–2518.

Rinsley, D. B. (1988). The dipsas revisited: Comments on addiction and personality. *Journal of Substance Abuse Treatment, 5,* 1–7.

Robins, L. N., & Regier, D. A. (1991). *Psychiatric disorders in America.* New York: Free Press.

Tolstoy, L. (1877/2001). *Anna Karenina* (R. Pevear & L. Volokhonsky, Trans.). New York: Viking.

Wise, R. A. (1988). The neurobiology of craving: Implications for the understanding and treatment of addiction. *Journal of Abnormal Psychology, 97,* 118–132.

Wurmser, L. (1984). The role of superego conflicts in substance abuse and their treatment. *International Journal of Psychoanalytic Psychotherapy, 10,* 227–258.

Wurmser, L. (1985). Denial and split identity: Timely issues in the psychoanalytic psychotherapy of compulsive drug users. *Journal of Substance Abuse Treatment, 2,* 89–96.

Ziedonis, D., & Kosten, T. (1993). Behavioral pathology. In J. Langenbucher, B. McCrady, W. Frankenstein, & P. Nathan (Eds.), *Addictions research and treatment.* New York: Pergamon Press.

Zinberg, N. E. (1970). *Drug, set, and setting.* New Haven, CT: Yale University Press.

4

Exploration in the Service of Relapse Prevention

A Psychoanalytic Contribution to Substance Abuse Treatment

Daniel S. Keller

Advances in substance abuse treatment over the past two decades have been stimulated largely by developments from within the cognitive-behavioral, 12-step/disease model, family therapy, and pharmacotherapeutic orientations. Increasingly, treatment as it is currently practiced relies on one or more of the therapeutic strategies deriving from these perspectives (Institute of Medicine, 1989). In particular, cognitive-behavioral approaches to addictions treatment (e.g., Marlatt & Gordon, 1985; Monti, Abrams, Kadden, & Cooney, 1989) have begun to demonstrate both effectiveness (e.g., Carroll, Rounsaville, & Gawin, 1991) and increasing use across theoretical orientations (Morgenstern & McCrady, 1992).

During precisely this same period, a number of fairly well-developed psychoanalytic models on the nature of substance use disorders have emerged (e.g., Khantzian, 1980; Krystal, 1975; Krystal & Raskin, 1970; Wurmser, 1978). In addition, several psychodynamically informed treatment approaches, which have been influenced to a greater or lesser degree by these models, have been generated (e.g., Galanter, 1993; Kaufman, 1994; Khantzian, Halliday, & McAuliffe, 1990). Yet by and large psychoanalytic ideas on substance abuse and its treatment have failed to find a place within the treatment techniques of most practitioners treating substance abusers (see Leeds & Morgenstern, Chapter 3, this volume).

This chapter examines the potential for a more robust psychoanalytic contribution to substance abuse treatment. To do so, I (1) review current psychoanalytic psychotherapy indicating why it needs substantial modification in the treatment of substance use disorders; (2) provide a rationale for integrating aspects of psychoanalytic technique with cognitive-behavioral treatment for addictive disorders; and (3) illustrate how such an integrated psychoanalytic/cognitive-behavioral approach to substance abuse treatment, in which selected exploration of the substance abuser's attitudes, defenses, conflicts, and feelings as they are revealed within the moment-to-moment process of therapy, may be used to facilitate engagement in treatment and cognitive-behavioral relapse prevention.

One final word of introduction: throughout the chapter "psychodynamic therapy" refers to the broad range of insight-oriented therapies based on psychoanalytic principles (e.g., Luborsky, 1984; Wallerstein, 1986) and not to orthodox or classical psychoanalysis per se (e.g., Greenson, 1967).

CONTEMPORARY PSYCHOANALYTIC PSYCHOTHERAPY

Psychoanalytic psychotherapy has undergone enormous development since Freud first invented it (e.g., Breuer & Freud, 1893–1895; Freud, 1894/1953, 1896/1953, 1905/1953). Yet until relatively recently these developments, many of which are now decades old, have not been fully understood and appreciated by therapists of other orientations (see Safran & Siegel, 1990, for a notable exception). It has been my impression that many nonanalytically oriented therapists often believe that psychoanalytic psychotherapy focuses almost exclusively on "deep" unconscious conflicts rooted in the distant past and that such conflicts can be resolved only through "id interpretations," generally of an oedipal cast. No doubt, at one time much analytic therapy was conducted along these lines as, for example, in Freud's (1905/1953) "Dora" case. Yet the old caricature of a silent, depriving, incognito analyst whose utterances are limited to foisting interpretations, such as "You wanted to kill your father," on an otherwise reluctant or suggestible patient is certainly much less true today than a century ago and is more likely to be found in a cartoon in the *New Yorker* magazine than in the Park Avenue consulting room of a New York City analyst. For one thing, psychoanalysts have long recognized that for interpretations of repressed unconscious material to have any therapeutic effect, they must be preceded by an analysis of the elaborate layering of the patient's characteristic ego defenses and resistances (e.g., Fenichel, 1941; Freud, 1923/1961; Greenson, 1967; Reich, 1933/1945). Much of what constitutes contemporary psychoanalytic therapy is an analysis of such resistances (Schafer, 1976). Moreover, nowadays the analytically oriented clinician tends to focus on the here-and-now experience of the patient as revealed in the moment-to-moment process of their psychotherapeutic relationship (Gill, 1982; Schlesinger, 1981, 1982). Transference and resistance, for example, are regarded as having as much to do with the patient's present experience of him- or herself, the therapist, and the therapeutic situation as they have to do with their infantile moorings. Further-more, contemporary psychodynamic clinicians are far less likely to regard a pa-tient's symptoms as the expression of a specific, circumscribed, drive–defense conflict the resolution of which is brought about by one fundamental pene-trating insight into archaic experience but rather as the expression of well-integrated aspects of the patient's personality or character that ramify through-out the patient's contemporary life. As Wheelis (1973) put it, "The symptom does not afflict the patient, it *is* the patient" (p. 17). Thus, the locus of change in psychoanalytic therapy is the person, not symptoms. Much of the work of therapy investigates and attempts to alter the contemporary characteristic ways that the patient acts, feels, and relates to others.

An open-ended exploration and understanding of the meanings of these phenomena are the stuff of psychoanalytic psychotherapy, broadly speaking. Such exploration tends to reveal attitudes, postures, stances, feelings, ways of relating to others, and ways of thinking about things of which the patient has had perhaps only a dim intimation but about which he or she has been con-fused, puzzled, disturbed, or perplexed—often over a period of many years. In the course of this exploration it is the therapist's task, in Shapiro's apt phrase, to "introduce the patient to himself" (1989, p. 10). In so doing, the patient may come to see that the very complaints that motivated him or her to seek treat-ment in the first place are brought about precisely through these characteristic yet obscure ways in which he or she thinks, feels, and relates. For example, a patient who wants a satisfying, intimate relationship but can never seem to find the right partner may come to discover a deep-seated fear of intimacy ex-pressed perhaps only as an oddly peculiar uncomfortable feeling, vaguely expe-rienced, followed by a curious loss of interest in the other when each new re-lationship "threatens" to become more intimate. Such an "insight" serves not merely as an end in itself but as yet another starting point for further explora-tion into yet other facets of the patient's experience. While the patient's fear of intimacy may have been forged initially in his earliest conflicts with parents—perhaps in how he learned to love—it is now likely that this and other uncon-scious conflicts have achieved a kind of autonomy, have become typical, char-acteristic modes of "being-in-the-world" (Binswanger, 1946). Insight into the *initial conflict* may be useful as a kind of basic formulation—a working hypoth-esis—but therapy must explore the myriad unknown ways in which this initial as well as other conflicts have been transmuted and now interpenetrate the pa-tient's contemporary life.

In order for the patient's characteristic ways of thinking, feeling, and relat-ing to emerge in therapy, the therapeutic situation is deliberately ambiguous. Apart from patients agreeing to communicate whatever occurs to them as best they can—the so-called basic rule of free association (Freud, 1900/1953, p. 102)—there are no rules or directives for patients to follow. In contrast, the therapist reveals relatively little about him- or herself. One of the results of such an ambiguous situation is that the patient's unconscious and preconscious fantasies as well as his or her defenses against them begin to emerge and, in particular, in relation to the therapist (i.e., the transference). *Transference* refers to the human inclination to distort one's experience of others based on fantasy rather than reality considerations and is potentially more likely under ambiguous circumstances. Transference distortions occur in all of us, as anyone who has gone on a job interview or out on a first date can attest. In therapy, transferences are at first more or less isolated reactions. As therapy develops, however, the patient's transference relationship to the therapist tends to blossom into what is known as a *transference neurosis* wherein the patient's prototypic pathology is "relived" or enacted. This provides the therapist the opportunity of working *in vivo* with the pathological aspects of the patient's personality. It is through the interpretation of the transference that the patient's pathological symptoms and character traits may be worked through and ultimately resolved. It is well beyond the scope of this chapter to discuss transference and its interpretation in any depth. The point I wish to make here is that the treatment situation is purposely designed to be ambiguous and nondirective so that these unconscious phenomena—especially the transference—may emerge.

Several important advances in psychoanalytic clinical theory which have evolved over the years deserve mention. These advances have had an enormous impact on contemporary technique and require a brief explication in order to understand many of the technical recommendations that follow in this chapter. First, in the early years in which psychoanalytic therapy was practiced, the central technical goal involved unearthing repressed wishes, that is, making the unconscious conscious. However, it was not long before analysts realized that in order for this to have a therapeutic effect, the patient's resistances—the dynamic, defensive forces that led to the repression in the first place—had to be analyzed first (Freud, 1912/1958). This fact as well as other considerations actually led Freud (1923/1961, 1926/1959) to revamp his entire model of the mind ushering in the beginning of psychoanalytic ego psychology. Thereafter, clinical work focused primarily on the patient's ego, not on the repressed unconscious (Fenichel, 1941; Greenson, 1967). In so doing, the therapist helps prepare the patient's ego to cope better with disturbing unconscious thoughts when they do emerge. In practice, this means that psychoanalytic therapists avoid attempting to "reach behind" the patient's resistances in order to "pull out" the unconscious material. Rather, resistances must be explored and worked through first. Greenson (1967), in his classic treatise on technique, summarized the technical rule that resulted from this change thusly: "Analyze resistance before content, ego before id, begin with the surface" (p. 137).

Second, when analysts began to focus on characterological patterns and traits (Reich, 1933/1945), the therapist's attention expanded to include not only *what* the patient said (i.e., the content of the patient's communications to the therapist) but *how* the patient communicated, that is, the manner, form, and style in which the patient interacted with the therapist (i.e., the process of the patient's communications). A thought followed by a silence, a shifting emotional attitude, a stilted way of talking, a forced facial expression—all these and a multitude of other ways of behaving may indicate important resistances and require that the therapist remain attuned as much to *how* the patient thinks, feels, and relates as to *what* the patient thinks, feels, and relates. As we shall see later, these technical skills may be employed usefully in substance abuse treatment.

Despite the fact that no other therapy has yet evolved that permits so full an exploration of the total personality, there remain significant problems in recommending such unmodified psychoanalytic therapy as the *central* form of treatment for addictive disorders. First, on the basis of present knowledge, it seems reasonably clear that once the addictive disorder has achieved sufficient severity and chronicity, extrapersonality factors—behavioral, cognitive, environmental, and biological—are essentially responsible for maintaining the disorder (Marlatt & Gordon, 1985; Wikler, 1973). This is not to say that unconscious conflicts may not have initially contributed to the development of the disorder, nor is it to suggest that aspects of personality functioning do not play their part as well in sustaining an addiction. However, at least in the early to middle phases of treatment—when relapse is most likely to occur—these latter psychological factors are better considered as relatively *peripheral* as contrasted with the central task of achieving and maintaining abstinence. Therapy, to be effective, requires behavior change because the disorder is governed by behavioral laws.

Second, psychoanalytic conceptualizations of addiction (e.g., Khantzian et al., 1990; Krystal & Raskin, 1970; Wurmser, 1985) regard substance abuse as essentially rooted in some form of *underlying*, psychological disorder (see Leeds & Morgenstern, Chapter 3, this volume) despite the growing consensus among researchers and clinicians regarding the multiple biological, behavioral, and environmental factors involved in the etiology of addiction. To be sure, these analytic theorists have contributed immensely to elucidating important personality dynamics and deficits in substance abusers such as severe superego pathology, poor affect tolerance and expression, and the like. Yet again, while attention to such personality factors is important, these factors are, in my opinion, relatively peripheral as compared with the centrality of behavior change. Indeed, as I try to show in the next section, recent psychodynamically informed approaches to addictions treatment include cognitive-behavioral skills-building components.

Third, cognitive-behavioral treatments have emerged that directly address these behavioral, cognitive, and environmental factors associated with the maintenance of addictive processes (e.g., Marlatt & Gordon, 1985; Monti et al.,

1989), and these therapies are beginning to demonstrate efficacy in controlled clinical trials (e.g., Carroll, Rounsaville, & Gawin, 1991; Institute of Medicine, 1989; Miller & Hester, 1986).

Fourth, as any clinician who works with substance abusers knows, the therapist must be active, directive, and prescriptive in working with such patients. However, dynamic therapy requires precisely the opposite. In order to foster exploration, in order to permit the patient's resistances to emerge, in order to nurture the transference, the therapist remains purposely nondirective and nonprescriptive. Yet to proceed this way with substance abusers before abstinence has been achieved and stabilized, the therapist risks entering into a collusion with the patient in which the patient's wish for a magic cure (i.e., that he or she needs to feel better before changing) is reinforced by the therapist's belief that insight into intrapsychic conflict must precede change in behavior.

RATIONALE FOR A COMBINED TREATMENT

Given this somewhat pessimistic preamble, it might be asked: Is there any role at all for psychoanalytic ideas in the treatment of substance use disorders? It should be clear from the foregoing that some form of cognitive–behavioral therapy is indicated in the treatment of addictive disorders, particularly those of sufficient severity and chronicity. This is so because, as noted above, the primary factors maintaining the addiction tend to be behavioral, cognitive, and environmental. Nevertheless, in my opinion, cognitive–behavioral therapy for addictions may be enhanced by attention to defenses, resistances, and unconscious conflicts as expressed in the psychotherapeutic process and relationship, traditionally the central focus of psychoanalytic psychotherapy. There are several reasons for this. First, cognitive–behavioral therapy is undertaken within an interpersonal context, no less so than psychodynamic therapy. This interpersonal relationship acquires significant meaning for patients if one wishes to pay attention to it (Safran & Siegel, 1990; Wachtel, 1977). A focus on the nuances of the interpersonal process in therapy may well influence relapse prevention and outcome. Second, substance abusers exhibit a broad range of unconscious defense mechanisms, which often contribute significantly to exposures to risky situations and irrational thoughts and feelings that also predispose to relapse (e.g., Kaufman, 1994; Krystal, 1975; Wurmser, 1978). An understanding of defenses may also assist in surmounting various difficulties in acquiring and maintaining skills. Third, like other people, substance abusers experience unconscious conflicts that may also lead to relapse if left unattended (Kaufman, 1994). Fourth, the psychodynamic makeup of an individual will often exert a significant influence on how a structured task such as skills acquisition is approached and performed (Rapaport, Gill, & Schafer, 1968).

In recent years a combined psychodynamic/cognitive-behavioral approach to the treatment of general psychiatric disorders has found growing acceptance from within both psychodynamic (e.g., Wachtel, 1977) and cognitive-behavioral perspectives (e.g., Safran & Siegel, 1990). Moreover, initial integrative efforts have already begun to appear in the substance abuse field as well. In a recent book, Kaufman (1994) has delineated what he refers to as a "pragmatic approach" to the psychoanalytic treatment of addicted persons. In Kaufman's view, previous psychodynamic approaches to the therapy of alcoholics and addicts have met with little success because they have failed to sufficiently promote abstinence before engaging in psychodynamic exploration of the patient's conflicts. He describes a three-phase treatment in which the better part of the first two phases (i.e., the first 1–2 years of therapy) is spent attempting to secure and stabilize abstinence principally through rigorous application of cognitive-behavioral relapse prevention and 12-step involvement. Psychodynamic therapy enters these phases only minimally, although a psychodynamic understanding of the patient is used to address patients with personality disorders and/or periodic intrapsychic conflicts that threaten sobriety. In the third phase, which Kaufman refers to as "advanced recovery," therapy becomes more traditionally psychodynamic in the sense that the transference is permitted to develop more freely and is analyzed through an understanding of the transference–countertransference paradigms that emerge. Kaufman suggests that the typical conflictual themes that characterize this phase of treatment in addicts are mourning the loss of alcohol or other drugs as well as issues around intimacy and autonomy. These too are resolved within an understanding of the transference relationship.

Galanter (1993) has also recently described a treatment for substance abuse that combines both psychodynamic therapy and cognitive-behavioral methods, which he calls "network therapy." Like Kaufman, Galanter believes that abstinence must be achieved and secured for therapy to be effective. Thus, the initial stages of his approach utilize cognitive-behavioral principles and techniques in order to achieve and maintain abstinence—but with a twist. The bulk of Galanter's cognitive-behavioral interventions are administered within the context of a network of supportive family members and friends who, along with the patient, meet regularly with the therapist. These network sessions, which augment the patient's concurrent individual treatment, focus on teaching the patient and his network the nature of craving as a classically conditioned response, identifying triggers and high-risk situations, and developing skills and strategies to prevent relapse. It is Galanter's contention that a patient's family and friends can be galvanized into a cohesive team in which network members actively partake in the patient's relapse prevention efforts, (e.g., in monitoring disulfiram [Antabuse] and executing avoidance strategies). In contrast to other forms of substance abuse treatment that involve family members (e.g., Stanton, Todd, & Associates, 1982), Galanter does *not* attempt to alter or restructure family systems, interpret "codependency," or in any way address network members' own psychopathology. Rather, when individual and/or group dynamics emerge, the therapist attempts to manage these as a good office manager might address staff difficulties.

Galanter (1993) does not expand at length on the nature of the patient's individual sessions because his volume is expressly concerned with the description of network therapy. However, in the early phase of treatment, psychodynamic conflicts or character traits are dealt with when they pose a threat to sobriety. For example, the network session of a patient who relapsed in the early phase of treatment focused on the cognitive and behavioral precipitants to the relapse and the development of more appropriate strategies. However, in the patient's next individual session, attention was devoted to his marked impulsive character style, which had also played a role in his relapse (Galanter & Keller, 1994). According to Galanter, once sobriety is stabilized, a more traditional psychodynamic treatment may unfold.

Although both Kaufman (1994) and Galanter (1993) have described innovative approaches in which the therapist utilizes techniques from both psychodynamic and cognitive-behavioral schools of thought, neither describes exactly how psychodynamic technique may be used to facilitate the cognitive-behavioral components of the treatment, though this is strongly implied in both. For instance, both recommend interpretation of unconscious conflict and character traits when these present a threat to abstinence. In the remainder of this chapter I attempt to illustrate more precisely how selected use of psychoanalytic technique may foster engagement in treatment and cognitive-behavioral relapse prevention.

INTEGRATED PSYCHOANALYTIC AND COGNITIVE-BEHAVIORAL THERAPY

An integrated model of psychodynamic and cognitive-behavioral therapy for substance abusers can be conceptualized as an admixture of supportive and expressive interventions (Schlesinger, 1969). In the early and middle phases of treatment, when the achievement and maintenance of abstinence are primary, the therapist will act in an essentially supportive, educative manner utilizing cognitive-behavioral techniques. However, when resistances, defenses, or unconscious conflicts pose a threat to treatment and/or sobriety, selective use of expressive–exploratory techniques are utilized. Conversely, in the advanced stage of treatment, when sobriety has been stabilized, a more expressive form of psychodynamic treatment may predominate in which unconscious conflicts are resolved within the traditional transference–countertransference matrix; however, selective reversion to supportive, cognitive-behavioral techniques is employed when abstinence is threatened.

In order to understand how cognitive-behavioral and psychodynamic components of this model interact, it may be helpful to briefly describe a purely didactic cognitive-behavioral approach to substance abuse treatment and then consider the central psychodynamic additions I am proposing here.

Cognitive-Behavioral Components

In general, the approach I am suggesting derives its cognitive-behavioral influence mainly from the relapse prevention model (RP) developed by Marlatt and Gordon (1985). Briefly, RP is essentially didactic and represents the supportive–educative emphasis of the integrated psychodynamic–cognitive-behavioral model. RP focuses on identification of a set of addiction-maintaining phenomena such as high-risk situations, conditioned cues for craving (triggers), and maladaptive thought processes operative within the patient's life—all of which increase the likelihood of relapse. In addition, RP addresses the substance abuser's general inclination to unwittingly expose him- or herself to such phenomena despite the effort to become sober (apparently irrelevant decisions). In this respect, as I try to show below, RP is quite compatible with psychodynamic clinical theory since such unwitting exposures are an illustration of unconscious motivation par excellence.

The RP approach is essentially psychoeducational in that it teaches patients to become aware of such addiction-related phenomena and assists them in developing coping skills and strategies that minimize the risk of exposure or the risk of using when exposure is unavoidable. In this respect the treatment is fairly straightforward, relying on common sense augmented by commitment to the change process. The goal is the achievement and maintenance of abstinence. Typical techniques might include avoidance of high-risk situations; understanding the nature of craving; strategies to endure craving, such as decision delay and self-monitoring; challenging maladaptive thoughts; drink refusal; and so forth (for a detailed discussion of these and related RP techniques for substance abuse treatment, see Marlatt & Gordon, 1985; Monti et al., 1989; Carroll, Rounsaville, & Keller, 1991; Kadden et al., 1992; and Morgan, Chapter 8, this volume).

Psychodynamic Components

In contrast to a purely didactic approach, the integrated psychodynamic–cognitive-behavioral model focuses selectively on the interpersonal process that develops between patient and therapist that may either facilitate or hinder skills acquisition and the attainment of abstinence. This interpersonal process can be viewed from a number of perspectives, but it may be most useful here to consider it from two interrelated vantage points: the working alliance and patient resistance. The *working alliance* (e.g., Greenson, 1967) refers to the ability of the patient to use his or her reasonable, observing ego to identify with the therapist's methods as they pursue mutually agreed-on treatment goals. In contrast, *resistance* refers to the expression of defense within the treatment situation. As such, there may be times when the patient's resistances may temporarily impede his or her ability to maintain a good working alliance with the therapist. Such resistances may be blatant, such as noncompliance with treatment procedures, but more often are subtle or "quiet," such as a slight shift in the patient's attitude or nonverbal activity discordant with the patient's verbal communications (Schlesinger, 1982). At such times, the therapist in the integrated model would explore such resistances by interpreting defenses, unconscious conflicts, emotional or attitudinal shifts in the patient's demeanor, or the interpersonal process itself. The purpose of the exploration is to identify what is unconsciously bothering the patient at that moment in time so that a good working alliance may be reestablished and skills acquisition may proceed.

Clinical Illustrations

Let us now examine how psychodynamic exploration of the psychotherapeutic process can enhance RP efforts. I will focus on the assessment, early/middle, and advanced phases of treatment, respectively. Clinical examples are used to illustrate how selective exploration of ambivalence, resistances, defenses, painful affects, unconscious conflicts, and distorted cognitions may facilitate an otherwise cognitive-behavioral RP approach to treatment.

ASSESSMENT PHASE: ADDRESSING AMBIVALENCE
AND RESISTANCE

It is not uncommon for clinicians to think of the assessment or evaluation phase as somewhat distinct from treatment. In this view, assessment is a kind of information-gathering phase wherein the therapist amasses relevant data, arrives at a diagnosis, and recommends a treatment on which both patient and therapist agree. To be sure, we do gather a great deal of information during the assessment phase. For example, we would like to know the patient's substance abuse history in detail. We pay particular attention to when, how, and under what circumstances the patient's use began; how it made the patient feel; and how the patient's use has increased over time. We also want to know the patient's most recent use and whether he or she has developed tolerance or exhibits signs and symptoms of withdrawal. Moreover, we pay very special attention to previous attempts at abstinence and previous relapses. In addition to all this, we want to assess the problems the patient's substance abuse has caused in significant life areas (e.g., legal, financial, occupational, and with significant others such as family and friends). Finally, we want to make a careful assessment of the presence of concurrent psychiatric disorders. All this is important, indeed crucial, information for arriving at an accurate diagnosis and for tailoring an appropriately individualized treatment plan.

In the assessment phase, however, additional attention to the *way* the patient communicates offers another opportunity and one which, from the psychoanalytic viewpoint, may actually facilitate information-gathering activities. It is the opportunity for *engaging* the patient in the treatment process. Simply because a patient has presented in our consulting room does not mean that the patient feels that treatment is an undertaking upon which he or she wishes to embark. Indeed, quite a number of substance abusers present for treatment under a variety of conditions of duress, such as the importunings of a spouse, an employer, or the legal system. And even patients who present more or less willingly usually have some reservations. Our primary question must be: Does substance abuse treatment make sense to *the patient*? Not to his spouse, not to his employer, not to the courts, but to him or her?

The fact is that *ambivalence* typically characterizes the motivation of most patients (not just substance abusers) upon entering treatment. Sometimes the ambivalence is relatively mild, and eliciting the array of negative consequences the substance use has engendered in the patient's life is enough to counteract the ambivalence, at least in the short run. At the other end of the spectrum, the patient may so disavow the need or desire for treatment that only external mandates ensure his or her participation. Usually, however, ambivalence is expressed more subtly. For example, the patient makes and keeps an initial appointment, but as we begin to query him his answers reveal hesitations of one sort or another. He "guesses" he has a problem despite a lifetime of unremitting drinking. Or, he may become more evasive or withholding about certain topics, thereby impeding our information gathering. The patient is physically present but not wholeheartedly psychologically present. Literally, he is in the office; figuratively, he has one foot in and one foot out the door.

The therapeutic task at this point is not to rid the patient of his ambivalence but to explore the curious obstacles he has put in his and our path. It may well be that the patient *does* feel the need for treatment but fears any number of implications it might entail.

For instance, a 34-year-old married alcoholic woman presents for an initial interview. Her mood is somewhat dysphoric and she states hesitantly that she "might" have a drinking problem, though her substance use history leaves little doubt that her problem is fairly severe. When I ask about her marriage, however, her dysphoria and hesitancy become intensified. Her answers are short, clipped, terse, and withholding. It is as if an invisible wall has gone up between us. I realize I have touched on a sore spot, but it is also clear that to proceed in this area *now* will likely only intensify her defensiveness. As we move on to other areas of her life, she begins to describe with much greater ease and animation a project she is involved with at work. I am struck by the difference in her overall psychological and emotional demeanor and say in a mildly upbeat way: "You know, as you talk about your project, you've really perked up." The patient reacts with a bit of a startle. She had not been aware of this significant shift in her mood until I had pointed it out to her. She continues to discuss her work a bit more and then falls silent. After a short period of quiet brooding, she openly begins to reevaluate her comparatively withholding attitude regarding her marriage. She then relates some serious difficulties in her marriage that are, not surprisingly, related to her drinking, which she now states has "really gotten out of control lately."

Let us consider this clinical illustration further. First, by temporarily abandoning the pursuit of information and by focusing on the shifting emotional attitude of the patient, she is assisted in looking at herself in a way she was unwilling to do earlier. She is "introduced to herself," to quote Shapiro (1989) again. It is also important to note that the intervention was directed toward something positive—in this case the greater ease with which she began to communicate. Had I commented, for example, on her hesitancy to discuss her marriage, she might have felt criticized. Or she might have grudgingly conceded the information I wanted. But it would not have been what *she* wanted to say at that point in time. It certainly would not have facilitated a good working alliance. Yet once she was able to acknowledge her concerns about her marriage, talking about her marital problems began to make sense to her and the previously held-back information emerged easily. Second, this therapeutic fragment tells us much more than the extent of her marital problems or the extent of her drinking. It tells us that the patient is able to look at herself productively, that she has a good "observing ego," and that other similar interventions may also be indicated in working with this patient, particularly her resistances. Third, she becomes *engaged* in the therapeutic process. Whereas she starts out the interview stating that she "might" have a problem, she ends up with a new stance: namely, that she believes she does in fact have an alcohol problem and that it is related to a significant area of her life. She now has reasons for wanting to enter treatment.

Often therapists are tempted to avoid exploration of just these sorts of sore spots and just as often rationalize the avoidance as an attempt to build a positive rapport. Actually, such avoidance usually diminishes rapport in the long run. The patient will feel, in some corner of her mind, that she has "bested" or "hoodwinked" the therapist and how good can such a therapist be who can have the wool pulled over his or her eyes so easily? This is especially true for substance abusers.

To return to the clinical illustration: I do not suggest that this *particular* intervention would work with every patient. Patients vary in their degree of ambivalence and in their manner of expressing it. But I do think that the therapist's general attention to the process—in this case the patient's emotional attitude in relating her difficulties—can significantly enhance information-gathering efforts. In the above case, I think that the therapist's process comment made a decisive difference in the outcome of the session.

EARLY AND MIDDLE PHASES OF TREATMENT

In the early and middle phases of treatment the achievement and maintenance of abstinence are the central focus of therapy. Although there is debate within the literature regarding the feasibility of "controlled" drinking, as a practical matter, patients with moderate to severe substance abuse problems (i.e., most alcoholics, cocaine addicts, and heroin addicts) generally need to learn how to abstain and maintain their abstinence for treatment to succeed (Kaufman, 1994). This does not mean that the patient *must* be abstinent during all points of treatment. However, abstinence and its maintenance should be the central goals toward which both patient and therapist are striving. Generally, the early and middle phases occupy the first 6–9 months. It is here that RP techniques are most often utilized.

As delineated in cognitive-behavioral approaches (e.g., Carroll, Rounsaville, & Keller, 1991; Kadden et al., 1992; Marlatt & Gordon, 1985), treatment for substance abuse during these phases involves (1) identification of high-risk situations and classically conditioned cues (triggers) for craving and the development of strategies to limit exposure to them, (2) development of skills to successfully endure cravings and other painful affects, (3) learning how to challenge or better manage maladaptive thoughts about using, (4) learning how to avoid using when one is in an otherwise unavoidable high-risk situation, (5) generating a basic emergency plan for coping with high-risk situations in which other skills are not working, (6) learning to detect various ways in which one is "setting oneself up," and (7) generating pleasurable sober activities and relationships to offset feelings of emptiness and loss after removal of substance use from the patient's repertoire. During this phase, slips, lapses, and relapses are not uncommon and are regarded as opportunities to fine-tune one's future efforts to achieve abstinence.

How might the use of psychoanalytic technique facilitate this skills-building phase? I would like to focus on how knowledge of psychological defenses; attention to resistance and transference; and the use of free association, empathic listening, countertransference reactions, and interpretation might influence how one can promote abstinence and skills acquisition when working with (1) cravings, (2) apparently irrelevant decisions, (3) common maladaptive cognitions, (4) negative affects, and (5) intrapsychic conflict.

Working with Cravings. It has often been pointed out in the literature (e.g., Marlatt & Gordon, 1985; Wikler, 1973) that craving for substances is a classically conditioned response elicited by exposure to stimuli that have been repeatedly paired with substance use. Such stimuli are often *external*—such as bars, drug paraphernalia, substance-abusing friends and acquaintances, neighborhoods in which use occurred, and so forth—or *internal*—such as irrational thoughts or painful affect states that one has learned to temporarily abolish through substance use. In RP, the therapist teaches the patient the nature of the craving response by explaining Pavlov's learning paradigm and then helps the patient to develop strategies for limiting exposure to these conditioned cues as well as other ways to manage cravings once exposures have elicited the craving response.

Nevertheless, due to the nature of unconscious psychological defense mechanisms, not all craving is noticed or regarded as craving by the patient. For example, one chronically relapsing patient in group therapy for cocaine addiction, through the use of projection, would see signs of craving in other group members, though not in himself, generally in the week prior to *his* relapses.

Therapists who work with addicted people have long been aware of the use of the defense mechanism of denial in substance abusers. However, there has been an unfortunate tendency to mislabel other defensive processes as "denial." One sometimes suspects that those who overuse the term "denial" are actually referring to a more general process, namely, resistance, which refers to the expression of all defenses within the treatment situation (Gill, 1982). Yet if we are going to help patients discover the many ways in which unconscious defenses operate so as to both express and disguise cravings, it is important to be as precise as possible. A good starting point is to study Anna Freud's (1936) classic articulation of this subject: *The Ego and the Mechanisms of Defense*. With respect to the use of defenses in substance abusers, Kaufman (1994) has provided an excellent discussion.

Although almost any defense mechanism may come into play, in my experience one of the most common defenses employed in the expression of craving is the defense of "displacement." *Displacement* refers to an unconscious mental process through which feelings toward a person or object are transferred or shifted to some other person or object and experienced in relation to this new person or object (Fenichel, 1945). For example, transference is quintessentially a displacement (Greenson, 1967). With respect to craving, substance abusers frequently displace the urge to drink or use substances onto some other activity that may be extremely high risk but that they do not experience as risky at all. It is important to stress that the displacement takes place *unconsciously*. If, for example, a patient experiences a sudden urge to pay off the money he owes his dealer, it is not necessarily the case that he is aware of the desire to use drugs. If one told the patient at this point, "You really want to use drugs," it would likely increase his defensiveness, perhaps through the use of a variety of rationalizations.

Let us consider the operation of displacement in craving and the technique utilized to interpret it. A 33-year-old male alcoholic has been sober for approximately 2 months after beginning treatment in an outpatient chemical dependency rehabilitation program in which he has been receiving a combination of RP augmented by various 12-step activities. During a group therapy session the patient, in the midst of relating to the group how well his recovery is going, casually adds that this upcoming weekend he is planning to go on the annual family fishing trip, which he eagerly looks forward to every year. He states this with a kind of avid enthusiasm and without the slightest trace of awareness that fishing trips are often high-risk situations because they are frequently accompanied by copious amounts of beer. Not too much time elapses before other group members inquire about the potential for beer to be present on the trip. The patient acknowledges that his uncle generally does bring four to six cases but states somewhat testily that he [the patient] is different now, he is in recovery, values his sobriety, and in any event is not going to drink. He adds that he "has" to go because it is also his uncle's birthday. The group becomes more confrontational (e.g., "You're in denial," "You're setting yourself up," "You're gonna drink, don't go"), which is followed by the patient, now somewhat angry, stating that his mind is made up, he is not going to drink, "I have to go!" After a brief silence, the patient looks up toward the therapist and asks what the latter thinks. The tone of the patient's voice sounds as if he expects the therapist to side with the group, but the therapist also senses a faint trace of honest curiosity in the way the patient asks the question. The therapist replies: "I think you want to go on this fishing trip *very* badly" and then adds somewhat ironically, "It sounds similar to a craving." The patient is slightly taken aback but then begins to mull over the therapist's comment. He has to admit that he had not thought about it that way but still believes he will not drink and reiterates his commitment to go on the trip. Nevertheless, his reiteration lacks the fire it had at the outset and seems somewhat empty, as if the patient were now only saving face. Two days later, at the next group therapy session, the patient informs the group that he has decided to forgo the fishing trip, adding that his recovery is more important.

I believe that this clinical vignette illustrates how the therapist's attention to the patient's displacement of craving from alcohol onto the fishing trip helps to facilitate the patient's RP efforts. It is important to note that the therapist does not say that the patient's desire to go on the trip masks his "real" desire to drink. Rather, the therapist states that the patient's desire to go contains an urgency that is similar to the urgency of a craving, something with which the patient is all too familiar and cannot reject out of hand. What makes the intervention effective is that it addresses what the patient is consciously experiencing (the urgency), not what is being hidden (the desire to drink), though it suggests a possible connection between this conscious experience and craving for alcohol in general. It is as if the patient must take this step first before he can even permit himself to entertain the possibility that he might actually want to drink on the fishing trip. The therapist addresses the defense rather than the motive underlying it.

It may be instructive to specify how a purely didactic RP approach might have differed from the one presented here. For instance, a didactically oriented RP therapist might have attempted to assist the patient in identifying the fishing trip as a high-risk situation in which cravings would emerge, in generating a list of pros and cons for going on the trip, and perhaps in utilizing the group to "brainstorm" or "problem-solve" a variety of alternative behaviors. From the psychodynamic point of view, however, such techniques are more likely to be effective when the patient is able to establish a good working alliance—that is, to identify with the therapist's methods and therapeutic goals. In this case, due to resistance, the patient was temporarily unable to identify with therapeutic behavior and goals he had largely embraced up to that point in the treatment. His resistance, as expressed in the displacement, had to be addressed first. He was then able to reestablish a good working alliance and was consequently able to "problem-solve."

Apparently Irrelevant Decisions. In working with substance abusers one is frequently impressed by the capacity of these patients to expose themselves to high-risk situations and conditioned cues with hardly the slightest awareness that they are headed for trouble. The patient who wanted to go on the fishing trip was certainly in that category. These sorts of setups are what Marlatt and Gordon (1985) have referred to as "apparently irrelevant decisions." Essentially, the patient makes a decision or set of decisions that does not appear to be related to the desire to drink or use drugs but in fact brings the patient ever closer to risky environments in which cues for craving are likely to abound. It is as if these apparently irrelevant decisions are linked together in a chain, the last of which is the actual decision to use. However, it is often the case that the only decision the patient is aware of making is this final decision. In RP the therapist attempts to demonstrate that the final decision is only the last link in the chain of decisions, and skills are then taught to interrupt such decision chains earlier when cues, craving, and risky situations are more easily avoided.

From the psychoanalytic perspective, one is impressed by the fact that such decisions, particularly the earlier ones, are experienced with varying degrees of unawareness. When one explores a chain of decisions, it is often difficult for the patient to remember very clearly what he or she was thinking and feeling at such decision points. From a psychodynamic perspective, such vaguely articulated cognitive and affective states often indicate that unconscious factors are operative.

In fact, one is quite struck by the phrase itself: "apparently irrelevant decisions." It sounds so strangely psychoanalytic. After all, it was apparently irrelevant *thoughts* that Freud instructed his patients to report when he explained the basic rule of free association (Freud, 1900/1953, p. 102). Let us consider how elicitation of the patient's associations may facilitate the articulation of a chain of apparently irrelevant decisions.

A 25-year-old single male cocaine abuser reports that he used cocaine during the interval between therapy sessions. Essentially, he had gotten off work and was driving home. Along the way he decided to take a different route and after awhile discovered that he was driving by a bar he used to frequent. He then decided to stop off, say hello, and have a soda. However, at the bar he told himself that as his problem was with cocaine, he could have a beer. After two beers he encountered a friend who "happened" to have a gram of cocaine—and the slip inevitably ensued. I would also like to note that the patient related these events in a bored, monotonous manner, which struck me as interesting.

In exploring the concept of apparently irrelevant decisions, the patient was able to see—somewhat intellectually—how his decisions to enter the bar and drink beer brought him closer to using cocaine. However, he reported that he was not aware of wanting to use cocaine until he ran into the friend. Moreover, he had greater difficulty connecting the events associated with the bar to taking a different route home. His experience of this action seemed limited to a sense of aimless drifting. I then asked whether he could recall what he was thinking or feeling around the time he decided to take the alternative route and he drew a blank. At this point I invited him just to let his thoughts flow and report what occurred to him. After a bit of silence, he reported that the word "relax" had popped into his mind, but it did not seem to have much significance. I then inquired, "What do you think of when you want to relax?" He paused for a moment, then broke out into a wide grin and said: "Gettin' high." Now the connection between the "apparently irrelevant" different route home and his ultimate decision to use had meaning. This also led him to recall that he had felt "uptight" at work that day and in fact had a fleeting thought about using, which he had brushed aside. When we explored what "uptight" meant (the patient tended to use this word somewhat indiscriminantly for many negative feelings), it turned out that he had felt bored. Thus, his uptight boredom led to a desire to "relax." Both the feeling and the cognition could now be used as red flags in the future.

Again let us attempt to distinguish the integrated approach from a purely didactic one. In the above case the didactic RP therapist might have attempted to educate the patient by explaining the concept of apparently irrelevant decisions and by illustrating how the patient's decisions appeared to be linked together. However, I doubt that such an approach alone would have produced in the patient the emotionally charged "aha" experience he had when we followed his associations. The concept now had experiential meaning and significance to him.

It has been my experience that apparently irrelevant decisions are often accompanied by just these sorts of obscure, fleeting, vaguely experienced words or feeling states that when fleshed out and explored help to reestablish the actual connections between the decisions. In this case, the word "relax" was a condensation of two thoughts into one, namely, "relax *and* get high." Obtaining the patient's associations was critical both in deciphering this condensed thought and in promoting RP skills.

Exploring Maladaptive Cognitions. It is quite common within the early and middle phases of treatment for patients to experience a variety of cognitions that may predispose them to slips, lapses, or relapses. For instance, a patient may tell himself that "It would be all right to have just one drink," or that "It's okay to hang out in the bar; I just want to visit my friends," or that "I'll keep some liquor in the house in case I have visitors." The tendency for patients to have these and a variety of similar thoughts is so common that Alcoholics Anonymous has developed the phrase "stinkin' thinkin'" to refer to this class of cognitions, which captures their essence quite nicely.

From a psychodynamic perspective, these and other similar cognitions suggest that psychological defenses are at work. Many will recognize the defense of rationalization in the above examples. Cognitive-behavioral treatments recommend a variety of techniques to combat such rationalizations, such as challenging the thought or weighing the costs and benefits of drinking or using. It has been my experience, however, that such techniques work best the *poorer* the rationalization. For example, the thought that "I can have just one" is not as good a rationalization as "I'll keep some liquor around the house for guests." In the former, the intention to drink is explicit and can be challenged directly, whereas in the latter the rationalization conceals the explicit intention to drink. While it is possible to challenge this latter thought, it may be met with a good deal of resistance. This is because effective rationalizations work precisely because they are *good* reasons. They are acceptable or "ego-syntonic" to the patient. In such cases, it may help to agree with the patient that there is some legitimacy in wanting to be a good host but point out that it becomes a problem in that it simultaneously permits alcohol to be available to him or her as well. Depending on the patient, one can even go a bit further and explain how rationalizations work and empathize with him or her as to how difficult it is to make such alterations in one's life, though it should also be stressed that such alterations are temporary and can be modified when sobriety is stabilized.

Not all maladaptive cognitions, however, are rationalizations. Another fairly commonly employed defense that produces maladaptive thoughts is the defense of reversal. In reversal, patients generally turn an unconscious feeling into its opposite before they can permit it to become conscious. In this respect, reversals are similar to reaction formations, although they differ in important respects (G. Mahl, personal communication, 1984). One often hears patients in early recovery wanting to "test" themselves by going to a bar. But what is it that these patients wish to test? Consciously, they may say they want to see whether they are strong enough to resume their normal activities without alcohol. However, in early recovery such tests are generally tests of weakness, not strength, and the therapist may wish to explore with the patient other indications of feeling weak. Or the therapist may by analogy suggest the idea of weakness. For example, I have told patients who wanted to test themselves that they remind me of someone who has just had major surgery and wants to work out.

Another illustration of reversal is often encountered in patients who want to "reward" themselves for their achievement of sobriety. One alcoholic patient, a sort of disheveled, sad sack of a man, during an assessment session described his longest period of sobriety, which had lasted a full year. When asked how he relapsed he said he had been feeling great about his success and had decided to "reward" himself. Unfortunately, but all too predictably, his "reward" led to heavy levels of drinking, loss of his job, and even homelessness. I responded to his statement that he had wanted to reward himself by suggesting, in a compassionate tone of voice, that his reward sounded more like a punishment. The patient, who had impressed me as both articulate and reflective, was startled, but the interpretation was on target and he began to view his behavior in this new light. Interestingly, over the course of treatment, in which the patient did quite well, the recognition that he punished himself by drinking helped him to avoid a number of slips.

Negative Affective States. Marlatt and Gordon (1985) have noted that empirical research supports the notion that negative emotional states frequently "trigger" relapses in substance abusers. Intolerance of negative affects and inability to verbalize them are at the heart of most contemporary psychoanalytic views on substance abuse (e.g., Khantzian, 1980; Krystal, 1975; Wurmser, 1978). There is some empirical evidence to support these psychoanalytic propositions. Keller and Wilson (1994) found that opiate and cocaine addicts were able to tolerate negative affects significantly less effectively than a group of matched normals. Taylor, Parker, and Bagby (1990) and Haviland, Shaw, MacMurray, and Cummings (1988) found significantly greater rates of *alexithymia*—the inability to verbally identify and differentiate affect states—in alcoholics. Recently, Keller, Carroll, Nich, and Rounsaville (1995) found high rates of alexithymia in a group of cocaine addicts.

Various means are available to the clinician in helping patients to tolerate negative affects more effectively. In some abusers, better articulation of affects tends by itself to promote affect tolerance. When affects are blended together or dedifferentiated they seem to be experienced as global, diffuse, overwhelming, and peremptory (Krystal, 1975). It is not that dissimilar from the way in which infants experience emotions. For example, when a baby feels frustration the emotion appears to radiate throughout its body from head to toe (Kernberg, 1975). The infant learns to manage and differentiate such emotions progressively better through its interactions with the primary caretaker and its own maturation (Greenspan, 1979; Stern, 1985). Ultimately, the toddler learns to label these emotions verbally. That is, the radiating effect of emotions in infancy appears to wane as the emotions become progressively more differentiated. Krystal and Raskin (1970) suggest that substance abusers may need a kind of remedial course in affect differentiation in therapy. They recommend a "pretreatment" phase prior to psychoanalytic psychotherapy in which the abuser is taught to identify and properly label affects.

Nevertheless, many affects that trouble addicts only become apparent during the course of treatment. If the therapist remains attuned to the patient's affective expression within the therapy hour, he or she may help the patient to articulate them. For example, let us return to the patient who took the alternate route home and ended up in a bar. As he recounted these events he sounded bored. This tone of voice in the therapy session impressed the therapist, who pointed it out to the patient, and it turned out that indeed the patient had been feeling bored at work but had not articulated it. Identifying the feeling in the here-and-now greatly facilitates patients in being able to identify it later on their own.

Another way in which therapists can facilitate affect identification is through the use of their own countertransference reactions to the patient. In psychoanalysis, countertransference has traditionally referred to the therapist's *neurotic* emotional reactions to the patient (e.g., Freud, 1910/1957; Gitelson, 1952; Reich, 1933/1945). More recently, the concept has been broadened so that countertransference refers to the therapist's total emotional reaction (Kernberg, 1965; Racker, 1957). Patients stir up powerful feelings in therapists, and this is certainly the case with substance abusers (Kaufman, 1994). There are a number of typical such countertransferences and Weiss (1993) recently provided an excellent discussion. One of the most frequent is through the use of the defense known as "projective identification" (Ogden, 1979). In projective identification, the patient rids some unwanted part of him- or herself such as a threatening affect, by inducing it in the therapist. It is as if the therapist becomes a "container" for feelings the patient has no other way of handling. The task for the therapist is to notice this in him- or herself, analyze its meaning, and then take appropriate action.

For example, a 40-year-old heroin addict with bipolar disorder and a borderline characterological organization had been in substance abuse treatment on and off for many years. He generally never did well in treatment, often decompensated, and required multiple hospitalizations. The treatment staff in the clinic where he usually received his substance abuse treatment tended to regard him with disdain and derision. Upon his most recent presentation, however, he was assigned a therapist who treated him with interest, concern,

and respect and after 18 months of hard work, he exhibited drastic and significant improvement. The therapy, unfortunately, was prematurely terminated
when the therapist accepted another position elsewhere. Although the patient
was assigned another therapist, he quickly deteriorated. One day he entered
the clinic for an appointment with his new therapist and as he walked by the
clinic secretary's desk he provocatively flipped up the bottom of his sportcoat
which revealed a pistol in his back pocket. Security was summoned and, as it
turned out, the gun was only a water pistol. Staff reactions, however, were intense, ranging from "We can't treat this guy" to "He's got to be discharged immediately" to recommendations for long-term psychiatric hospitalization. The
fact that for much of the past 18 months the patient had been functioning extremely well and that he had just suffered a major loss appeared to evaporate
into thin air. However, staff members eventually were able to recognize their
own extreme responses as intense countertransference reactions induced by
the patient's provocative behavior. The patient had acted out his feeling that
without his first therapist he was worthless and untreatable. He, however, could
not say this. He had to get the staff to say it for him. He was briefly hospitalized and returned to substance abuse therapy.

Use of Empathy and Interpretation of Conflict. Empathy is one of the key
tools the clinician has at his or her disposal. It is through the act of empathic
listening that the therapist gains access to the emotional life of the patient.
Greenson (1960) has referred to empathy as a kind of "emotional knowing" (p.
418). One often has the impression that clinicians, especially beginners, think
that empathy means listening supportively and sympathetically. These are indeed good therapist qualities, but they are not the same thing as empathy.
Empathic listening is a specific attempt to understand the patient's emotional
experience and convey this to the patient.

In psychodynamic terms, the act of empathic listening involves several
steps (Greenson, 1960). First, the therapist temporarily suspends his or her observing functions in order to become a participant in the patient's emotional
life, to see what it feels like to be the patient. The therapist makes a partial,
temporary, "trial identification" (Fliess, 1942). Second, on the basis of this temporary identification, the therapist oscillates back into the role of observer and
on a cognitive level attempts to articulate the meaning(s) of the emotion for
the patient. Third, the therapist may communicate these "findings" to the patient in the form of a clarification or interpretation (Greenson, 1960).

It is important to note that the experience of oscillating back and forth
between observer and participant is not based on a conscious attempt to follow
this step-by-step breakdown of the empathic process. One does not say, "I am
now going to empathize with the patient. First, I will adopt the role of participant. . . . " Rather, it seems to take place rather quickly, almost automatically,
and only in retrospect does the empathic act appear to be sequenced.

Empathy may be used as (1) a gauge by which the therapist measures his emotional understanding of the patient, (2) a method for helping patients clarify and articulate their feelings more precisely and accurately, and (3) as a means for the patient to feel understood. It may also be used to facilitate the exploration of unconscious conflicts. Though RP for substance abuse focuses on behavior change that supports abstinence, it may be necessary from time to time to obtain insight into unconscious conflicts that might threaten the patient's abstinence if left unattended. Let me illustrate how empathic listening may be utilized toward this end.

A 22-year-old female college student with a history of alcohol and marijuana abuse has been sober approximately 6 months. Her recovery is generally stable although she has recently been musing over the possibility of controlled drinking in the future. The patient began drinking and using marijuana as a teenager in response to feelings of depression, but I subsequently learned that her use also coincided with an experimental homosexual relationship. The patient formerly thought of herself as heterosexual but shortly after beginning treatment had "come out" and now considers herself a lesbian. Despite the fact that she feels generally good about her choice, she has been grappling with a number of troubling implications of such a sexual orientation, not the least of which is telling her parents.

At the beginning of the therapy session in question she complains that she has been feeling sad for the past several months and does not know why. She is sober, her relationship with her girlfriend is in good shape, her grades have improved significantly; it just puzzles her that she should be feeling sad when "everything is going so well." She goes on to discuss a number of other things and midway through the session mentions that she has been teaching Sunday school at her church, which she has found to be enormously rewarding. I comment that this is certainly good news and add that I had not realized she had been teaching. I then asked her, essentially out of curiosity, how long she had been at it and she says "about 2 months." I then say, "You know that's interesting since it corresponds roughly to the time you've been feeling sad." The patient nods in agreement and then recalls that in fact she had first noticed feeling sad at the Sunday school. I am both struck and puzzled by this development. Why should she be saddened by this? I inquire as to her thoughts on the matter and as she begins to speak I find myself beginning to imagine being her in the Sunday school, looking out at a group of children. I see her now in a new light. In my office, I see her as a petite young woman just barely out of her teens. But in the Sunday school she is now a grown woman teaching little children and as I continue to imagine being her, looking out at the little children, I experience a kind of wistful sadness. I then imagine her thinking, "I love working with these children and I feel sad because as a lesbian I may not be able to have my own." At an appropriate moment, I tell her, "And you've been feeling sad with the children at Sunday school because it's sort of an unconscious reminder that it may be much more difficult to have your own children." The interpretation hit home. Whether she could become a mother as a lesbian had indeed been a troubling thought, one she had barely allowed herself to think. Nor had she connected it to the sadness she experienced in working with the children at Sunday school. We then raised the possibility that her thoughts about controlled drinking might also be related to these sad feelings, as painful feelings often trigger the desire to use. We were not able to reach a decisive conclusion, but the *patient* suggested intensifying her recovery program with extra group therapy and more Alcoholics Anonymous meetings.

In addition to explicating the empathic process, this clinical example illustrates several other points. First, the therapist helps the patient to articulate and establish meaning and significance for a previously inexplicable emotional experience. Second, the patient and therapist are able to connect these feelings with thoughts that might, if they are permitted to develop, lead to a slip or relapse. Third, the therapist does not explore in any great detail the unconscious determinants either now or in the past, of her conflicts regarding her sexual orientation. The exploration of the conflict takes place at the surface and its purpose is to promote relapse prevention.

Resistance and Transference. In psychoanalysis and psychoanalytic psychotherapy it is the analysis of resistance and transference that become the central focus of treatment. It may have struck the reader as somewhat peculiar that this chapter has thus far devoted relatively little attention to these variables. Actually, this is only apparently so at least with respect to resistance. In psychoanalytic clinical theory, resistance is defined as defense expressed within the treatment situation (Freud, 1912/1958; Gill, 1982; Greenson, 1967). In an important sense, virtually everything we have thus far encountered regarding an exploration of the patient's cravings, apparently irrelevant decisions, distorted cognitions, affects, and conflicts are examples of working with resistances.

As noted earlier, far too often there is a tendency to think of resistance in its most egregious or blatant forms such as gross noncompliance. These "noisy" resistances do occur, especially in the treatment of substance abusers. But as Schlesinger (1982) pointed out, it is far more often the case that we deal with "quieter" resistances, which demand attention to the therapeutic process. For example, a patient talks so fast he does not have time to hear himself think, let alone to mull over the implications of what he has said. Or, as in the case of the alcoholic woman we considered in the section on assessment, a patient's communications take on a relative withholding quality. The technique we have been describing for meeting these and other resistances deals with the resistance as it is presented and refrains from reaching behind the defense, as it were, in order to pull out the material it conceals.

From the standpoint of utilizing this sort of psychodynamic technique to promote relapse prevention through cognitive–behavioral skills acquisition, we pay *selective* attention to the patient's resistances. Thus, we want to examine those resistances that may lead to a slip or relapse. However, many resistances that might become the focus of therapy in standard psychodynamic treatment are passed over in this form of treatment. Indeed, some may be reinforced if they lead to relapse prevention and skills acquisition. For example, obsessional defenses that might be the principal source of resistance and central focus in the psychotherapy of certain patients often facilitate a substance abuser in creating distance from painful affects or in engaging in skills acquisition assignments. In the treatment described here I would support such defensive–resistive activity.

Transference, as defined earlier, refers to the patient's propensity to develop a fantasy-based relationship to the therapist. In standard psychoanalytic psychotherapy, the transference is allowed to flourish and the therapist's quiet, neutral, generally incognito manner creates a certain amount of ambiguity, which further augments the transference potential in the patient. In psychodynamically informed RP, however, we seek to *minimize* the transference potential in the patient. Treatment is essentially focused around reality factors and goals are well defined. That the therapist is more active, "real," and gives advice and support also tends to attenuate the transference. RP, as described here, also capitalizes on but leaves unanalyzed an important aspect of the positive transference: namely, the patient's capacity to form a moderately dependent relationship on a generally helpful therapist.

Nevertheless, this does not mean that transference reactions do not occur that require our attention. For instance, some substance abusers unconsciously attempt to cast the therapist into the role of a policeman, which, if successfully elicited, makes the patient feel justified in using. Some insight into how the patient does this may be helpful to avert a relapse. In addition, transference fantasies usually become intensified at termination and should always be explored as the termination phase is also a risky time for a substance abuser. The general principle here is the same as with other psychodynamic phenomena: We explore psychodynamically if the problem, feeling, conflict, or behavior increases the chances of relapse.

ADVANCED PHASE OF TREATMENT

Advanced recovery is a subject that occupies relatively less space in the literature than recovery in the early and middle phases of treatment. This is due in part to the recalcitrant fact that stable abstinence is so difficult to achieve (Institute of Medicine, 1989) relative to remission rates for other psychiatric disorders. Moreover, not all addicted individuals elect to continue psychotherapy once abstinence has been secured, often preferring to continue in 12-step or other self-help treatment.

Nevertheless, some individuals do wish to continue in treatment and psychodynamic therapy may be of value (Kaufman, 1994). In the model of treatment delineated in this chapter as well as in other similar models (e.g., Kaufman, 1994), the advanced phase of treatment may become progressively more psychoanalytic in nature. In this respect, the therapist takes on a more neutral, exploratory role, which permits the patient's transference potential to emerge, the analysis of which may help to resolve a number of underlying conflicts. To a certain extent, some things the patient has learned in the earlier stages of treatment can actually facilitate this analysis. For example, I once treated a female alcoholic who, in resisting exploration of how she participated (unconsciously) in provoking arguments with her lover, eventually reminded herself, "If I could set myself up to drink, maybe I am setting up these arguments too." On the other hand, the essentially supportive, advice-giving, more "real" role that the therapist has adopted in the earlier treatment phases may hinder the patient from being able to tolerate the more depriving role the therapist assumes in psychodynamic treatment (Kaufman, 1994). In such cases, it may be necessary to refer the patient to a new therapist.

Owing to considerations of space, a full exposition of the advanced phase of psychoanalytic treatment with substance abusers is not possible. However, I would like to touch on three basic areas that generally become the focus of this latter phase: (1) exploration of critical affects, (2) the examination of unconscious conflicts, and (3) reconstructing and adjusting to a substance-free life.

As has been previously noted, substance abusers find managing and tolerating negative affects extremely difficult. In the advanced stage, further work in this area is possible. First, the abuser can be helped to express such emotions as guilt, shame, and rage. These are often extremely difficult to express in the transference as the patient, by this time, is often exceedingly grateful for the therapist's previous help (Kaufman, 1994). Often, it is more useful to explore such feelings through an examination of their expression to significant others in the patient's life. In this way, the transference can be interpreted within the "metaphor" of the significant other (Schlesinger, 1982). Assisting the patient to give expression to such affect also permits the therapist to help the patient learn to endure and tolerate the feelings without using (Khantzian et al., 1990). Gradually, greater self-regulation of emotional states may be achieved.

Kaufman (1994) has suggested that the central conflictual issues that characterize the advanced phase of treatment are intimacy and autonomy. Psychodynamically, substance abusers have developed an intense "object relationship" with their drug (Krystal, 1978). In a certain sense, this object relationship has served as a substitute for intimate relations with people. One frequently hears, for example, addicts describe their drug as "the best lover I've ever had," or some variation on this theme. For such people, intimacy with others carries the dual unconscious meaning of a kind of blissful merging and a simultaneous terrifying engulfment with the other (see Krystal, 1978; Leeds & Morgenstern, Chapter 3, this volume). What the addict needs, therefore, is to become capable of tolerating intimacy with people while simultaneously building a more autonomous sense of self, and it is through the analysis of the transference relationship to the therapist during the advanced stage of treatment that these conflicts may be more fully resolved.

Finally, the substance abuser must learn to adjust to a substance-free life. Cognitive-behavioral clinicians (e.g., Marlatt & Gordon, 1985) have suggested that such "lifestyle modification" can be accomplished by helping abusers substitute sober pleasurable activities for their substance-abusing ones. Often those activities abusers found pleasurable *prior* to the onset of their substance abuse are of great value. For example, one patient who had been an amateur artist but had given up the avocation during her many years of cocaine addiction was helped to resume this activity by encouraging her to paint cravings and other painful affects.

However, no matter how many sober pleasurable activities the therapist can promote in his or her patients, the fact is that for many patients life without alcohol or drugs is experienced as an arid, desiccated, empty existence. It is helpful to remember that the substance abuser is not merely someone with an alcohol or drug problem but a person who has *become* an alcoholic or addict. By the time he or she has reached the therapist's office, the "behavior" has become a way of life, has insinuated itself into areas the patient may not have even realized until sobriety has been achieved. Giving up the substance use may be initially experienced as gratifying but later on experienced as giving up too much. A kind of mourning process must take place, not only over the loss of the substance but over of a way of life.

In addition, substance abusers must learn finally to renounce immediate blissful gratification and accept life's inevitable frustrations. Freud, in a much-quoted passage, once remarked that the essential achievement of psychotherapy consisted of "transforming hysterical misery into common unhappiness" (Breuer & Freud, 1893–1895, p. 305). Yet it appears that "common unhappiness" is precisely what substance abusers find so intolerable. The normal aches and pains and frustrations of everyday life, which most of us accept as given, are for them deeply and profoundly disturbing. In this respect, a key aspect of the advanced phase of treatment is to nurture in the patient a kind of stoical acceptance that life's ordinary difficulties *are* tolerable and do not preclude the more enduring gratifications of love and work.

Summary and Conclusions

This chapter has focused on how psychodynamic therapy may contribute to cognitive-behavioral relapse prevention treatment of substance use disorders. It has emphasized that by focusing on the moment-to-moment process of psychotherapy, selected use of psychoanalytic technique may facilitate engagement in treatment, achieving abstinence, and preventing relapse. Several implications for the future development of substance abuse treatment are indicated. First, the treatment model suggested here is based on a cognitive-behavioral approach that has begun to demonstrate efficacy in controlled trials and the accrued clinical wisdom of psychodynamic technique whose efficacy is largely anecdotal. Such a model, therefore, needs to be tested under controlled conditions, particularly with reference to matching appropriate patients to this treatment type. Second, greater attention needs to be paid to the training of substance abuse therapists and, in particular, with reference to the process of psychotherapy, to the psychodynamics of the patient, and to the nuances of the interpersonal relationship that develops in treatment. Much of this can *only* be achieved through intensive personal supervision, which ought to be incorporated into existing training programs. Third, there is a paucity of articles in the clinical substance abuse literature that attempt to describe the therapeutic process through which techniques are actually administered. More are needed. This chapter has been an attempt to begin to address that need.

ACKNOWLEDGMENT

I wish to thank Drs. Jon Morgenstern, Edward Paul, Sally Satel, and Laurence Westreich for their many helpful comments and suggestions on an earlier version of the manuscript.

REFERENCES

Binswanger, L. (1946). The existential analysis school of thought. In R. May, E. Angel, & H. F. Ellenberger (Eds.), *Existence.* New York: Basic Books, 1958.

Breuer, J., & Freud, S. (1893–1895). Studies on hysteria. *Standard Edition, 2,* vii–309. London: Hogarth Press, 1955.

Carroll, K. M., Rounsaville, B. J., & Gawin, F. H. (1991). A comparative trial of psychotherapies for ambulatory cocaine abusers: Relapse prevention and interpersonal psychotherapy. *American Journal of Drug and Alcohol Abuse, 17,* 229–247.

Carroll, K. M., Rounsaville, B. J., & Keller, D. S. (1991). Relapse prevention strategies in the treatment of cocaine abuse. *American Journal on Drug and Alcohol Abuse, 17,* 249–265.

Fenichel, O. (1941). *Problems of psychoanalytic technique.* Albany, NY: The Psychoanalytic Quarterly.

Fenichel, O. (1945). *The psychoanalytic theory of neurosis.* New York: Norton.

Fliess, R. (1942). The metapsychology of the analyst. *Psychoanalytic Quarterly, 11,* 211–227.

Freud, A. (1936). *The ego and the mechanisms of defense.* New York: International Universities Press, 1966.

Freud, S. (1894/1953). The neuro-psychoses of defense. *Standard Edition, 3,* 43–68. London: Hogarth Press.

Freud, S. (1896/1953). Further remarks on the neuro-psychoses of defense. *Standard Edition, 3*, 159–185. London: Hogarth Press.

Freud, S. (1900/1953). The interpretation of dreams. *Standard Edition, 4 & 5*. London: Hogarth Press.

Freud, S. (1905/1953). Fragment of an analysis of a case of hysteria. *Standard Edition, 7*, 3–122. London: Hogarth Press.

Freud, S. (1910/1957). The future prospects of psycho-analytic therapy. *Standard Edition, 11*, 139–151. London: Hogarth Press.

Freud, S. (1912/1958). The dynamics of transference. *Standard Edition, 12*, 97–108. London: Hogarth Press.

Freud, S. (1923/1961). The ego and the id. *Standard Edition, 19*, 12–66. London: Hogarth Press.

Freud, S. (1926/1959). Inhibitions, symptoms, and anxiety. *Standard Edition, 20*, 87–174. London: Hogarth Press.

Galanter, M. (1993). *Network therapy for alcohol and drug abuse.* New York: Basic Books.

Galanter, M., & Keller, D. S. (1994). *Network therapy for substance abuse: A therapist's manual.* Unpublished manuscript, New York University, New York, NY.

Gill, M. (1982). *Analysis of transference* (Vol. 1, Psychological Issues, 353). New York: International Universities Press.

Gitelson, M. (1952). The emotional position of the analyst in the psycho-analytic situation. *International Journal of Psycho-Analysis, 33*, 1–10.

Greenson, R. R. (1960). Empathy and its vicissitudes. *International Journal of Psycho-Analysis, 41*, 418–424.

Greenson, R. R. (1967). *The technique and practice of psychoanalysis.* New York: International Universities Press.

Greenspan, S. I. (1979). *Intelligence and adaptation: An integration of psychoanalytic and Piagetian developmental psychology* (Psychological Issues, 47–48). New York: International Universities Press.

Haviland, M. G., Shaw, D. G., MacMurray, J. P., & Cummings, M. A. (1988). Validation of the Toronto Alexithymia Scale with substance abusers. *Psychotherapy and Psychosomatics, 50*, 81–87.

Institute of Medicine. (1989). *Prevention and treatment of alcohol problems. Opportunities for research: Report of a study.* Washington, DC: National Academy Press.

Kadden, R., Carroll, K. M., Donovan, D., Cooney, N., Monti, P., Abrams, D., Litt, M., & Hester, R. (1992). *Cognitive-behavioral coping skills therapy manual: A clinical research guide for therapists treating individuals with alcohol abuse and dependence* (NIAAA Project MATCH Monograph Series, Vol. 3, DHHS Publication No. ADM 92–1895). Rockville, MD: National Institute on Alcohol Abuse and Alcoholism.

Kaufman, E. (1994). *Psychotherapy of addicted persons.* New York: Guilford Press.

Keller, D. S., Carroll, K. M., Nich, C., & Rounsaville, B. J. (1995). Alexithymia in cocaine abusers: Response to psychotherapy and pharmacotherapy. *American Journal on Addictions, 4*, 234–244.

Keller, D. S., & Wilson, A. (1994). Affectivity in cocaine and opiate abusers. *Psychiatry, 57*(4), 333–347.

Kernberg, O. F. (1965). Notes on countertransference. *Journal of the American Psychoanalytic Association, 13*, 38–56.

Kernberg, O. F. (1975). *Borderline conditions and pathological narcissism.* New York: Jason Aronson.

Khantzian, E. J. (1980). An ego–self theory of substance dependence. In D. J. Lettieri, M. Sayers, & H. W. Wallace (Eds.), *Theories of addiction* (NIDA Research Monograph No. 30, DHHS Publication No. ADM 80–967). Washington, DC: U.S. Government Printing Office.

Khantzian, E. J., Halliday, K. S., & McAuliffe, W. E. (1990). *Addiction and the vulnerable self: Modified dynamic group therapy for substance abusers.* New York: Guilford Press.

Krystal, H. (1975). Affect tolerance. *Annual of Psychoanalysis, 3,* 179–219.

Krystal, H. (1978). Self-representation and the capacity for self-care. *Annual of Psychoanalysis, 6,* 209–246.

Krystal, H., & Raskin, H. A. (1970). *Drug dependence: Aspects of ego functioning.* Detroit, MI: Wayne State University Press.

Luborsky, L. (1984). *Principles of psychoanalytic psychotherapy: A manual for supportive-expressive treatment.* New York: Basic Books.

Marlatt, G. A., & Gordon, J. R. (Eds.). (1985). *Relapse prevention: Maintenance strategies in the treatment of addictive behaviors.* New York: Guilford Press.

Miller, W. R., & Hester, R. K. (1986). The effectiveness of alcoholism treatment: What research reveals. In W. R. Miller & R. K. Hester (Eds.), *Treating addictive behaviors: Processes of change.* New York: Plenum Press.

Monti, P. M, Abrams, D. B., Kadden, R. M., & Cooney, N. L. (1989). *Treating alcohol dependence: A coping skills training guide.* New York: Guilford Press.

Morgenstern, J., & McCrady, B. S. (1992). Curative factors in alcohol and drug treatment: Behavioral and disease model perspectives. *British Journal of the Addictions, 87,* 901–912.

Ogden, T. H. (1979). On projective identification. *International Journal of Psycho-Analysis, 60*(3), 357–373.

Racker, H. (1957). The meanings and uses of countertransference. *Psychoanalytic Quarterly, 26,* 303–357.

Rapaport, D., Gill, M. M., & Schafer, R. (1968). In R. Holt (Ed.), *Diagnostic psychological testing.* New York: International Universities Press.

Reich, W. (1933/1945). *Character analysis.* New York: Orgone Press.

Safran, J. D., & Siegel, Z. V. (1990). *Interpersonal process in cognitive therapy.* New York: Basic Books.

Schafer, R. (1976). The idea of resistance. In *A new language for psychoanalysis.* New Haven, CT: Yale University Press.

Schlesinger, H. J. (1969). Diagnosis and prescription for psychotherapy. *Bulletin of the Menninger Clinic, 33,* 269–278.

Schlesinger, H. J. (1981). The process of empathic response. *Psychoanalytic Inquiry, 1*(3), 393–416.

Schlesinger, H. J. (1982). Resistance as process. In P. Wachtel (Ed.), *Resistance: Psychodynamic and behavioral approaches.* New York: Plenum Press.

Shapiro, D. (1989). *Psychotherapy of neurotic character.* New York: Basic Books.

Stanton, M. D., Todd, T. C., & Associates. (1982). *The family therapy of drug abuse and addiction.* New York: Guilford Press.

Stern, D. (1985). *The interpersonal world of the infant.* New York: Basic Books.

Taylor, G. J., Parker, J. D., & Bagby, R. M. (1990). A preliminary investigation of alexithymia in men with psychoactive substance dependence. *American Journal of Psychiatry, 147*, 1228–1230.

Wachtel, P. (1977). *Psychoanalysis and behavior therapy.* New York: Basic Books.

Wallerstein, R. S. (1986). *Forty-two lives in treatment: A study of psychoanalysis and psychotherapy.* New York: Guilford Press.

Weiss, R. (1993). Countertransference issues in treating the alcoholic patient: Institutional and clinician reactions. In J. D. Levin & R. Weiss (Eds.), *The dynamics and treatment of alcoholism.* New York: Jason Aronson.

Wheelis, A. (1973). *How people change.* New York: Harper & Row.

Wikler, A. (1973). Dynamics of drug dependence. *Archives of General Psychiatry, 28*, 611–616.

Wurmser, L. (1978). *The hidden dimension.* New York: Jason Aronson.

Wurmser, L. (1985). Denial and split identity: Timely issues in the psychoanalytic psychotherapy of compulsive drug users. *Journal of Substance Abuse Treatment, 2*, 89–96.

5

Theoretical Bases of Family Approaches to Substance Abuse Treatment

Barbara S. McCrady
Elizabeth E. Epstein
Rene D. Sell

Mental health professionals have accorded the family a central role in the etiology, maintenance, and treatment of a variety of psychological and psychiatric disorders. Theoretical models of etiology have ranged from the notion of the schizophrenogenic mother (reviewed in Broderick & Schrader, 1981) to the heritability of depressive disorders (reviewed in Hammen, 1991). Maintenance models have conceived of individual symptoms as indicators of dysfunction in the family system (reviewed in Barton & Alexander, 1981) or have focused on inept family management skills as important factors maintaining child behavior problems (Patterson, 1986). Family-based treatments have evolved from a variety of theoretical models, ranging from treatments to teach spouses to model and reinforce appropriate eating behavior as part of treatment for obesity (Brownell, Heckerman, Westlake, Hayes, & Monti, 1978), to family educational models for schizophrenics (reviewed in Konstantareas, 1990), to family systems models for treatment of eating disorders (Dare, Eisler, Russell, & Szmulker, 1990).

The family also has been an integral part of the conceptualization of the etiology, maintenance, and treatment of substance use disorders since at least the 1880s when families petitioned judges to have their family members institutionalized for alcoholism, and then participated in treatment and aftercare planning (McCrady, 1998). This chapter describes the historical roots of family approaches to conceptualizing the etiology, maintenance, and treatment of psychoactive substance use disorders, with a special emphasis on alcohol abuse and dependence. The chapter then presents key theoretical elements that serve as the basis for family-based treatment approaches, which will be described in Chapter 6 by Fals-Stewart, O'Farrell, and Birchler.

HISTORICAL OVERVIEW

Psychodynamic Models

In the 1930s, many alcoholics received treatment in state mental hospitals. Social workers in those facilities began to interview the spouses (most often, wives) of the alcoholic patients, and began to observe the significant distress that these women experienced. Lewis (1937) was the first to publish observations of this distress. Other authors continued to note that the women were anxious, depressed, and that the women reported experiencing a variety of psychosomatic symptoms. Theoretical models began to develop to attempt to explain these observations. The earliest model, the disturbed personality hypothesis, derived from the psychodynamic models that predominated at the time, postulated that wives of alcoholics were disturbed women who resolved their own neurotic conflicts through their marriages to alcoholic men. Although some authors postulated one primary underlying conflict (e.g., with aggression or dependence), Whalen (1953) hypothesized four different kinds of conflicts that could be resolved through marriage to an alcoholic and provided colorful names for each of these types of wives of alcoholics. She suggested conflicts with aggression ("Punitive Polly"), control ("Controlling Catherine"), masochism ("Suffering Susan"), and ambivalence ("Wavering Winifred").

A corollary to the disturbed personality hypothesis was the decompensation hypothesis. Central to psychodynamic models is the notion that neurotic conflicts serve as a defense against more basic or primitive conflicts. If defenses are removed, an individual would be expected to exhibit these more primitive conflicts and decompensate. Thus, it was hypothesized that if a married alcoholic successfully stopped drinking, his wife would decompensate and exhibit more severe psychopathology. MacDonald (1956) studied 18 women hospitalized in a state mental hospital, all of whom were married to alcoholics. He reported that 11 of these women had husbands who had decreased drinking recently, suggesting these observations as support for the decompensation hypothesis.

Stress and Coping Models

In the 1950s, alternative models began to develop. Jackson (1954) interviewed women who were attending Al-Anon meetings, and developed a stress and coping model. She suggested that living with an alcoholic is stressful, and that most of the symptoms wives of alcoholics experienced were common to families living with long-term stressors such as a chronically ill family member or a family member away in combat. She also suggested that families go through "stages" in coping with alcoholism, and that each stage is characterized by different psychological phenomena. Jackson suggested that family denial of the problem characterized the earliest stage of family coping, followed, in sequence, by attempts to control the problem, feeling hopeless and chaotic, attempting to maintain stable family functioning with the alcoholic present, attempting to escape from the problem through marital separation, organizing and maintaining the family without the alcoholic present, and a final adjustment phase if the alcoholic stopped drinking. Kogan and Jackson (1965) later tested this stress and coping model by comparing the psychological characteristics of women whose husbands were actively drinking, women whose husbands had stopped drinking, and women whose husbands had never had drinking problems. They reported that women whose husbands were actively drinking were significantly more distressed than women in the comparison groups, who were indistinguishable from one other. Many years later, Moos and his colleagues (Moos, Finney, & Gamble, 1982) reported results of a longitudinal study that followed alcoholics and their families for 2 years from the beginning of treatment, and compared their functioning to sociodemographically matched community controls. The results of this prospective design supported Jackson's model: spouses whose alcoholic partners successfully resolved their drinking problems were indistinguishable on measures of psychological distress from spouses in the community control sample at follow-up. Follow-up results from research on behavioral couple therapy (BCT) for alcohol dependence provides further support for Jackson's model that readjustment occurs in the relationship if the alcoholic stops drinking. Maisto, McKay, and O'Farrell (1998) compared self-reported marital adjustment in couples where men were abstinent in the year following BCT with couples where men continued to drink following treatment. Results showed that both husbands and wives perceived their marriages as better adjusted when the alcoholic partner had stopped drinking.

Jackson's stress and coping paradigm views wives of alcoholics as actively attempting to cope with their spouses' drinking and the stresses associated with chronic drinking. Wives of alcoholics often try to facilitate change as well. In their review of the literature, Hurcom, Copello, and Orford (2000) describe a three-factor model of spouse coping that holds across cultures. The first factor represents engagement with the drinker: using assertive, controlling, emotional, and supportive behaviors to change the husband's drinking. The second major style of spouse coping Hurcom and colleagues described is tolerance of the drinking, including self-sacrifice and inactivity by the wife of the alcoholic. The third factor identified is withdrawal, where the wife avoids the drinker and engages in independent activities. Avoidant or withdrawing coping styles appear to have particularly negative consequences for the family, and they are associated with higher rates of depression in the nonalcoholic spouse, higher alcohol intake by the nonalcoholic spouse, and more arguments between the partners. Avoidance and withdrawal coping also are associated with poorer drinking outcomes for the alcoholic, whereas assertive anti-alcohol messages by the female spouse are associated with a reduction in drinking levels in the male spouse (reviewed in Hurcom et al., 2000). Thus, a confrontational yet supportive coping style seems likely to lead to better drinking outcomes.

Advances have been made in the methods used to assess coping skills in the spouses of alcoholics. Rychtarik and colleagues (Rychtarik, Carstensen, Alford, Schlundt, & Scott, 1988; Rychtarik & McGillicuddy, 1997) developed the Spouse Situation Inventory (SSI) for this purpose. The SSI is a role-play interview in which wives are asked to imagine themselves in prescribed situations related to their partner's drinking, and to respond exactly as they would with their partner in that situation. The wives' responses are rated on a 6-point scale of effectiveness using developed scoring criteria. The SSI was administered to 472 women with alcoholic partners. Women who demonstrated highly skilled responses to their partner's drinking reported lower levels of drinking for themselves and their partners in the previous 6 months (Rychtarik & McGillicuddy, 1997). More effective coping, as measured by the SSI, also was associated with the partner's recognition of the problem, but not associated with the wife's level of depression.

Family Systems Models

By the 1970s, family systems models began to influence the alcohol field. In a series of studies, Steinglass and his colleagues observed the behavior of alcoholics hospitalized on an experimental unit, noting repetitive, patterned interactions between an alcoholic father and son, alcoholic brothers (Steinglass, Weiner, & Mendelson, 1971), and alcoholics and their husbands or wives (Steinglass, Davis, & Berenson, 1977), as well as significant differences in their patterns of interaction when sober and when intoxicated. These observations led to the hypothesis that alcohol performed certain positive functions in a family, by stabilizing family roles, allowing for the expression of affect, allowing for greater intimacy among family members, or allowing for the exploration of topics that the family might avoid when sober. This set of positive functions was called the "adaptive consequences of alcoholism" (Davis, Berenson, Steinglass, & Davis, 1974). After these initial observational studies, Steinglass later studied alcoholic families in their homes as well as in the laboratory. He reported observable differences among families with an alcoholic family member who was drinking, abstinent, or in transition from one drinking status to

another. Families with a sober alcoholic were most flexible in their functioning, having a balance between time together and time apart when at home
(Steinglass, 1981) and showing more flexibility in solving structured tasks in
the laboratory (Steinglass, 1979). Drinking families showed the most rigidity of
family roles and interactions, while transitional families were intermediate in
their functioning.

Wolin and Bennett (Wolin, Bennett, Noonan, & Teitelbaum, 1980) provided a second family systems perspective on alcoholism, focusing primarily
on the intergenerational transmission of alcoholism. Their work examined the
family "rituals" that characterize all families: how families vacation, have dinner, celebrate holidays, and so on. They observed three types of ritual patterns
in alcoholic families: *intact rituals* that were maintained despite drinking,
subsumptive ritual patterns that were modified to incorporate the drinking, and
disrupted rituals that were not maintained in the face of the drinking. They reported that those families whose rituals were maintained intact were least
likely to have offspring who became alcoholic, while those families whose rituals were most disrupted were most likely to have alcoholic offspring. A more
detailed review of family ritual research appears below.

Family systems theory has contributed a number of constructs to the
conceptualization of family functioning. Families are assumed to be governed
by the law of *homeostasis*. All systems are assumed to operate to try to maintain
balance, stability, and equilibrium. Factors that threaten to change the functioning of a family threaten that homeostasis, and the family system is assumed
to function to try to avoid change. Thus, family systems models would assume,
if an alcoholic family has functioned as a stable family unit with a drinking
member, that introducing sobriety into the system would threaten homeostasis. A variety of aspects of the family's structure and functioning (*organization*)
all serve to maintain homeostasis. Family members have defined *roles* that
guide their actions. Roles may range from "caretaker" to "bad child," but these
roles are well defined and are assumed to be difficult to modify over time.
Families also have unwritten family *rules* that govern the functioning of the
family. These rules are not necessarily explicit or deliberate (e.g., the oldest
child takes out the garbage), but are more likely to be implicit and unspoken
(e.g., never talk about Mommy's drinking). Families also have a variety of
boundaries that define relationships within the family and between the family
and the rest of the world. Boundaries define alliances between family members, the degree to which information is available to different family members,
the degree to which family members have influence in the decision making of
the family, the degree to which outsiders are welcomed into the family, and the
degree to which the family seeks interaction with outside persons and social
institutions.

The acquisition or loss of roles can change the overall functioning of the
family system as well as individual members' drinking patterns. Hajema and

Knibbe (1998) assessed changes in drinking patterns following changes in familial and social roles among a community sample of 1,327 Dutch men and women. Adult men who got married reduced their drinking overall, and those who became parents decreased the frequency of their heavy drinking. The greatest reduction in drinking occurred for men after gaining employment and becoming a parent during the same period. Women also reduced the frequency of heavy drinking after becoming a parent, but did not alter their drinking after any other role acquisitions. The only significant change in drinking following a role loss was for women, who showed an increase in heavy drinking following any loss of the spouse role (through divorce or death). These results suggest that gaining or losing roles other than familial roles may not lead to changes in drinking, but becoming a spouse or a parent has a significant impact on overall drinking and heavy alcohol consumption in a community sample. Hajema and Knibbe suggest that changes in drinking patterns occur because gaining familial roles places additional constraints on drinking and makes it more rewarding not to drink.

Drinking can serve various functions within a family system, and these unique functions have implications for the quality of the marital relationship. Roberts and Leonard (1998) identified five distinct drinking patterns among a community sample of newlywed couples. Using cluster analysis techniques, Roberts and Leonard classified 85% of the husbands and wives as having drinking partnerships where they predominantly drank together and at compatible levels. These couples made up four of the five drinking types: (1) light social drinking couples; (2) light intimate drinking couples (i.e., infrequently drink at home); (3) heavy out-of-home drinking couples (i.e., marked by elevated quantity); and (4) frequent intimate drinking couples (i.e., frequently drink at home). The fifth type of couple, the husband heavy drinker category, made up 14% of all newlyweds and was marked by husbands who drank more than their wives. The drinking classifications were unrelated to the husband's or wife's age, number of children, or the length of the relationship. Heavy out-of-home drinkers, however, were less likely to have children than any of the other types of couples, and the wives in these couples were less likely to be employed full time. The light intimate drinking couples had lower incomes than other couple types, and 42% of the husband heavy drinkers had a wife who was pregnant.

Roberts and Leonard (1998) found that couples with compatible drinking styles generally reported more marital intimacy than couples with elevated male drinking levels, with the exception of the heavy out-of-home drinkers. Heavy out-of-home drinking was characterized by marital conflict, alcohol dependence, risky drinking styles, and increased adverse consequences for both the husband and the wife. Husband heavy drinking couples also suffered relationship problems, and the wives in these partnerships reported higher levels of depression than any of the other wives.

Behavioral Models and Marital Interaction Research

The fourth major group of family theoretical models to evolve were behavioral models. Model development began with an observational study of the interactions between alcoholic men and their wives in a structured problem-solving task (Hersen, Miller, & Eisler, 1973). Careful coding of behavior during the interactions revealed that the wives looked at their husbands more when the husbands were discussing alcohol than when they were discussing a more neutral topic. Becker and Miller (1976) found that alcoholic husbands spoke more during alcohol-related conversations, while wives spoke more when discussing other topics. These researchers hypothesized that discussing alcohol was reinforced in the couple's interaction, either by increased attention from the spouse or increased talking and dominance of the conversation by the alcoholic.

Later interactional research focused on the relationships between drinking and marital communication. Billings, Kessler, Gomberg, and Weiner (1979) made alcohol available to alcoholic couples and then observed their interactions. Although half the couples did not drink at all, and most of those who did drank only one or two drinks, they found that alcoholics spoke more when drinking. Frankenstein, Hay, and Nathan (1985) administered a standard alcohol dose to all alcoholics in their marital communication study. They found that alcoholics spoke more when intoxicated than when sober, that couples emitted more positive verbal behaviors in drinking than sober sessions, and that spouses were more positive verbally in the alcohol session. They also reported that alcoholics asked more questions when drinking, and that objective raters and the couples themselves rated the alcoholic as more dominant when drinking than when sober (Frankenstein, Nathan, Sullivan, Hay, & Cocco, 1985).

Jacob and his colleagues initially reported findings contradictory to other interactional studies, finding that alcoholic couples became more negative when drinking, and that the wives of male alcoholics expressed more disagreements during drinking than during sober sessions (Jacob, Ritchey, Cvitkovic, & Blane, 1981). However, in later studies they identified two subtypes of alcoholics: steady, at-home drinkers, and binge, out-of-home drinkers. In the steady, at-home drinkers, alcohol consumption was associated with positive familial consequences, but drinking was associated with negative consequences for the binge, out-of-home drinkers (Dunn, Jacob, Hummon, & Seilhamer, 1987; Jacob, Dunn, & Leonard, 1983). In later research, Leonard and Jacob (1997) continued to report differences in interaction based on drinking style. They found that wives of episodic drinkers were more likely to reciprocate negativity from their husbands in a drinking session than in a nondrinking session. The reverse was true of steady drinkers' wives and control group wives, who both were less negative when their husbands were drinking than not. However, when the episodic husbands used problem-solving behaviors during the interaction, their wives' negativity was tempered. It may be that wives of episodic alcoholics are more reactive to their husbands' mood and behaviors, especially when the men are drinking, because binge drinking is less predictable and causes greater disruption and stress for the family system (Leonard & Jacob, 1997).

Couples also appear to have different interactional patterns depending on the gender of the alcoholic. Haber and Jacob (1997), in a study comparing verbal and nonverbal partner interactions in male alcoholic, female alcoholic, and concordant (both spouses alcoholic) couples, found that alcohol may have adaptive effects for female alcoholic couples. The female alcoholic couples were the least positive of all couples in the study, overall. They exhibited more negative interactions than male alcoholic couples when not drinking, but less negative interactions when they were drinking. Alcohol seemed to temper the conflicted marital situation for female alcoholic couples, but the same was not true of male alcoholic couples and concordant alcoholic couples. Male alcoholic couples were no more negative than control couples in the drink and no-drink conditions. The concordant couples, in which the male and the female spouse both had alcohol problems, were just as negative as the female alcoholic couples when not drinking, but were even more negative when they were drinking. Alcohol intoxication may have a maladaptive effect for concordant couples, increasing negativity in an already conflicted marital situation.

Taken as a whole, these interactional studies suggest that interactions of alcoholic couples change when alcohol is present or is discussed, and that these changes have a variety of positive features that may reinforce and maintain the drinking in some couples, and negative features that may complicate the marital relationship for others.

Family Disease Models

The family has been a focus of the disease model almost from the beginning of Alcoholics Anonymous (AA). The primary publication of AA, *Alcoholics Anonymous* (Alcoholics Anonymous, 1976) includes a chapter with advice to family members in each edition. Early AA meetings, held in members' homes, often included husbands and wives together in the meetings. Al-Anon began in 1949 as an organization to assist the family and friends of alcoholics. The contemporary family focus of disease model approaches began with Cork's (1969) book on children of alcoholics, followed by Black's (1982) and Wegsheider's (1981) books about children in alcoholic families and the adult sequelae of their early experiences. Later authors began to focus on the partners of alcoholics, and attempted to describe their problems (e.g., Beattie, 1987; Cermak, 1986). Although controlled research related to disease model conceptualizations is limited, these models have had a substantial impact on both treatment and popular thinking.

Contemporary disease model approaches describe alcoholism as a "family disease." Family members are seen as suffering from a disease, just as is the alcoholic. The "disease" of the family member is called "codependence." *Codependence* has been described as a "recognizable pattern of personality traits, predictably found within most members of chemically dependent families" (Cermak, 1986, p. 1). Cermak proposed several specific symptoms of codependence: (1) investing self-esteem in controlling self and others in the face of serious adverse circumstances, (2) assuming responsibility for meeting the needs of others before one's own, (3) experiencing anxiety and distortions of boundaries around issues of intimacy and separation, (4) being enmeshed in relationships with persons with personality disorders or alcohol or drug problems, (5) having at least three from a list of 10 other signs and symptoms, including, (a) using denial as a primary coping strategy, (b) having constricted emotions, (c) experiencing depression, (d) being hypervigilant, (e) displaying compulsive behavior, (f) experiencing anxiety, (g) being a substance abuser, (h) being a victim of physical or sexual abuse, (i) having stress-related illnesses, and (j) being in a relationship with a substance abuser for more than 2 years without seeking help.

Families members who are codependent are assumed to engage in a variety of behaviors that "enable" the substance abuser. *Enabling* refers to patterns of behavior that perpetuate the substance use, either by making it easier for the person to use or by providing positive responses to use and avoiding negative or limit-setting responses. Although clinical descriptions of codependency are common, empirical support for the concept is lacking. Correlational studies find relationships between hypothesized codependency characteristics and depression, problems with reality testing, and a history of sexual abuse (Carson & Baker, 1994). Studies comparing subjects in relationships with substance-abusing partners to normal controls find that the prior group is higher on stress due to the substance abuse, higher on other life stressors, and lower on measures of relationship functioning (Wright & Wright, 1990). One study reported that subjects who had an alcoholic father are more likely to want to help an exploitive person (Lyon & Greenberg, 1991). To date, although there is substantial literature demonstrating that spouses of substance abusers experience distress when their partner is actively using, there are no compelling empirical data to support the full construct of codependency.

Current Status of Family Theory

Three models dominate contemporary family substance abuse treatment: family disease models, family systems models, and behavioral models. Research now examines constructs derived from more than one of these models, and the focus has shifted away from large theories to a focus on more specific realms related to family functioning and alcoholism: biology, affect, cognition, behavior, and the environment, and how these interact. Three spheres currently dominate family research in substance abuse: the role of the family in etiology, maintenance, and the change process.

Most treatments provide some amalgam of the three dominant models. For example, contemporary family disease models emphasize codependency, alcoholism as a disease, and family members learning to focus on changing themselves—all concepts deriving from disease models. At the same time, many disease model treatment programs that include the family also emphasize communication, dysfunctional family roles, and family equilibrium—all concepts derived from family systems theory.

Similarly, family systems models examine the functions the substance use serves for the family, and attempt to change family roles, rules, and boundaries. At the same time, the treatment focuses on communication, problem solving, and direct behavioral treatments to facilitate abstinence.

Behavioral family models examine family behaviors as antecedents to substance use and as reinforcing consequences, and utilize treatments to modify antecedents and consequences of substance use. Behavioral therapists also examine repetitive relationship themes, communication, and the functions that alcohol may play in maintaining the stability of the relationship.

The next section describes how the historical trends in understanding substance use and family functioning, and the terminology of behavioral, systemic, and disease model approaches, are integrated into our model for conceptualizing the functioning of families with substance abuse.

KEY ELEMENTS IN THEORY

Etiology of Substance Abuse

The etiology of substance abuse is generally thought to be a complex developmental phenomenon (Hill, 1994; Schuckit, 1998) with multiple determinants. Not only are there multiple environmental and biological pathways to substance abuse, but there appears to be substantial variability in the expression of substance abuse among substance abusers (Babor et al., 1992; Hesselbrock, 1986). Several models of alcoholism posit an ongoing interaction among environmental and genetic (including family-of-origin, extrafamily social network, and societal) factors in a developmental framework (Devor, 1994; Schuckit, 1999; Tarter & Vanyukov, 1994). It is important to be cognizant of the complex nature of substance abuse and to be aware of its many faces, in both the identified patient and in his or her family members. A family therapist who adopts a simplistic model of substance abuse and does not consider empirical findings on variation in the presentation of substance use problems will lose a great deal of valuable information to help conceptualize the case and develop treatment strategies. The following section briefly reviews the literature on familial transmission of substance and related psychiatric disorders. Then more proximate factors in the etiology and maintenance of substance abuse are reviewed.

It is rarely the case that only one family member is substance-dependent. Rather, family studies indicate that alcoholism has a high rate of familial transmission (Bierut et al., 1998; Merikangas, 1990). Furthermore, alcoholism rates are elevated in family members of alcoholic probands (identified patients) but not of other substance abusers (Hill, 1994), indicating that "alcoholism (versus abuse of other drugs) breeds true." However, other evidence (Cowley et al., 1992) suggests that offspring of alcoholics experience a heightened euphoriant effect from benzodiazepines.

Adoption and twin research suggest that transmission of substance abuse involves some genetic mediation (Cadoret, O'Gorman, Troughton, & Heywood, 1985; Kendler, Heath, Neale, Kessler, & Eaves, 1992; see also Hesselbrock, 1995). Further, rates of psychopathology are elevated in alcoholics (see below), and since these disorders are also transmitted in families, one can expect to see elevated rates of comorbid psychopathology in family members of substance abusers. Finally, *assortative mating* has been noted for substance abuse (Hall, Hesselbrock, & Stabenau, 1983a, 1983b)—that is, many female substance abusers marry alcoholic or drug-abusing males. This pattern has implications both for the severity of pathology in the family and for increased risk of substance abuse by the children. Thus, family therapy with substance abusers is complicated by the probability that several family members may have current or past problems, including non-substance-related psychopathology, similar to those of the identified patient. Many spouses of alcoholics, whether substance-abusing or not, have dealt with substance abuse problems in their parents or other close relatives.

Research on the (postnatal) role of the family of origin of the drinker and the spouse in the etiology of substance abuse problems has focused on family contact and interactions such as family rituals and behavior around drinking patterns. Bennett and Wolin (1990) reported that transmission of alcoholism is more probable if there is continuing interaction between alcoholic parents and their adult offspring. Also, adult males are more likely to develop alcoholism if there is continuing contact between them and the alcoholic parents of their spouses. Bennett, an anthropologist, attributes this transmission to an acceptance of alcohol as part of the "family culture" and an inculturation effect on the offspring. Wolin and Bennett's group (Wolin, Bennett, Noonan, & Teitelbaum, 1980) found that among 25 families with a family history of alcoholism, those who kept family rituals such as dinnertime and celebration of holidays, even during heavy drinking periods, showed less alcoholism among their offspring. Furthermore, among 68 adult married couples from an alcoholic family of origin, deliberate and planned family rituals seemed to protect against transmission of alcoholism into their own families (Bennett, Wolin, Reiss, & Teitelbaum, 1987). Both of these studies have been quoted widely and treatment interventions have been based on these findings (Steinglass, Bennett, Wolin, & Reiss, 1987). One might ask if the families most severely affected by alcohol were the ones with the most disrupted households and associated psychopathology, and whether the severity of the alcohol problem, not the "symptom" of disrupted family rituals, was responsible for increased transmission of alcoholism to the offspring. Bennett et al. (1987) checked for this possibility and found that the severity of alcoholism in the family of origin of the "transmitter" versus the "nontransmitter" families was not different, and concluded that transmission was not due to the severity of the parental alcoholism. Steinglass et al. (1987) nevertheless note that the degree to which alcoholic families uphold and keep their family rituals is best used as a "marker," or a measure of family identity, regardless of whether it is "mechanistic" or not in transmission.

Family behavior around drinking patterns has also been implicated in the transmission of alcoholism. Steinglass et al. (1987) report that the most important factor in cross-generation continuance of drinking is whether a family rejects or accepts intoxication during family rituals. Nontransmitter families did not tolerate the "intrusion of intoxicated behavior" (p. 321) during rituals, whereas transmitter families did not automatically and consistently reject the intoxicated family member from participating in the family ritual. That is, families that deliberately forbid intoxication and demanded sobriety as a prerequisite for participation were less likely to experience transmission of alcoholism to the offspring.

Maintenance of Substance Abuse

Just as etiology is multiply determined, so is maintenance. In this chapter we adopt a cognitive–behavioral–systemic framework to describe current factors maintaining drinking, regardless of etiological underpinnings. Using this approach, we assume that genetic vulnerability, environmental influences, and other etiological factors are not immutable. That is, we separate current antecedents from historical factors, and believe that distal causes of the drinking do not prohibit an individual from changing problematic behavior. This model views maintenance as a complex interplay of environmental, biological, social, cognitive, and familial factors. Drinking occurs in response to multiple stimuli, which may include craving, affective states, and interpersonal events (e.g., a fight with one's spouse). Drinking behaviors are necessarily followed by one or more consequences, some immediate and some long term. In order for the drinking to be maintained, there are positive consequences associated with use (e.g., it relieves stress, increases positive affect, stops withdrawal symptoms).

The cognitive–behavioral–systemic model of maintenance emphasizes the role of family interaction patterns and problems as both antecedent to and consequences for alcohol use. These family interactions maintain drinking both directly and indirectly, both intentionally and without the family's awareness of the process. Several basic assumptions are put forth: (1) external antecedents to drinking have a lawful relationship to subsequent alcohol consumption, through repeated associations with reinforcement or anticipation of reinforcement; (2) cognitive and affective events mediate the relationship between external antecedents and drinking; (3) drinking is maintained by physiological, psychological, and/or interpersonal consequences; and (4) reciprocal interactions between the drinker and his or her environment determine repetitive, stressful intra- and interpersonal behavioral patterns (Epstein & McCrady, 2002; McCrady, 2001).

ANTECEDENTS TO USE

A variety of antecedent events and stimuli may precede drinking, and these may include individual, dyadic, or other factors. Antecedents may be features of the physical environment (e.g., a bar or a beer commercial), certain times of the day, or interpersonal events. Here, we focus specifically on familial antecedents to drinking. Contemporary research points to specific types of familial antecedents associated with drinking. The role of negative affect and expectancies about specific effects of alcohol on negative affect seem central to understanding events antecedent to drinking.

Specific spouse coping behaviors form one class of drinking antecedents. The three-factor model of spouses' coping styles discussed previously has been tested to determine how spouse coping behaviors affect the alcoholic's drinking (described in Hurcom et al., 2000). Wives often withdraw from their drinking husbands because they believe withdrawal will encourage their husbands' abstinence, but empirical studies show that the opposite may be true. Research by Moos, Finney, and Cronkite (1990) and, earlier, by Orford et al. (1975) found that avoidance and withdrawal behaviors led to poorer drinking outcomes, while assertive and engaged spouse coping styles correlated with reductions in the male spouse's drinking. Thus, family treatment programs should perhaps emphasize assertive but supportive communication to address concerns about the drinking, rather than withdrawal.

A second class of familial antecedents are negative interactions. The cognitive–behavioral–systemic model of maintenance is based in part on a series of findings that alcoholic families are more negative, conflicted, and estranged than control families (Rotunda & O'Farrell, 1997). These negative familial qualities point to a series of interactional deficits that characterize communication and behaviors in an alcoholic family. The presence of these negative interactions is a source of stress for alcoholic families, and probably serves as one antecedent to drinking and relapses.

Demand–withdraw interactions are a specific type of negative communication style characteristic of alcoholic families (Shoham, Rohrbaugh, Stickle, & Jacob, 1998). Demand–withdraw interactions are defined by one partner pursuing and demanding while the other partner distances, defends, and withdraws. This type of interaction is quite common in alcoholic partnerships where the nondrinking spouse criticizes and requests change from the alcoholic spouse, who then withdraws, leading to an ongoing demand–withdraw cycle. This cycle may maintain problem drinking, as it leads to more and more stress and marital dissatisfaction for both partners, and the stress and dissatisfaction in turn become antecedents to further drinking.

Other types of negative communication styles also are common in alcoholic marriages, and help perpetuate the drinking and problems in the relationship. Because lower marital satisfaction predicts higher levels of drinking following treatment (Moos et al., 1990), understanding the sources and patterns of dissatisfaction is important for understanding the maintenance of alcoholism. Expressed emotion, one form of negative communication that has received considerable attention in the alcohol and family literature (O'Farrell, Hooley, Fals-Stewart, & Cutter, 1998), probably represents an important antecedent to drinking. Expressed emotion in alcoholic families has been defined to consist of criticism, hostility, and emotional overinvolvement directed at the alcoholic spouse. High expressed emotion (in spouses of alcoholics), as compared to low expressed emotion, is related to lower marital satisfaction as well as to higher rates of relapse, shorter time to relapse following couple alcohol treatment, and a higher percentage of drinking days in the year following treatment. The nonalcoholic spouse's criticism and disappointment, when directed at the alcoholic spouse, may lead to more marital stress, dissatisfaction and, ultimately, more drinking. Alternatively, a more severe drinking problem may lead to more expressed emotion as well as to a greater probability of relapse.

Specific relationship problems, such as sexual dissatisfaction and dysfunction, may be another source of stress and a possible antecedent to drinking. This may be an especially problematic source of conflict because there tend to be large discrepancies in sexual satisfaction between partners in an alcoholic relationship (O'Farrell, Choquette, Cutter, & Birchler, 1997). In research comparing sexual problems and sexual satisfaction in alcoholic couples, nonalcoholic conflicted couples, and nonalcoholic happily married couples (O'Farrell et al., 1997), wives of alcoholic husbands reported more sexual difficulties and less sexual satisfaction compared to the nonconflicted couples. Although their wives expressed dissatisfaction, alcoholic husbands reported the same high level of sexual satisfaction as husbands in nonconflicted couples. This discrepancy in sexual satisfaction and awareness of sexual problems between the husband and the wife may be a source of conflict, negative interactions, and discontented feelings for the couple. As part of the cognitive–behavioral–systemic model of maintenance, any interaction that elicits negative affect or stress is likely to contribute to the maintenance of the drinking.

CONSEQUENCES OF USE

Positive reinforcers for drinking can occur at the intrapersonal or the interpersonal level. At the individual level, for instance, alleviation of withdrawal symptoms or temporary euphoria to replace a depressed mood may reinforce drinking. The spouse and other family members also may unwittingly supply positive consequences of drinking, for instance, by taking care of the intoxicated family member, pampering him or her when sick from drinking too much, or protecting the drinker from negative consequences at work (e.g., calling in sick for the drinker).

As noted in the review of contemporary research on behavioral models, for certain couples, drinking also may be associated with an increase in positive interactions. It is assumed that interactions within a relationship have a *reciprocity* in that the behavior can best be understood in its interactional context. "Reciprocity" refers to the pattern of behaviors that occur between two people in which the behavior of one partner cues the behavior of the other partner, which in turn cues further behavior of the first partner. Behavioral marital research has focused heavily on positive and negative reciprocity, finding that distressed couples in general have a higher rate of negative reciprocity (negative behavior begets negative behavior), while nondistressed couples have higher rates of positive reciprocity (positive behavior begets positive behavior). However, female alcoholic couples and concordant alcoholic couples have been shown to differ from male alcoholic couples in their interactional styles when alcohol is present (Haber & Jacob, 1997). For female alcoholic couples with nonalcoholic spouses, drinking appears to decrease conflict and regulate affect, a perhaps desirable consequence that reinforces and perpetuates drinking.

The effect of alcohol on family and marital interaction is complex, but negative consequences are often quite prominent. Family members may avoid or criticize the drinker. In some cases, family members find it difficult to tolerate the drinking or the behavior of the intoxicated individual, and verbal or even physical assaults ensue. Typically, these negative consequences serve only to exacerbate the problem: the drinker may leave the house and drink elsewhere or may learn to drink in secret. In either case, a pattern of lying on the alcoholic's part and of hypervigilance and mistrust on the spouse's part may result, severely damaging family functioning. Finally, since the alcoholic with a moderate to severe problem spends an inordinate amount of time seeking, consuming, or recovering from the effects of alcohol, he or she typically is unable to contribute fully to the daily functioning of the household. The nonalcoholic spouse and children must then take on more responsibilities, leading to increased resentment and stress. All of this may serve to deepen the unpleasantness in the home and cue the alcoholic to spend more time out of the home and drinking.

Marital violence is one potential negative consequence associated with alcoholism in the family system. Among a community sample of newlywed couples, the husband's drinking during the first year of marriage was found to predict marital violence in subsequent years (Quigley & Leonard, 2000). Later violence appeared to be mediated by the drinking status of the wife; if the wife was a heavy drinker, the husband's drinking was no longer predictive of violence. The highest levels of marital violence were seen in couples where the husband was a heavy drinker and the wife was not. Violence was not seen in couples where the wife was a heavy drinker and the husband was not. Leonard and Quigley (1999) observed that the husband's drinking was more likely to result in physical violence than in verbal aggression. In fact, it was three times more likely that physical aggression involved the husband's drinking than did verbal aggression. Wives reported that their husbands were drinking in 9.5% of verbal aggression episodes, 27.3% of moderate aggression episodes (e.g., throw something; push, grab, or shove; slap), and 43.3% of severe physical aggression episodes (e.g., kicked, hit with fist, beat up).

Marital violence is strongly related to alcoholism. Stopping drinking following behavioral couple therapy for alcoholism is associated with a significant reduction in such violence (Murphy & O'Farrell, 1996). Conversely, relapse after behavioral couple therapy is associated with continued marital violence. Maritally violent alcoholics are likely to be binge drinkers, have negative communication styles with their spouses, have a history of antisocial behaviors, have more consequences associated with their drinking, and feel less confident about dealing with interpersonal conflict without drinking (Murphy & O'Farrell, 1996).

To summarize, problem drinking is maintained by many intersecting factors, and involves the individual's intra- and interpersonal state, antecedent cues, and positive and negative consequences on the individual and family level. This complexity results in a spiral effect: reciprocal interactions between the drinker and his or her social environment typically tend to worsen the drinking and drinking-related consequences over time, and dysfunctional patterns of individual and family interactions become overlearned and "automatic" through repetition. Families experiencing substance abuse may also be experiencing other individual and family problems.

Relationship between Substance Abuse and Other Psychopathology

As mentioned above, research indicates that rates of psychopathology are elevated in substance-abusing populations. Estimates of lifetime drug use disorders comorbid with alcohol dependence are as high as 80% (Carroll, 1986; Ross, Glaser, & Germanson, 1988). Comorbid antisocial personality disorder rates among male alcoholics range from 23% (Morgenstern & Langenbucher, 1994) to 53% (Ross, Glaser, & Stiasny, 1988), depending on the recruitment site (e.g., rates tend be higher in Veterans Administration populations) and the diagnostic instrument used. For mood disorders, Ross, Glaser, and Germanson (1988) cited rates of 23% and 60% for depressive disorders and anxiety disorders, respectively, in men, and 35% and 67%, respectively, for women.

The relationship between substance abuse and psychopathology is complex. Simple models do exist—for instance, the classic disease model contends that psychopathology in both the identified patient and his or her family members is a result of chronic substance abuse, and abates after the abuser is able to maintain sobriety. There is no empirical evidence to support this hypothesis. Indeed, several studies indicate that a substantial proportion of psychopathology is primary (i.e., it predates substance abuse) (Epstein, Ginsburg, Hesselbrock, & Schwarz, 1994). Khantzian (Khantzian & Khantzian, 1984) is a proponent of an alternative theory, that substance abusers use alcohol and drugs to self-medicate preexisting conditions. For instance, narcotic addicts, according to this view, are not seeking euphoria but are attempting to alleviate the dysphoria associated with intense affect and drive states such as rage and depression. Further research is needed to evaluate this view and in general to untangle the relationship between substance use and psychopathology.

Family systems models view psychopathological symptoms as serving particular functions in the family interaction. In general, psychopathological symptoms are an integral part of and help to maintain the "family identity." Since, according to family systems models, stability and predictability are important to maintain a homeostatic balance (Steinglass et al., 1987), behaviors and interactions, including psychopathology, become incorporated into the system. For instance, in a family where the husband is alcoholic, a child who behaves badly at school can serve as a focus for the nonalcoholic spouse. In this way, rather than concentrating on her unhappiness and frustration with her husband and thus jeopardizing the stability of the marital relationship and the viability of the family as a whole, she concerns herself with the poor behavior of the child. In this way, the psychopathology of the child serves as a distraction from the alcoholism in the family.

Regardless of the etiology of individual psychopathology in the family, one point is clear: it must be assessed in terms of severity, need for treatment, and impact on the family functioning and maintenance of substance abuse. For instance, if in the context of family therapy it becomes apparent that the alcoholic father is suffering symptoms of a major depression, strategies must be devised to address the depression. Does it persist for at least 2 weeks after the individual becomes sober? Is it so severe that it is interfering with the individual's ability to stop drinking? Is the individual a suicide risk? If the answer to any of these questions is yes, then the therapist needs to consider a referral for a medication evaluation or for other treatment specific to the depression. Sometimes, character disorder either in the spouse or in the substance abuser interferes with couple treatment and must be addressed as well.

Impact of Family Involvement on Treatment Engagement and Outcomes

A number of researchers have examined whether the actions of family members can influence substance abusers to seek treatment. Although the traditional perspective of Al-Anon emphasizes the inability of families to influence the alcoholic, research provides a different perspective. The "intervention" is a family-involved approach in which several family members and close friends work closely with a counselor, eventually confronting the drinker/drug user with the consequences of his or her substance use, and requesting that the individual seek help. Research with families of alcoholics (e.g. Liepman, 1993; Miller, Meyers, & Tonigan, 1999) suggests that the majority of families who consider an intervention do not follow through. However, among those families that do follow through, more than 80% of drinkers who are the focus of the intervention seek treatment. A second approach has combined counseling to support the family member with behavioral strategies to rearrange consequences of drinking/drug use to increase the user's experience of negative consequences to motivate the person to change. Earlier research on this model (unilateral family therapy [UFT]; Thomas & Ager, 1993) reported that more than 60% of drinkers sought treatment or decreased their drinking after the spouse had participated in UFT. Later research with a somewhat more explicit contingency management approach (community reinforcement and family training [CRAFT]; Miller et al., 1999) also found that the majority of drinkers entered treatment after family involvement in CRAFT. CRAFT has been reported to be significantly more effective than Al-Anon or interventions in getting drinkers to seek treatment. All three, however, were equally effective in alleviating distress in family members (Miller et al., 1999). A meta-analysis of studies of the family role in initiation of treatment found an average effect size for entering treatment of 1.83, a statistically significant increase (Edwards & Steinglass, 1995).

A second role for families is in facilitating retention in substance abuse treatment. Liddle and Dakof (1995) reviewed the efficacy of family-based treatments for adolescent substance abusers. In general, they found that family treatment was more effective than alternative strategies in retaining substance-abusing adolescents and their families in treatment. More recent research (e.g., Marques & Formigoni, 1998) supports Liddle and Dakof's earlier findings. With adults, behavioral contracting with a family member for compliance with specific aspects of treatment, such as attendance at aftercare or use of disulfiram, has been demonstrated to enhance compliance (Keane, Foy, Nunn, & Rychtarik, 1984). Numerous correlational studies (e.g., Connor et al., 1998) have found better retention and treatment completion for alcoholics and substance abusers whose families participate in treatment.

A third important finding is the impact of family-involved treatment on family functioning and the functioning of the children. Here, research supports the positive impact of family-involved therapy on the marital relationship (e.g., Fals-Stewart et al., 2000; McCrady, Stout, Noel, Abrams, & Nelson, 1991), family functioning (McKay, Longabaugh, Beattie, Maisto, & Noel, 1993), and the functioning of the children (O'Farrell & Feehan, 1999). O'Farrell and his colleagues (O'Farrell & Murphy, 1995; O'Farrell, Van Hutton, & Murphy, 1999) studied the specific impact of conjoint therapy on domestic violence in couples with a male alcoholic, and reported a significant decrease in domestic violence among treated couples.

Data on the specific impact of family-involved treatment on drinking or drug use are less consistent than data on the positive changes in family functioning. A meta-analysis of alcohol treatment studies (Edwards & Steinglass, 1995) found mixed results, with evidence that family-involved behavioral therapies, particularly those that involved both the family and other social systems, had a significant positive effect, but that family systems treatment did not have statistically significant effects. A larger meta-analysis of studies of family-involved treatment for other substance use disorders (Stanton & Shadish, 1997) found better outcomes for family-involved treatment than for individual therapy, peer group therapy, or family psychoeducational interventions. Research is unambiguous, however, in supporting family-involved treatment with relapse prevention. Two separate studies found that relapse prevention strategies, when integrated with behavioral couple therapy (BCT), resulted in less frequent drinking (O'Farrell, Choquette, & Cutter, 1998) and shorter relapses (McCrady, Epstein, & Hirsch, 1999). Cost-effectiveness studies of BCT suggest that BCT, compared to treatment without the partner involved, is more cost-beneficial in effecting positive outcomes and reducing social costs associated with a substance use disorder (Fals-Stewart, O'Farrell, & Birchler, 1997), and is associated with decreased health care and legal costs after treatment for alcohol use disorders (O'Farrell et al., 1996).

Therapeutic Tasks Required for Treatment to be Successful

There are at least three different reasons to involve families in treatment: (1) to help the user change his or her substance use, (2) to change family members' own behavior and patterns of coping, or (3) to modify dysfunctional patterns of interaction. As reviewed in the previous section, empirical studies support treatment interventions in each of these domains.

Helping the individual change his or her substance use includes a range of therapeutic tasks that involve the family. The first family-related therapeutic task is treatment engagement. Family members may be engaged in treatment prior to the user (as in the UFT or CRAFT model). During this phase, family members learn to rearrange the consequences of substance use so that the user experiences greater negative consequences for using and greater positive consequences for either not using or for help seeking. Family behaviors may include feedback, allowing naturally occurring consequences to unfold, or making specific requests for change. A second therapeutic task that may involve the family is facilitating therapeutic compliance. Here, behavioral-contracting procedures appear to be particularly effective, both for treatment attendance and for compliance with medication. A third family role is to assist in user-focused cognitive-behavioral treatment. During treatment, the family provides valuable information to help identify antecedent stimuli for use, organismic mediating variables, and consequences of use. Family members may play an active role in helping the user to identify high-risk situations, cognitions and affects associated with use, and reinforcing as well as negative consequences.

Family members also play an important role in effecting change in the substance use. Most contemporary family models first focus on stabilizing abstinence or nonproblem use before addressing family functioning. A variety of behavioral techniques may be used to achieve this goal, and pharmacological adjuncts may be considered as well. Family members can be educated about necessary individual change efforts, and can learn ways to support and participate in these changes.

Treatment may also focus on the individual difficulties of family members. At times, family members may be sufficiently distressed that they need separate treatment to manage their own life difficulties. As noted above, however, the distress of family members often is linked directly to the active substance use, and will abate as the use decreases or stops. Family members, however, may have dysfunctional coping styles, so another task of treatment is to facilitate the development of more effective coping responses such as reacting to the substance use rather than the user, being assertive and clear in reactions to the use, decreasing control behaviors, and detaching from alcohol- or drug-related interactions.

The third major area of therapeutic work involves modifying patterns of family interaction; improving communication and problem-solving skills; and considering family themes, rules, and roles that interfere with effective family functioning. Specific family problems, such as financial, child, or sexual problems, may serve as antecedents to alcohol or drug use, and may respond to direct family-level interventions. In addition, recent research (reviewed above) has identified several patterns of interaction that appear particularly toxic, including polarized demand–withdrawal interactions and hostile and critical expressed emotion from family members. The clinician is also challenged to identify ways in which alcohol or other substance use may serve to stabilize family interactions, by, for example, decreasing negative interactions (particularly in women and in certain subtypes of alcoholics), or by facilitating regulation and dampening down of negative affect. Modification of family interactions to facilitate more effective means of dealing with intense affect in the family may be a particularly crucial family-level intervention.

Finally, recent research on domestic violence has identified the high probability of some level of physical aggression in families where a member is abusing alcohol or drugs. Therapists must address this issue through a direct assessment, development of appropriate safety plans, and utilization of effective treatments for domestic violence.

Therapy often requires the clinician to be flexible in the planning and sequencing of therapy. Therapeutic plans may involve a dynamic interplay among different levels of intervention at different points in the therapy.

ADVANTAGES AND DISADVANTAGES OF A FAMILY-BASED APPROACH

There are several advantages to a family-based approach to conceptualizing and treating substance use disorders. Most important is the strong empirical base for the theoretical models and for treatments derived from family models. Family models also direct the theoretician's attention to the environmental contexts in which alcohol and other drug use occur, and direct the clinician to consider maintaining factors beyond the individual. Family involvement is associated with better engagement, greater compliance with treatment, and better treatment outcome. By directing attention to the family, the clinician increases the probability that the identified client will comply with treatment and have a successful outcome. In addition, ample research supports the negative impact that substance use has on the functioning of the rest of the family, thus involving the family in treatment may ease familial distress. Family models provide a framework for conceptualizing the interrelationships between substance use and family functioning, and can be used as a guide for treatment with any part of the family that is available for treatment.

One disadvantage of family models is their greater complexity. Theoreticians must account for multiple interactive relationships, and clinicians must be able to attend to the complexities inherent in dealing with several individuals and the interactions among them. Working with families requires specialized skills and training.

Family models also have some limits from a theoretical perspective. The models lack a conceptualization of the limits of family treatment. The models do not address the complexities introduced by families with multiple substance-abusing members, families with members with other kinds of psychopathology, or families characterized by an extremely high degree of disorganization or destructive interactions. The models also give no explicit attention to the relative importance of the needs of various family members. For example, although the presence of a supportive spouse might increase the probability of a successful treatment outcome, continuing in a relationship might have adverse consequences for the non–substance-abusing partner. Family models also have no explicit theory to facilitate decision making about the focus of intervention (e.g., individual, familial, or other social systems).

SUMMARY AND CONCLUSIONS

In summary, family models have evolved over the past 60 years into contemporary models that emphasize the multiple determinants of psychoactive substance use disorders, the multiple factors that maintain these disorders, and the complex interrelationships between the substance user and his or her familial and other interpersonal environments. A rich body of empirical literature provides strong support for family-based models and for the effectiveness of treatments based on these models. Research knowledge is limited by its relative lack of attention to gender, culture, racial, and sexual orientation issues among subjects, although current research is beginning to attend at least to gender issues. The practicing clinician will be confronted repeatedly with family issues among substance-abusing clients, and with concerned family members, and should incorporate family models into everyday clinical practice.

ACKNOWLEDGMENTS

Preparation of this chapter was supported in part by Grant Nos. R37 AA07070 and T32 AA07569 from the National Institute on Alcohol Abuse and Alcoholism. We are grateful to Jean Schellhorn for her expert assistance with the preparation of the manuscript.

REFERENCES

Alcoholics Anonymous. (1976). *Alcoholics Anonymous: The story of how many thousands of men and women have recovered from alcoholism* (3rd ed.). New York: Alcoholics Anonymous World Services.

Babor, T. F., Dolinsky, Z. S., Meyer, R. E., Hesselbrock, M., Hofmann, M., & Tennen, H. (1992). Types of alcoholics: Concurrent and predictive validity of some common classification schemes. *British Journal of the Addictions, 87,* 23–40.

Barton, C., & Alexander, J. F. (1981). Functional family therapy. In A. S. Gurman & D. P. Kniskern (Eds.), *Handbook of family therapy* (pp. 403–443). New York: Brunner/Mazel.

Beattie, M. (1987). *Co-dependent no more.* Minneapolis, MN: Hazelden.

Becker, J. V., & Miller, P. M. (1976). Verbal and nonverbal marital interaction patterns of alcoholics and nonalcoholics. *Journal of Studies on Alcohol, 37,* 1616–1624.

Bennett, L. A., & Wolin, S. J. (1990). Family culture and alcoholism transmission. In R. L. Collins, K. E. Leonard, & J. S. Searles (Eds.), *Alcohol and the family: Research and clinical perspectives* (pp. 194–219). New York: Guilford Press.

Bennett, L., Wolin, S. J., Reiss, D., & Teitelbaum, M. A. (1987). Couples at risk for transmission of alcoholism: Protective influences. *Family Process, 26,* 111–129.

Bierut, L. J., Dinwiddie, S., Begleiter, H., Crowe, R. R., Hesselbrock, V. M., Nurnberger, J. I. Jr., Schuckit, M. A., & Reich, T. R. (1998). Familial transmission of substance dependence: Alcohol, marijuana, and cocaine. *Archives of General Psychiatry, 55,* 982–988.

Billings, A. G., Kessler, M., Gomberg, C. A., & Weiner, S. (1979). Marital conflict resolution of alcoholic and nonalcoholic couples during drinking and nondrinking sessions. *Journal of Studies on Alcohol, 40,* 183–195.

Black, C. (1982). *It will never happen to me!* Denver: M.A.C.

Broderick, C. B., & Schrader, S. S. (1981). The history of professional marriage and family therapy. In A. S. Gurman & D. P. Kniskern (Eds.), *Handbook of family therapy* (pp. 5–35). New York: Brunner/Mazel.

Brownell, K. D., Heckerman, C. L., Westlake, R. J., Hayes, S. C., & Monti, P. M. (1978). The effect of couples training and partner cooperativeness in the behavioral treatment of obesity. *Behaviour Research and Therapy, 16,* 323–333.

Cadoret, R. J., O'Gorman, T. W., Troughton, E., & Heywood, E. (1985). Alcoholism and antisocial personality: Interrelationships, genetic and environmental factors. *Archives of General Psychiatry, 42,* 161–167.

Carroll, J. F. X. (1986). Treating multiple substance abuse clients. *Recent Developments in Alcoholism, 4,* 85–103.

Carson, A. T., & Baker, R. C. (1994). Psychological correlates of codependency in women. *International Journal of the Addictions, 29,* 395–407.

Cermak, T. (1986). *Diagnosing and treating co-dependence.* Minneapolis: Johnson Institute Books.

Conner, K. R., Shea, R. R., McDermott, M. P., Grolling, R., Tocco, R. V., & Baciewicz, G. (1998). The role of multifamily therapy in promoting retention in treatment of alcohol and cocaine dependence. *American Journal of Addictions, 7,* 61–73.

Cork, M. (1969). *The forgotten children.* Toronto: Addiction Research Foundation.

Cowley, D. S., Roy-Byrne, P. P., Godon, C., Greenblatt, D. J., Ries, R., Walker, R. D., Samson, H. H., & Hommer, D. W. (1992). Response to diazepam in sons of alcoholics. *Alcoholism: Clinical and Experimental Research, 16*(6), 1057–1063.

Dare, C., Eisler, I., Russell, G. F. M., & Szmulker, G. I. (1990). The clinical and theoretical impact of a controlled trial of family therapy in anorexia nervosa. *Journal of Marital and Family Therapy, 16,* 39–58.

Davis, D. I., Berenson, D., Steinglass, P., & Davis, S. (1974). The adaptive consequences of drinking. *Psychiatry, 37,* 209–215.

Devor, E. (1994). A developmental/genetic model of alcoholism: Implications for genetic research. *Journal of Consulting and Clinical Psychology, 62*(6), 1108–1115.

Dunn, N. J., Jacob, T., Hummon, N., & Seilhamer, R. A. (1987). Marital stability in alcoholic-spouse relationships as a function of drinking pattern and location. *Journal of Abnormal Psychology, 96,* 99–107.

Edwards, M. E., & Steinglass, P. (1995). Family therapy treatment outcomes for alcoholism. *Journal of Marital and Family Therapy, 21,* 475–509.

Epstein, E. E., Ginsburg, B., Hesselbrock, V., & Schwarz, J.C. (1994). Alcohol and drug abusers subtyped by antisocial personality disorder and primary or secondary depressive disorder. *Annals of the New York Academy of Sciences, 708,* 187–201.

Epstein, E. E., & McCrady, B. S. (1998). Alcohol behavioral couples therapy: Current status and innovations. *Clinical Psychology Review, 18,* 689–711.

Epstein, E. E., & McCrady, B. S. (2002). Couple therapy in the treatment of alcohol problems. In A. S. Gurman & N. S. Jacobson (Eds.), *Clinical handbook of couple therapy* (3rd ed., pp. 597–628). New York: Guilford Press.

Fals-Stewart, W., O'Farrell, T. J., & Birchler, E. E. (1997). Behavioral couples therapy for male substance-abusing patients: A cost outcomes analysis. *Journal of Consulting and Clinical Psychology, 65,* 789–802.

Fals-Stewart, W., O'Farrell, T. J., Feehan, M., Birchler, E. E., Tiller, S., & McFarlin, S. (2000). Behavioral couples therapy versus individual-based treatment for male substance-abusing patients: An evaluation of significant individual change and comparison of improvement rates. *Journal of Substance Abuse Treatment, 18,* 249–254.

Frankenstein, W., Hay, W. M., & Nathan, P. E. (1985). Effects of intoxication on alcoholics' marital communication and problem solving. *Journal of Studies on Alcohol, 46,* 1–6.

Frankenstein, W., Nathan, P. E., Sullivan, R. F., Hay, W. M., & Cocco, K. (1985). Asymmetry of influence in alcoholics' marital communication: Alcohol's effects on interaction dominance. *Journal of Marital and Family Therapy, 11,* 399–411.

Haber, J. R., & Jacob, T. (1997). Marital interactions of male versus female alcoholics. *Family Process, 36,* 385–402.

Hajema, K.-J., & Knibbe, R. A. (1998). Research report: Changes in social roles as predictors of changes in drinking. *Addiction, 93,* 1717–1727.

Hall, R. L., Hesselbrock, V. M., & Stabenau, J. R. (1983a). Familial distribution of alcohol use: I. Assortative mating of alcoholic probands. *Behavior Genetics, 13*(4), 373–382.

Hall, R. L., Hesselbrock, V. M., & Stabenau, J. R. (1983b). Familial distribution of alcohol use: II. Assortative mating in the parents of alcoholics. *Behavior Genetics, 13*(4), 361–372.

Hammen, C. L. (1991). Mood disorders (unipolar depression). In M. Hersen & S.

M. Turner (Eds.), *Adult psychopathology and diagnosis* (2nd ed., pp. 170–207). New York: Wiley.

Hersen, M., Miller, P. M., & Eisler, R. M. (1973). Interactions between alcoholics and their wives: A descriptive analysis of verbal and nonverbal behavior. *Quarterly Journal of Studies on Alcohol, 34*, 516–520.

Hesselbrock, M. (1986). Alcoholic typologies: A review of empirical evaluations of common classification schemes. *Recent Developments in Alcoholism, 4*, 191–206.

Hesselbrock, V. (1995). The genetic epidemiology of alcoholism. In H. Begleiter & B. Kissin (Eds.), *The genetics of alcoholism* (pp. 17–39). New York: Oxford University Press.

Hill, S. (1994). Etiology. In J. Langenbucher, B. McCrady, W. Frankenstein, & P. Nathan (Eds.), *Annual review of addictions research and treatment* (Vol. III, pp. 127–148). Elmsford, NY: Pergamon Press.

Hurcom, C., Copello, A., & Orford, J. (2000). The family and alcohol: Effects of excessive drinking and conceptualizations of spouses over recent decades. *Substance Use and Misuse, 35*, 473–502.

Jackson, J. (1954). The adjustment of the family to the crisis of alcoholism. *Quarterly Journal of Studies on Alcohol, 15*, 562–586.

Jacob, T., Dunn, N. J., & Leonard, K. (1983). Patterns of alcohol abuse and family stability. *Alcoholism: Clinical and Experimental Research, 7*, 382–385.

Jacob, T., Ritchey, D., Cvitkovic, J. F., & Blane, H. T. (1981). Communication styles of alcoholic and nonalcoholic families when drinking and not drinking. *Journal of Studies on Alcohol, 42*, 466–482.

Keane, T. M., Foy, D. W., Nunn, B., & Rychtarik, R. G. (1984). Spouse contracting to increase Antabuse compliance in alcoholic veterans. *Journal of Clinical Psychology, 40*, 340–344.

Kendler, K. S., Heath, A. C., Neale, M. C., Kessler, R. C., & Eaves, L. C. (1992). A population-based twin study of alcoholic women. *Journal of the American Medical Association, 14*, 1877–1882.

Khantzian, E. J., & Khantzian, N. J. (1984). Cocaine addiction: Is there a psychological predisposition? *Psychiatric Annals, 14*(10), 753–759.

Kogan, K. L., & Jackson, J. (1965). Stress, personality and emotional disturbance in wives of alcoholics. *Quarterly Journal of Studies on Alcohol, 26*, 486–495.

Konstantareas, M. M. (1990). A psychoeducational model for working with families of autistic children. *Journal of Marital and Family Therapy, 16*, 59–70.

Leonard, K. E., & Jacob, T. (1997). Sequential interactions among episodic and steady alcoholics and their wives. *Psychology of Addictive Behaviors, 11*, 18–25.

Leonard, K. E., & Quigley, B. M. (1999). Drinking and marital aggression in newlyweds: An event-based analysis of drinking and the occurrence of husband marital aggression. *Journal of Studies on Alcohol, 60*, 537–545.

Lewis, M. L. (1937). Alcoholism and family casework. *Social Casework, 35*, 8–14.

Liddle, H. A., & Dakof, G. A. (1995). Family-based treatment for adolescent drug use: State of the science. In E. Rahdert et al. (Eds.), *Adolescent drug abuse: Clinical assessment and therapeutic interventions*. (National Institute on Drug Abuse Research Monograph No. 156, pp. 218–254). Rockville, MD: U.S. Department of Health & Human Services Public Health Service, National Institutes of Health.

Liepman, M. R. (1993). Using family influence to motivate alcoholics to enter treatment: The Johnson Institute Intervention approach. In T. J. O'Farrell (Ed.), *Treating alcohol problems: marital and family interventions* (pp. 54–77). New York: Guilford Press.

Lyon, D., & Greenberg, J. (1991). Evidence of codependency in women with an alcoholic parent: Helping out Mr. Wrong. *Journal of Personality and Social Psychology, 61*, 435–439.

MacDonald, D. E. (1956). Mental disorders in wives of alcoholics. *Quarterly Journal of Studies on Alcohol, 17*, 282–287.

Maisto, S. A., McKay, J. R., & O'Farrell, T. J. (1998). Twelve-month abstinence from alcohol and long-term drinking and marital outcomes in men with severe alcohol problems. *Journal of Studies on Alcohol, 59*, 591–598.

Marques, A., & Formigoni, M. (1998). Family intervention influences adherence and outcome in psychotherapeutic treatment for alcohol/drug dependents. *Alcoholism: Clinical and Experimental Research, 22*, 964.

McCrady, B. S. (1998, January). *The man who painted his wife: A history of family approaches to alcohol treatment.* Paper presented at the Eighth International Meeting on the Treatment of Addictive Behaviors, Santa Fe, NM.

McCrady, B. S. (2001). Alcohol use disorders. In D. H. Barlow (Ed.), *Clinical handbook of psychological disorders* (3rd ed., pp. 376–433). New York: Guilford Press.

McCrady, B. S., Epstein, E. E., & Hirsch, L. S. (1999). Maintaining change after conjoint behavioral alcohol treatment for men: Outcomes at six months. *Addiction, 94*, 1381–1396.

McCrady, B. S., Stout, R., Noel, N., Abrams, D., & Nelson, H. F. (1991). Effectiveness of three types of spouse-involved behavioral alcoholism treatment. *British Journal of Addiction, 86*, 1415–1424.

McKay, J. R., Longabaugh, R., Beattie, M. C., Maisto, S. W., & Noel, N. E. (1993). Does adding conjoint therapy to individually focused alcoholism treatment lead to better family functioning? *Journal of Substance Abuse, 5*, 45–59.

Merikangas, K. R. (1990). The genetic epidemiology of alcoholism. *Psychological Medicine, 20*, 11–22.

Miller, W. R., Meyers, R. J., & Tonigan, J. S. (1999). Engaging the unmotivated in treatment for alcohol problems: A comparison of three strategies for intervention through family members. *Journal of Consulting and Clinical Psychology, 67*, 688–697.

Moos, R. H., Finney, J. W., & Cronkite, R. C. (1990). *Alcoholism treatment: Context, process and outcome.* Oxford, UK: Oxford University Press.

Moos, R. H., Finney, J. W., & Gamble, W. (1982). The process of recovery from alcoholism: II. Comparing spouses of alcoholic patients and matched community controls. *Journal of Studies on Alcohol, 43*, 888–909.

Moos, R. H., & Moos, B. S. (1984). The process of recovery from alcoholism: III. Comparing functioning of families of alcoholics and matched control families. *Journal of Studies on Alcohol, 45*, 111–118.

Morgenstern, J., & Langenbucher, J. (1994, August). *Comorbidity: Recent findings and their implications for understanding and treating addictive disorders.* Symposium presentation at the Annual Meeting of the American Psychological Association, Los Angeles.

Murphy, C. M., & O'Farrell, T. (1996). Marital violence among alcoholics. *Current Directions in Psychological Science, 5*, 183–186.

O'Farrell, T. J., Choquette, K. A., & Cutter, H. S. (1998). Couples relapse prevention sessions after behavioral marital therapy for male alcoholics: Outcomes during the three years after starting treatment. *Journal of Studies on Alcohol, 59*, 357–370.

O'Farrell, T. J., Choquette, K. A., Cutter, H. S., & Birchler, G. R. (1997). Sexual satisfaction and dysfunction in marriages of male alcoholics: Comparison with nonalcoholic martially conflicted and nonconflicted couples. *Journal of Studies on Alcohol, 58*, 91–99.

O'Farrell, T. J., Choquette, K. A., Cutter, H. S., Brown, E., Bayog, R., McCourt, W., Lowe, J., Chan, A., & Deneault, P. (1996). Cost–benefit and cost-effectiveness analyses of behavioral marital therapy with and without relapse prevention sessions for alcoholics and their spouses. *Behavior Therapy, 27*, 7–24.

O'Farrell, T. J., & Feehan. M. (1999). Alcoholism treatment and the family: Do family and individual treatments for alcoholic adults have preventive effects for children? *Journal of Studies on Alcohol, 13*(Suppl.), 25–129.

O'Farrell, T. J., Hooley. J., Fals-Stewart, W., & Cutter, H. Q. (1998). Expressed emotion and relapse in alcoholic patients. *Journal of Consulting and Clinical Psychology, 66*, 744–752.

O'Farrell, T. J., & Murphy, C. M. (1995). Marital violence before and after alcoholism treatment. *Journal of Consulting and Clinical Psychology, 63*, 256–262.

O'Farrell, T. J., Van Hutton, V., & Murphy, C. M. (1999). Domestic violence before and after alcoholism treatment: A two-year longitudinal study. *Journal of Studies on Alcohol, 60*(3), 317–321.

Orford, J., Guthrie, S., Nicholls, P., Oppenheimer, E., Egert, S., & Hensman, C. (1975). Self-reported coping behavior in wives of alcoholics and its association with drinking outcome. *Journal of Studies on Alcohol, 36*, 1254–1267.

Patterson, G. R. (1986). Performance models for antisocial boys. *American Psychologist, 41*, 432–444.

Quigley, B. M., & Leonard, K. E. (2000). Alcohol and the continuation of early marital aggression. *Alcoholism: Clinical and Experimental Research, 24*, 1003–1010.

Roberts, L. J., & Leonard, K. E. (1998). An empirical typology of drinking partnerships and their relationship to marital functioning and drinking consequences. *Journal of Marriage and the Family, 60*, 515–526.

Ross, H. E., Glaser, F. B., & Germanson, T. (1988). The prevalence of psychiatric disorders in patients with alcohol and other drug problems. *Archives of General Psychiatry, 45*, 1023–1031.

Ross, H. E., Glaser, F. B., & Stiasny, S. (1988). Sex differences in the prevalence of psychiatric disorders in patients with alcohol and drug problems. *British Journal of Addiction, 83*, 1179–1192.

Rotunda, R. J., & O'Farrell, T. J. (1997). Marital and family therapy of alcohol use disorders: Bridging the gap between research and practice. *Professional Psychology: Research and Practice, 28*, 246–252.

Rychtarik, R. G., Carstensen, L. L., Alford, G. S., Schlundt, D. G., & Scott, T.

(1988). Situational assessment of alcohol-related coping skills in wives of alcoholics. *Psychology of Addictive Behaviors, 2,* 66–73.

Rychtarik, R. G., & McGillicuddy, N. B. (1997). The Spouse Situation Inventory: A role-play measure of coping skills in women with alcoholic partners. *Journal of Family Psychology, 11,* 289–300.

Schuckit, M. A. (1998). Biological, psychological, and environmental predictors of the alcoholism risk: A longitudinal study. *Journal of Studies on Alcohol, 59,* 485–494.

Schuckit, M. A. (1999). New findings in the genetics of alcoholism. *Journal of the American Medical Association, 281,* 1875–1876.

Shoham, V., Rohrbaugh, M. J., Stickle, T. R., & Jacob, T. (1998). Demand–withdraw couple interaction moderates retention in cognitive-behavioral versus family-systems treatments for alcoholism. *Journal of Family Psychology, 12,* 557–577.

Stanton, M. D., & Shadish, W. R. (1997). Outcome, attrition, and family-couples treatment for drug abuse: A meta-analysis and review of the controlled, comparative studies. *Psychological Bulletin, 122,* 170–191.

Steinglass, P. (1979). The alcoholic family in the interaction laboratory. *Journal of Nervous and Mental Disease, 167,* 428–436.

Steinglass, P. (1981). The alcoholic family at home: Patterns of interaction in dry, wet, and transitional stage of alcoholism. *Archives of General Psychiatry, 38,* 578–584.

Steinglass, P., Bennett, L. A., Wolin, S. J., & Reiss, D. (1987). *The alcoholic family.* New York: Basic Books.

Steinglass, P., Davis, D. I., & Berenson, D. (1977). Observations of conjointly hospitalized "alcoholic couples" during sobriety and intoxication: Implications for theory and therapy. *Family Process, 16,* 1–16.

Steinglass, P., Weiner, S., & Mendelson, J. H. (1971). Interactional issues as determinants of alcoholism. *American Journal of Psychiatry, 128,* 275–280.

Tarter, R. E., & Vanyukov, M. (1994). Alcoholism: A developmental disorder. *Journal of Consulting and Clinical Psychology, 62*(6), 1096–1107.

Thomas, E. J., & Ager, R. D. (1993). Unilateral family therapy with spouses of uncooperative alcohol abusers. In T. J. O'Farrell (Ed.), *Treating alcohol problems: Marital and family interventions* (pp. 3–33). New York: Guilford Press.

Wegsheider, S. (1981). *Another chance: Hope and health for the alcoholic family.* Palo Alto, CA: Science and Behavior Books.

Whalen, T. (1953). Wives of alcoholics: Four types observed in a family service agency. *Quarterly Journal of Studies on Alcohol, 14,* 632–641.

Wolin, S. J., Bennett, L. A., Noonan, D. L., & Teitelbaum, M. A. (1980). Disrupted family rituals: A factor in the intergenerational transmission of alcoholism. *Journal of Studies on Alcohol, 41,* 199–214.

Wright, P. H., & Wright, K. D. (1990). Measuring codependents' close relationships: A preliminary study. *Journal of Substance Abuse, 2,* 335–344.

6

Family Therapy Techniques

William Fals-Stewart
Timothy J. O'Farrell
Gary R. Birchler

Any review of the development and applications of the family treatment model for addictions over the last half century reveals a rapid progression in the acceptance of family-involved therapy as a critical component of treatment for alcoholism and drug abuse. For example, the treatment literature from the 1950s and early 1960s primarily conceptualized substance abuse as an individual problem that was best treated on an individual basis (e.g., Jellinek, 1960). However, during the 1960s this view was gradually supplanted by what is now the prevailing clinical wisdom that family members can play a central role in the treatment of alcoholics and drug abusers (Stanton & Heath, 1997). By the early 1970s, couple and family therapies were described by the National Institute on Alcohol Abuse and Alcoholism as "one of the most outstanding current advances in the area of psychotherapy of alcoholism" (Keller, 1974, p. 161). By the late 1970s, family therapy for substance abuse was embraced by the majority of substance abuse treatment programs and community mental health settings (e.g., Coleman & Davis, 1978; Kaufman & Kaufman, 1992). During the last two decades, family-based assessment and intervention has become widely viewed as part of standard care for alcoholism and drug abuse. In fact, many have argued that the only reason not to include family members in the treatment of a substance-abusing patient is refusal by the patient or members of the family to be involved (e.g., O'Farrell, 1993b).

In addition, the popular literature on families and substance abuse has grown into its own cottage industry of sorts, with a wide range of books describing codependency, enabling, and adult children of alcoholics appearing on bookstore shelves. Thus, the role of family factors in the etiology and maintenance of addictive disorders and the application of family therapy in substance abuse treatment has indeed come a long way.

Historically, the family interventions used to treat alcoholism grew out of marital treatment approaches and focused primarily on the spousal system. In contrast, family-based treatments for drug abuse evolved from systemic family therapy approaches, focusing on the entire family, which might include the patient's spouse, children, parents, siblings, and so forth. More recently, this distinction has blurred, with both alcoholism and drug abuse treatment programs often providing a wide array of family therapy services for the patients and their family members. Moreover, many family therapists who work with substance-abusing patients have broadened the definition of what constitutes "family members" to include other members of the substance user's social network, including employers, close friends, and concerned others in the intervention (Kaufman, 1985).

The purpose of the present chapter is to provide an overview of different systems of family therapy commonly used in the treatment of alcoholism and drug abuse, with an emphasis on a description of the treatment techniques identified with each of these systems. Because a variety of theories of family functioning have influenced the family treatment of alcoholism and drug abuse, family-based interventions that are used with substance users are very diverse, varying in large part as a function of the theoretical underpinnings out of which the approach evolved. To organize this review, we focus on the use of family-involved treatments and their respective intervention techniques during three different stages of the treatment process: (1) family therapy for substance users resistant to seeking help; (2) family-involved treatment to aid recovery when the substance user has sought help; and (3) family therapy to assist in the maintenance of treatment gains.

FAMILY-BASED METHODS TO INITIATE CHANGE AMONG SUBSTANCE USERS RESISTANT TO SEEKING TREATMENT

It is likely that many, if not most, substance users, seek treatment in response to some form of external pressure, as exerted by a spouse, other family members, a physician, the legal system, and so forth (e.g., Hasin, 1994; Krampen, 1989). Thus, in many instances, one or more family members or concerned significant others recognizes the need for some form of intervention to help the substance user reduce or eliminate his or her substance misuse and the destructive behaviors that often co-occur with excessive drinking or drug use. As such, it is often a family member of a substance user who is the first person to come to the attention of the substance abuse treatment system. With the possible exception of coercion from the legal system, pressure to enter treatment by a family member or concerned significant other is the most powerful inducement for substance users to enter and engage in treatment (Stanton, 1997).

Several family-based intervention methods have been developed to motivate resistant substance users to enter some form of treatment, in addition to helping improve the spouse's or other family members' coping. Perhaps the five most well-known approaches are (1) the Johnson Institute Intervention; (2) A Relational Intervention Sequence for Engagement (ARISE); (3) Unilateral Family Therapy (UFT); (4) Pressure to Change (PTC); and (5) Community Reinforcement and Family Training (CRAFT). Although these interventions share a common goal, the techniques used within each vary considerably, particularly with respect to the level of coercion prescribed.

The Johnson Institute Intervention

Without question, the most well known of these family–involved motivational techniques is the Johnson Institute Intervention (Faber & Keating-O'Connor, 1991; Liepman, 1993), which was originally developed as a method to motivate resistant alcoholics to enter treatment, but has been applied more broadly to individuals with other psychoactive substance use disorders. The Johnson Institute Intervention, or the "intervention" as it is most commonly called, involves three to four educational and rehearsal sessions, conducted by a trained therapist, to prepare family members and the most meaningful support network members (e.g., employers, neighbors, friends) for a confrontation meeting. More specifically, once contact has been made by a concerned significant other, the therapist conducts an initial assessment of the nature and severity of the substance use problem, as well as the composition and structure of the substance user's social network. The therapist then makes a determination as to which of those family members and concerned significant others should participate in the intervention meeting.

Those who agree to be involved in the intervention are brought together initially to meet with the therapist, thereby forming the intervention team. The members of the team are given an orientation about the intervention process. Intervention participants are asked to list specific incidents and behaviors by the substance user that have affected them directly and have been the consequence of the drinking or drug use. They also practice the delivery of their feedback and are provided coaching and corrective feedback by the therapist. The members of the intervention team need to (1) agree about what treatment is necessary for the substance user, (2) firmly insist that the substance user enter into and engage in the treatment prescribed, (3) outline the specific consequences for the substance user if he or she fails to engage in the recommended treatment, and (4) follow through on these consequences if the substance user decides not to engage in treatment as recommended.

The intervention team is then convened and the substance user is brought to this meeting, typically not knowing the agenda of the group. Once the substance user is in their midst, members then share their concerns and feelings; these are to be presented in a sincere, nonjudgmental fashion. The intervention team members also express their hope that the substance user will enter treatment, outline the consequences if the substance user refuses, and openly discuss the desired outcome of both the intervention itself and the recommended treatment. A referral to treatment is then made. Often, at a later date, the members of the intervention team meet with the therapist to go through a debriefing and discuss a plan for change for the family members and others in the substance user's social network to follow.

Some have raised a number of ethical concerns about the Johnson Institute Intervention (e.g., Faber & Keating-O'Connor, 1991; Miller, Meyers, & Tonigan, 1999). For example, confidentiality is certainly an issue, given that the substance user does not participate in the decision about who becomes part of the intervention team and what information is disclosed during the intervention meeting. Additionally, there is the potential for significant negative and harmful aftereffects of the intervention, particularly in the instance where the referral to treatment is refused by the substance user and the consequences of this decision are imposed. Also, the therapist who is overseeing the intervention may have a conflict of interest, particularly in circumstances in which the recommended treatment for the substance user is to be provided at a facility where the therapist is employed.

A Relational Intervention Sequence for Engagement

In part, as a response to the aforementioned concerns about the Johnson Institute Intervention approach, A Relational Intervention Sequence for Engagement (ARISE; Garrett, Landau-Stanton, Stanton, Stellato-Kabat, & Stelleto-Kabat, 1997) was developed as a somewhat less coercive alternative to motivate resistant substance users to engage in treatment. ARISE is a hierarchically ordered three-stage family-based approach designed to encourage reluctant substance users to seek help, with each stage involving greater family involvement, greater therapist involvement, and more coercion. In the first stage, a concerned significant other contacts the treatment agency to obtain information about treatment options. The therapist, during one or more telephone sessions, assesses the nature and severity of the substance user's problem, the circumstances surrounding it, and the social support system of the substance user.

The network of concerned significant others in the substance user's life is also contacted and asked to attend at least an initial meeting at the clinic; they may be asked to attend additional meetings as needed. These meetings are designed to (1) review efforts of those in the network to engage and confront the substance user, (2) develop strategies to motivate the substance user to engage in treatment, and (3) prepare members of the network to handle possible crises as they arise. The goal of these sessions is to mobilize the members of the social network in support of treatment for the substance user.

Although these sessions may provide members of the network enough information and coaching to allow them to motivate the substance user to enter treatment, it is most likely that the process will move to the second stage, which involves an informal intervention with a therapist present. Again, concerned significant others in the substance user's social network are encouraged to attend this meeting (or meetings, as the need arises); the substance user is also asked to attend, although these meetings can still be conducted without the substance user present. In these meetings, the members collectively consider possible approaches that might be used to motivate the substance user to enter treatment.

If, after repeated attempts, the substance user remains unwilling to seek help, the process moves to the third and final stage, which involves use of an intervention similar to that used in the Johnson Institute Intervention approach. Thus, the ARISE model advocates use of less coercive steps early in the process and gradually proceeds to the use of greater counselor and family involvement if the lower intensity steps are not successful in motivating the substance user to engage in treatment.

The Unilateral Family Therapy Approach

Unilateral Family Therapy (UTF) is an extensive multifaceted method that consists of weekly individual counseling for 4–6 months with the spouse of the treatment-resistant substance user (Thomas, 1994; Thomas & Ager, 1993). In the early phases of UFT, the non-substance-abusing spouse is (1) educated about addiction, (2) trained to monitor her or his substance-abusing partner's drinking or drug use (or provide current, specific information on the amount of substance use), (3) introduced to methods to enhance relationship adjustment (e.g., engaging in behaviors that both partners find pleasing), and (4) taught to identify and cease enabling behaviors (e.g., making excuses for the drinker's behavior when he or she is intoxicated, drinking with the alcoholic).

The next phase of UFT involves "abuser-directed interventions" aimed at influencing the substance-using partner to enter substance abuse treatment, to reduce substance use, or both. These include methods to train spouses to support sobriety (e.g., initiating non-substance-use activities, such as going to a movie) and scheduling a physician's appointment for an examination to determine the nature and severity of the substance use. If these nonconfrontational approaches are not sufficient to change the substance user's drinking or drug use, a programmed confrontation and a programmed request are used. The *programmed confrontation* entails training the spouse and sometimes other family members to confront the substance user, usually in the presence of a trained treatment provider. It is carried out only if the spouse is willing to follow through with strong contingent consequences if the substance user refuses to enter treatment or change his or her substance-using behavior. A *programmed request* differs from a programmed confrontation in that there is evidence of readiness on the part of the substance user to respond favorably to such a request (i.e., for the substance user to enter treatment) and an unwillingness of the spouse to carry out a strong consequence if the substance user fails to comply with the request.

If the substance user ultimately enters treatment, the final phases of UFT involve methods to foster maintenance of treatment gains and helping to prevent relapse. These interventions include spouse support, in which the non-substance-abusing spouse refrains from enabling and continues behaviors designed to enhance relationship satisfaction and support sobriety. In addition, UFT trains spouses in the basic tenets of Marlatt and Gordon's (1985) relapse prevention procedure. This includes helping the substance user to identify high-risk situations, temptation resistance training, and handling relapses if they do occur.

The Pressure to Change Approach

Barber and colleagues (e.g., Barber & Crisp, 1995; Barber & Gilbertson, 1998) developed the Pressure to Change (PTC) approach for partners living with heavy drinkers who deny their alcohol problem and refuse treatment. PTC makes use of learning theory to train partners in coping responses that are designed to empower the non-substance-abusing partner and provide incentive for the alcoholic partner to change.

PTC involves five to six structured counseling sessions to instruct the non-substance-abusing partner in how to use five gradually increasing levels of pressure on the drinker to seek help or moderate his or her drinking. During the course of these five levels, the partner (1) receives feedback from the therapist about the seriousness of the drinker's problem and education on PTC; (2) plans incompatible activities during times when the drinker usually drinks (e.g., taking children to an amusement park, going to dinner with friends or relatives who do not drink); (3) responds to drinking by withdrawing reinforcers and to drinking-related crises by suggesting treatment; (4) establishes a contract with the drinker in which the partner agrees to exchange some reinforcer for sobriety; and (5) if prior steps have been unsuccessful, the partner confronts the drinker by outlining the negative effects of the drinking and making a simple, direct request that the drinker seek change or seek help.

The Community Reinforcement and Family Training Approach

The Community Reinforcement and Family Training (CRAFT) approach is an outgrowth of the Community Reinforcement Approach (CRA) for alcoholism (e.g., Azrin, 1976; Meyers, Smith, & Miller, 1998) and, as with CRA,

CRAFT interventions draw heavily on learning theory. In CRAFT, a family member or, more generally, a concerned significant other (CSO), participates in a multifaceted intervention designed to encourage the substance-abusing family member to stop drinking or using drugs and to enter treatment. CRAFT consists of several sequential steps. The CSO is asked to determine the severity of the substance use problem (by measuring the quantity and frequency of use) and outline the biopsychosocial problems the substance use and its concomitant behavior have caused. The CSO is given an overview of the CRAFT approach, the procedures involved, and his or her role in implementing different aspects of the intervention. The CSO is also asked to complete two functional analyses. The first is to identify the substance user's triggers for using alcohol or drugs and the consequences of such use. The second is to ascertain the substance user's triggers for more prosocial behaviors and their resulting consequences.

CSOs are trained in several family-initiated treatment procedures. These include teaching CSOs methods to effectively use positive reinforcement and negative consequences to discourage drug use or drinking by the family member. For example, positive reinforcement might include engaging in pleasant activities (e.g., discussing enjoyable topics, giving gifts) when the substance user is not drinking or using drugs. In addition, the CSO would expressly note that the reinforcement is being given because the substance user is not drinking or using drugs. Negative consequences for intoxication might include withhold reinforcements, explaining why, and ignoring the substance user during periods of intoxication. Emphasis is also placed on teaching the CSO methods to decrease stress in general and increase positive aspects of his or her own life, which might include establishing new friendships, engaging in positively rewarding activities outside of the relationship with the substance user, or joining a therapy group.

A unique aspect of CRAFT is its emphasis on identifying dangerous situations as behavioral changes are introduced at home. The CSO is instructed on how to identify potentially violent situations so that he or she can take immediate action before getting hurt. The therapist helps the CSO construct the sequence of events that lead to violence and teaches him or her to identify significant "cues" before physical violence begins. The CSO develops a specific plan for leaving these situations until it is safe to return.

CSOs are also instructed in the most effective ways to suggest treatment to the substance user, particularly during times when the substance user may be highly motivated to enter treatment (e.g., after engaging in embarrassing behavior when drinking, after becoming violent with a family member when intoxicated). The groundwork is also established for having treatment available immediately once the substance user has agreed to enter treatment, regardless of time of day or day of the week.

FAMILY-INVOLVED TREATMENT ONCE THE SUBSTANCE USER HAS ENTERED TREATMENT

The goal of the interventions described in the preceding section is to encourage and support the substance user's entry into treatment. Regardless of the impetus for seeking help, once the substance user has entered treatment, family therapy interventions are often used as a primary or adjunctive component of the treatment armamentarium of addictions therapists. The family treatment model will typically dictate the degree of spouse or family member involvement, ranging from little involvement (e.g., providing assessment information only) to being an equal partner in the treatment process (e.g., couple therapy).

Although several systems of family therapy have been used with substance-abusing patients, three theoretical perspectives have come to dominate family-based conceptualizations of substance use and thus have become the basis for the treatment strategies most often used with substance users (Gondoli & Jacob, 1990; O'Farrell, 1995). The best known of these and the most widely used is the *family disease approach*, which views alcoholism and other drug abuse as an illness of the family, suffered not only by the substance user, but also by family members. The *family systems approach* applies the principles of general systems theory to families, with particular attention paid to ways in which families maintain a dynamic balance between substance use and family functioning and whose interactional behavior is organized around alcohol or drug use. *Behavioral approaches* assume that family interactions serve to reinforce alcohol- and drug-using behavior. We next review the treatments that have evolved from these systems in more detail, emphasizing the hallmark therapy techniques identified with each approach.

The Family Disease Approach

From this perspective, alcoholism and drug abuse are thought of or viewed as a "family disease" that affects all (or nearly all) family members. Family members of substance users are viewed as suffering from the disease of "codependence," which is a term that is often used to describe the process underlying the various problems observed in the families of individuals who abuse psychoactive substances. Little consensus exists as to how the term should be defined or operationalized. However, one fairly popular definition has been put forth by Schaef (1986), who argues that *codependence* is a disease that parallels the addiction disease process and is marked by characteristic symptoms (e.g., external referencing, caretaking, self-centeredness, control issues, dishonesty, frozen feelings, perfectionism, and fear). The hallmark of codependency is *enabling*, which, as the term implies, is defined as any set of behaviors that perpetuates the psychoactive substance use. These include making it easier for the alcoholic or drug abuser to engage in substance use, or shielding the substance user from the negative consequences often associated with drinking or drug taking.

Although the problem of substance abuse exists within the family, the solution from this perspective is for each family member to recognize that he or she has a disease, to detach from the substance user, and to engage in his or her own program of recovery. Thus, the family disease approach typically involves separate treatment for family members without the substance user present. Treatment often consists of psychoeducational groups about the disease concept of addiction and codependency; referrals to Al-Anon, Al-Ateen, or Adult Children of Alcoholics groups; and individual and group therapy to address various psychological issues. Family members are taught that there is nothing they can do to help the substance user to stop using other than to cease enabling. In general, the family disease approach advocates that family members should not actively intervene to try to change the substance user's drinking or drug use, but should detach and focus on themselves to reduce their own emotional distress and improve their own coping (Al-Anon Family Groups, 1981; Laundergan & Williams, 1993).

Family Systems Models

The family systems model views the acquisition and use of alcohol or other drugs as a major organizing principle for patterns of interactional behavior within the family system. A reciprocal relationship exists between family functioning and substance use, with an individual's drug and alcohol use being best understood in the context of the entire family's functioning. According to family systems theory, substance abuse in either adults or adolescents often evolves during periods in which the individual family member is having difficulty addressing an important developmental issue (e.g., leaving the home) or when the family is facing a significant crisis (e.g., marital discord). During these periods, substance abuse can serve to (1) distract family members from their central problem or (2) slow down or stop a transition to a different developmental stage that is being resisted by the family as a whole or by one of its members (Stanton, Todd, & Associates, 1982).

From the family systems perspective, substance use represents a maladaptive attempt to deal with difficulties that develop a homeostatic life of their own and regulate family transactions. The substance use itself serves an important role in the family. Once the therapist understands the function of the substance use for the family, the therapist can then explain how the behavior has come about and the function it serves. In turn, treatment is aimed at restructuring the interaction patterns associated with the substance use, thereby making the drinking or drug use unnecessary in the maintenance of the family system functioning.

To accomplish this aim, a variety of therapy techniques are used by family systems therapists; these techniques fall into two broad categories. The first, *joining*, consists of techniques designed to promote therapeutic alliance and increase the therapist's leverage within the family. The therapist alternates between joining that supports the family system and its members and joining that challenges the system. This involves making a connection with each family member engaged in treatment and instilling a sense of confidence that the therapist has a firm commitment to working together with the family members on identified problems. In the joining process, the therapist typically solicits from each family member his or her perception of the problems in the family and his or her feelings about the issues raised. By attending to each person's views, the therapist conveys the message that each family member's viewpoint is important and promotes the view that differences in perception about the identity, nature, and severity of problems are acceptable. The therapist attempts to communicate to each family member that he or she (1) understands the family member's perceptions of the problems and (2) has a clear idea about how to address the issues raised by the family member.

The process of joining involves the therapist promoting areas of strength in the family, supporting a threatened member of the family, and using the family member's methods of communicating (e.g., humor, touching) to introduce new ideas and concepts (Minuchin, 1974). Of course, joining is an ongoing process, which is ultimately supported and reinforced as the therapist demonstrates his or her understanding and helpfulness throughout the course of treatment.

Unlike joining, the second category of intervention techniques, *restructuring*, involves challenging the family's homeostasis and takes place through modifications in the family's bonding and power alignments among individuals and subsystems in the family (e.g., Haley, 1976; Minuchin, 1974). Several different techniques are used in the process of restructuring, including contracting, enactment, reframing, restructuring, and marking boundaries. *Contracting* is an agreement to work on agreed-upon issues, with an emphasis on helping the substance user with his or her problems prior to expanding to and probing other issues. The contract is developed at the end of the first interview and is always maintained throughout treatment. As part of the contract, the family must choose to develop a family system that is conducive to abstinence by the substance user and agree to pursue the contract after it has been agreed upon as part of the initial evaluation.

Enactment involves the therapist eliciting recurring behavioral sequences (which the therapist can often observe by requiring family members to talk to each other about problems in sessions while being carefully observed by the therapist vs. directing their communications to the therapist) and interrupting and destabalizing the behavioral exchanges. *Reframing* requires the therapist to help family members understand the interrelatedness of their behaviors and to see and understand how the substance use (and any other dysfunctional behavior) serves an important function in the family. *Restructuring* is comprised of shifting family interaction patterns and establishing new, healthier behaviors (e.g., changing seating arrangements to strengthen the role of parents in the family, restating problems in solvable form, teaching methods of communication and problem solving that preclude triangulation or conflict avoidance). *Marking boundaries* is accomplished by clearly delineating individual and subsystem boundaries. For example, the parental subsystem should be protected from intrusion by children and other adults who may be inside or outside the family. To strengthen the parental subsystem, sessions with parents that exclude other family members should be held.

The family systems approach has been adopted widely in treatment settings. The highly influential work of Peter Steinglass (e.g., Steinglass, Bennett, Wolin, & Reiss, 1987) has demonstrated the application of family systems approaches with adult alcoholic patients and their families. In addition, the pivotal work of Stanton, Todd, and colleagues (1982) demonstrated the effectiveness of family systems approaches with heroin-dependent patients. Szapocznik and colleagues (e.g., Szapocznik, Kurtines, Foote, Perez-Vidal, & Hervis, 1983; Szapocznik et al., 1988) have demonstrated the effectiveness of family systems therapy with adolescent substance users.

The Behavioral Approach

Behavioral family therapy treatment models draw heavily on operant and social learning theories to understand the behavior of the substance user in the family context. Substance use is viewed as a behavior learned in the context of social interactions (e.g., observing peers, parents, role models in the media) and reinforced by contingencies in the individual's environment (Akers, Krohn, Lanza Kaduce, & Radosevich, 1979). Thus, from a family perspective, substance use is maintained, in part, by the antecedents and consequences that are operating in the family environment.

Following from the operant and social learning principles, treatment emphasizes contingency management designed to reward sobriety, reduce negative reinforcement of drinking or drug use, and increase prosocial behaviors that may be incompatible with substance use. The substance user and involved family members are trained in methods to increase positive interactions, improve problem solving, and enhance communication skills. Use of these newly developed skills serves to reduce the likelihood of continued drinking or drug use by the substance-using family member.

Family-based behavioral treatment models have been used most frequently with alcoholic and drug-abusing couples. Three general reinforcement patterns are typically observed in substance-abusing families: (1) reinforcement for substance-using behavior in the form of attention or caretaking, (2) shielding the substance user from experiencing negative consequences related to his or her drinking or drug use, and (3) punishing drinking behavior (e.g., McCrady, 1986). In turn, behaviorally oriented treatment generally focuses on changing spousal or family interactions that serve as stimuli for abusive substance use or trigger relapse, improving communication and problem-solving abilities, and strengthening coping skills that reinforce sobriety.

Behavioral couple therapy (BCT) works directly to increase relationship factors conducive to abstinence. A behavioral approach assumes that family members can reward abstinence—and that alcoholic and drug-abusing individuals from happier, more cohesive relationships with better communication have a lower risk of relapse. The substance-abusing patient and the spouse are seen together in BCT, typically for 15–20 outpatient couple sessions over 5–6 months. Generally, couples are married or have been cohabiting for at least 1 year, have no current psychosis, and one member of the couple has a current problem with alcoholism and/or drug abuse. The couple starts BCT soon after the substance user seeks help.

BCT sees the substance-abusing patient with the spouse to build support for sobriety. The therapist arranges a daily *Sobriety Contract* in which the substance user states his or her intent not to drink or use drugs that day (in the tradition of "one day at a time" from Alcoholics Anonymous), and the spouse expresses support for the patient's efforts to stay abstinent. For alcoholic patients who are medically cleared and willing, daily Antabuse ingestion witnessed and verbally reinforced by the spouse can also be part of the Sobriety Contract. The spouse records the performance of the daily contract on a calendar provided by the therapist. Both partners agree not to discuss past substance use or fears about future substance use at home to prevent substance-related conflicts that can trigger relapse, but reserve these discussions for the therapy sessions.

At the start of each BCT session, the therapist reviews the Sobriety Contract calendar to see how well each spouse has done his or her part. If the Sobriety Contract includes 12-step meetings or urine drug screens, these are also marked on the calendar and reviewed. The calendar provides an ongoing record of progress that is rewarded verbally at each session. The couple performs the behaviors of their Sobriety Contract in each session to highlight its importance and to let the therapist observe how the couple does the contract.

Using a series of behavioral assignments, BCT increases positive feelings, shared activities, and constructive communication because these relationship factors are conducive to sobriety. *Catch Your Partner Doing Something Nice* has each spouse notice and acknowledge one pleasing behavior performed by his or her partner each day. In the *Caring Day* assignment, the partners plan ahead to surprise their spouses with a day when they do some special things to show their caring. Planning and doing *shared rewarding activities* is important because many substance abusers' families have stopped the kind of shared activities that are associated with positive recovery outcomes (Moos, Finney, & Cronkite, 1990). Each activity must involve both spouses, either by themselves or with their children or other adults—and can be done at or away from home. Teaching *communication skills* can help the alcoholic and spouse deal with stressors in their relationship and in their lives, and this may reduce the risk of relapse.

Relapse prevention is the final activity of BCT. At the end of weekly BCT sessions, each couple completes a *Continuing Recovery Plan* that is reviewed at quarterly follow-up visits for an additional 2 years.

To a lesser extent, behavioral family therapy has also been used with adolescent substance users. For example, Azrin, Donohue, Besalel, Kogan, and Acierno (1994) describe a behaviorally oriented family treatment consisting of weekly groups that parents attended once per month. Therapists in these groups used modeling, rehearsal, and self-monitoring techniques with the participating families and gave written homework assignments that were reviewed during sessions. The principle techniques used in these sessions included (1) stimulus control methods (e.g., increasing time spent in safe vs. risky situations), (2) urge control (e.g., interrupting internal stimuli that served as precursors to substance use and substituting other stimuli); and (3) social control methods, which emphasized assistance from the parents in providing safe activities. These groups also provide training in problem-solving procedures, communication skills, and anger management.

OTHER FAMILY THERAPY APPROACHES WHEN THE SUBSTANCE USER ENTERS TREATMENT

Although the family therapies arising from the disease, behavioral, and family systems models are the most widely used in substance abuse clinical and/or research settings, there are three other family-based treatment models that are also highly influential in the substance abuse treatment community. *Social network therapy*, based on a social systems model (e.g., Galanter, 1999), uses a variety of family interventions in support of a treatment plan targeted at the substance user as the primary patient. *Ecological approaches* are based on the notion that substance use and other behavior problems arise in the context of many sources of influence from multiple systems in the substance user's life. In turn, interventions are used to modify these multiple systems of influence to create an ecological environment for the substance user that is conducive to abstinence. Finally, *psychodynamic approaches* view substance use, in part, as a family problem and work toward achieving what is often referred to as "second-order change." In other words, the goal of psychodynamic therapy is to change the entire family system of the substance user to ensure that dysfunction does not occur in other family members once the symptoms of the substance user have been addressed and alleviated.

The Social Network Therapy Approach

Social network therapy, which is most closely associated with the work of Mark Galanter (Galanter, 1999), is an approach to substance abuse treatment in which selected family members and friends are enlisted to provide ongoing support for the substance user and to promote behavior change. Network members are viewed as part of the therapist's treatment team, but are not the expressed targets of treatment interventions. The aim of social network therapy is the achievement of abstinence with relapse prevention for the substance user, and the development of a drug- and alcohol-free lifestyle. The network (i.e., supportive family members and concerned significant others) is considered an important resource, both to the substance user in his or her attempt to achieve and maintain abstinence and to the treatment provider helping the substance user achieve this objective. The emphasis of treatment is placed squarely on the substance user, with the network serving a supporting role for the therapist and the identified patient.

In social network therapy, the network is chosen from among family members and concerned significant others who have a long-standing relationship with the substance user. The network formed is used to (1) obtain an accurate, multifaceted substance use history of the substance user, (2) exert social pressure on the substance user to engage in the treatment process and to facilitate the substance user's compliance with treatment directives (e.g., disulfiram therapy, detoxification), and (3) increase positive social support for the substance user during and after treatment. In addition, members of the network are provided some counseling regarding how they can better cope with having a substance user in their social sphere.

Typically, the substance user is involved in individual counseling to assist him or her with elimination of alcohol or drug use, while the network members meet with the therapist to reach the network's aforementioned objectives. Thus, the substance user may be attending individual counseling once or twice a week in which the family and concerned significant others are not involved, while the network members may also meet concurrently with the treating therapist on a weekly basis. Additionally, family sessions may occur on a regular basis without the substance user early in the treatment course, particularly when the substance user is engaged in a detoxification or residential treatment program. However, eventually the substance user is involved in the network meetings.

The network meetings have three key agendas. First, the network assists in helping the substance user maintain abstinence. The substance user and the

network members should report at the outset of each session any events related to use of alcohol or other drugs. The substance user and network members make plans with the therapist on how to sustain abstinence. Cues to conditioned alcohol- and/or drug-seeking behavior are also examined. Second,
the network members commit to staying involved in the treatment and to attending scheduled sessions, with the additional understanding that they may be
asked to become more involved during times of crisis. Third, the network
members help with any and all aspects of the treatment as necessary to assure
the substance user's stability, including providing a stable, substance-free resi-
dence, encouraging avoidance of substance-abusing friends, encouraging attendance at 12-step meetings, and taking prescribed medications, such as
disulfiram or other pharmacological agents (e.g., naltrexone). The individual
counseling received by the substance user focuses on achieving abstinence,
with an emphasis on identifying cues for drug seeking that can be used to understand the potential for relapse, and to investigate areas of conflict. It is important to explore the emotional, circumstantial, or substance-related events
that bring substance use to mind. The ultimate objective of the individual
therapy is for the substance user to adopt a drug-free lifestyle in which abstinence will be embedded.

The Ecological Approach

In ecological treatment models, interventions are directed at assessing multiple
influences on the substance user and implementing treatments that influence
change in multiple systems, including the intrapersonal variables of the substance user, the interpersonal system of the family and larger social network,
and the extrapersonal system, such as the school and community at large.
These approaches have much in common with family systems methods, but
are broader in scope, focusing not only on the individual, but also on the family and extrafamilial factors (e.g., peer, school, and neighborhood) that may influence drinking and drug use.

    Perhaps the most well-known ecological model-based treatment is multi-
systemic family therapy (Henggeler et al., 1991), which is a treatment approach
used with adolescent substance users. Multisystemic family therapy typically
includes sessions or part of sessions held conjointly with the adolescent substance user and other family members. Individual sessions with the adolescent
substance user focus on decision making, emotion regulation, and other
intrapersonal factors that may be related to substance-using behavior. Interestingly, the therapeutic techniques used as part of multisystemic family therapy
are drawn from other treatment models, including family systems therapy,
behavioral approaches, and therapeutic approaches from the general counseling
interventions. Therapists work to evaluate the factors in the adolescent's ecological environment that contribute to the substance use and may work to im-

plement interventions at comparatively broad levels (e.g., in the school system, the juvenile delinquency programs) to affect change.

The Psychodynamic Approach

As argued by Kaufman (1995), psychodynamic approaches are not typically used with substance users because these individuals usually require more active, limit-setting emphasis on the here-and-now than is normally associated with psychodynamic techniques. However, psychodynamic therapy remains very influential and many of the methods that therapists employ with families can trace their roots to psychodynamic theory.

In psychodynamic therapy, the emphasis is on uncovering and working with unconscious material. In the context of family treatment, this is done by uncovering unconscious interpersonal processes, exposing and working through forbidden feelings (e.g., anger, resentment), and helping family members gain insight into how they support each other's defensive structure. In the context of psychodynamic family therapy, the therapist listens for evidence of unconscious material that may be supporting family members' defensive structures. The therapist also obtains a detailed family history to understand how difficulties of the past may be being replayed in the present. The family history is also important to understand how destructive repetitive behaviors observed in a patient's family of origin may recur with current family members, both within the family and in future generations. For example, "projective identification" is a process whereby one family member unintentionally elicits certain behaviors from other family members. Thus a father may cease his substance use, but the unconscious process that led to his excessive drinking or drug use may be passed to his son or daughter, leading to a transgenerational repetition of these destructive behaviors.

During the course of sessions, the therapist provides interpretations to members of the family, discerns repetitive destructive patterns of behavior, and assigns tasks that can change these patterns. In addition, the therapist works to overcome resistance (i.e., behaviors, feelings, patterns, or interpersonal styles) that prevent change. In families of substance users, key resistance behaviors often involve failure to perform functions that would allow the substance user to stay drug- or alcohol-free. Resistance is often overcome in the context of a therapy contract, with each family member agreeing to overcome resistance. Resistances such as bringing up the past, blaming, and scapegoating can be discouraged by the therapist if this is part of the therapy contract.

MAINTAINING BEHAVIOR CHANGE AFTER TREATMENT

Once a substance user has entered and successfully completed treatment, the next and perhaps most important stage of recovery is maintaining treatment gains during the posttreatment period. Thus, to assist with maintaining stable, long-term recovery, substance users often become involved in some form of aftercare after they complete primary treatment (Donovan, 1998). Given that family treatment methods have been developed to encourage substance users to enter treatment and have been used as part of primary treatment, it should come as no surprise that family-based interventions have also been developed to help stabilize long-term recovery. The two primary family-involved approaches used in the aftercare period are *behavioral continuing care contracts* and *couple relapse prevention*.

Behavioral Continuing Care Contracts

Ossip-Klein and Rychtarik (1993) describe the use of behavioral contracts to increase attendance at aftercare meetings once a more intensive primary intervention has been completed. The contract itself is negotiated between the patient, family member, and therapist as the substance user approaches the end of some form of intensive treatment (e.g., inpatient hospitalization, day treatment) and prepares to move on to less-intensive continuing care. The therapist provides an appointment calendar for continuing care sessions and helps negotiate an attendance contract between the patient and the family member. As part of the contract, the patient agrees to (1) post the appointment calendar in a prominent place in the home, (2) attend all aftercare sessions (barring any emergent, unforseen circumstances that reasonably preclude attendance), and (3) call to reschedule any appointments that must be missed. In exchange for adherence to this part of the contract, the family member agrees to provide a mutually negotiated and rewarding incentive within a week of the appointment.

Couple Relapse Prevention

Relapse prevention sessions have also been incorporated into the behaviorally oriented couple treatment approaches described by McCrady (1989, 1993) and O'Farrell and colleagues (O'Farrell, 1993a; O'Farrell, Choquette, & Cutter, 1998). As part of both of these programs, the first phase involves helping the substance user and his or her partner maintain the positive treatment gains they garnered during the course of couple therapy, in terms of reduced substance use and increased relationship satisfaction. Thus, the partners may be encouraged to continue with the negotiated Sobriety Contract, engagement in relationship-enhancing behaviors (e.g., Shared Rewarding Activities, Caring Days), and attendance at self-help meetings. The partners also develop a relapse prevention plan, which includes (1) identifying high-risk situations, (2) discerning early warning signs of relapse, (3) developing and practicing coping skills to deal with these situations, and (4) outlining a specific plan to deal with relapse if it does occur. Couple-based relapse prevention sessions are conducted with the partners with decreasing frequency during the year after completion of the primary couple intervention.

CASE EXAMPLE

To illustrate some of the procedures and techniques we have described thus far, we now provide a case example based on the case of a married couple treated by the first author. Although selected background data has been changed to protect these partners' confidentiality, the methods used and outcomes obtained have not been altered. To illustrate the communication patterns often observed in these types of couples, a partial transcript of a structured conflict resolution discussion between the partners is also provided.

Stephen L was a 37-year-old white male who was referred to outpatient substance abuse treatment by his physician, who had determined that Stephen met criteria for alcohol dependence. Stephen agreed to be evaluated by the physician only after a confrontation with his wife, Ellen, who had consulted with a local treatment provider about her husband's abusive drinking. During a detailed psychosocial assessment conducted as part of his intake assessment at the outpatient clinic, Stephen described an extensive history of problematic alcohol use. He reported that, in his early 20s, he drank nearly every day, usually consuming six to eight beers on each occasion. By his mid-20s, he began drinking greater quantities of alcohol on weekends (i.e., eight to 10 drinks on Fridays after work and Saturday evenings), holidays, and special occasions (e.g., birthdays, anniversaries). He had suffered two blackouts and had been arrested on one occasion for driving while intoxicated.

Stephen reported that he had entered a 28-day inpatient treatment program about 3 years before the present evaluation and had stayed sober for roughly 1 year after treatment. He reported that financial problems, arguments with his wife, and stress at work contributed to his relapse. He also noted that, during the last 2 years, he drank daily, but that there had been a steady increase in daily alcohol consumption over that time period, starting at two to three drinks daily, but rising more recently to six to eight drinks each day. Stephen admitted that he drove his car while intoxicated on "too many nights to count," although he had so far been able to avoid being caught by the police. The assessment revealed that Stephen met criteria for alcohol dependence. Although he had used marijuana occasionally in his early 20s, Stephen did not abuse drugs other than alcohol.

Stephen was asked if he was willing to participate in a marital assessment with his wife, Ellen. Although Stephen acknowledged that he was reluctant to participate, he reported that Ellen very much wanted to be involved in the treatment in some capacity. He signed a release of confidentiality form to allow his therapist to discuss the possibility of participation with Ellen. She agreed to come to the clinic with Stephen; the assessment procedures to be used were described to the partners. It was also emphasized that this was only an assessment and participation in this evaluation did not commit either the couple or the therapist to treatment. Both partners agreed to complete the assessment.

During the assessment, the therapist collected background data from Ellen and information about the couple's marriage. Ellen was a 33-year-old white female who was employed part time as a teller in a local bank. She reported that she had never abused alcohol or used other drugs. Stephen and Ellen married after dating for 1 year. Ellen reported that she knew Stephen drank "heavily," but was not aware of the extent of his drinking until he entered inpatient treatment.

Both partners described their relationship as unstable and mentioned that they had recently discussed divorce. Both had set up separate bank accounts and Ellen had discussed her situation with a divorce attorney. Stephen added that Ellen would state that she wanted a divorce every time the partners had a disagreement. Stephen's primary complaint was that Ellen "is never satisfied and throws the past in my face all the time!" Ellen reported that Stephen spent money "they could not afford to give up" to buy drinks for his friends after work. Because of limited income, the partners reported that they could not afford to have and support a child, although both wanted to have children.

Ellen said she felt "neglected" because Stephen spent so much time drinking with his friends. From her report, the partners rarely spoke, showed little affection toward each other, and had not spent time engaging in recreational activities they enjoyed (e.g., going to the movies, eating out). Neither partner reported any episodes of physical aggression, although both acknowledged that Stephen was verbally abusive on several occasions when he was drunk.

As part of the assessment, the partners were asked to discuss a problem they both agreed existed in their relationship while the therapist observed. The topic the partners chose was "financial problems." As part of this conflict resolution task, the partners were asked to describe the problem and work toward a solution. The following is a partial transcript of the partners' discussion, occurring about 3 minutes after the task was initiated:

ELLEN: Why is it that you spend all of our money on your friends, going out getting loaded, and not saving one f★★king dime for our future? You are never home, never here . . .

STEPHEN: Why would I want to stay home? When I'm there, you give me s★★t about drinking, bringing up every thing I've ever done wrong. I go out, and you complain about that. That's it . . . you just b★★ch.

ELLEN: That's how you see it, but I want you to stop drinking and care about me more than you care about your drinking buddies, who really don't give a damn about you anyway.

STEPHEN: I've tried to stop . . . you know I have . . . but even when I stop, you just bark at me about why I didn't do it before. Do you know how much that sucks? How long you gonna carry that cross?

ELLEN: For a while. Can you blame me? You come home drunk, go to sleep, go to work . . . we don't talk, we don't have sex . . . I swear, I don't know you at all anymore.

STEPHEN: I know, but at least I went to the doctor as you wanted and came here. I don't like it either.

ELLEN: I know you say you have stopped drinking, but I don't believe it and have never believed it. You do nothing around the house, you don't fix the car, lift a finger for anything.

STEPHEN: Christ, I stop drinking and you don't believe me and call me a liar. I drink and I am a drunk and a liar. F★★k the house, f★★ck the car . . .

ELLEN: Don't you see . . . I sit alone all the time. Please just stop. I want to get our lives back.

STEPHEN: Yeah, me too . . . that's why I'm in this place. But I am not here to have this turn into a place where you can just yell at me and I take . . . I won't take it, be warned. I'd rather start over with someone who doesn't know the past and can't use it as a weapon.

ELLEN: It won't take a rocket scientist to figure out your past, no matter who you are with.

This exchange revealed not only significant deficits in these partners' communication patterns, but also deficits in their relationship commitment, caring, and ability to resolve conflict. Although the agreed topic was "financial problems," they engaged in what is often called "kitchen sinking," that is, introducing several other conflict areas without addressing the problem at hand. This communication sample reveals the deleterious effects of alcohol and related concomitant behaviors on the marriage, with Stephen's drinking appearing to interfere greatly with important relationship activities (e.g., saving money, talking to each other, sex).

The partners agreed to participate in BCT. Early sessions involved introducing and following through with a negotiated Sobriety Contract, which included five primary components: (1) Stephen agreed to take disulfiram (for which he was medically evaluated) while being observed by Ellen; (2) the couple agreed to a positive verbal exchange at the time when Stephen took the disulfiram (i.e., Stephen reporting he had stayed sober during the last day and promising to remain sober for the ensuing day and Ellen thanking him for remaining sober); (3) Ellen agreed not to bring up negative past events concerning Stephen's drinking; (4) Stephen agreed to attend AA meetings daily; and (5) the partners agreed they would not threaten to divorce or separate while at home and would, for the time being, bring these thoughts into the sessions.

The partners reported Stephen's use of disulfiram was very helpful to both of them; Stephen did not entertain the idea of drinking while taking disulfiram, and Ellen, because she observed Stephen take the disulfiram, trusted he was not drinking (for the first time in many months) and thus had much greater peace of mind. The positive verbal exchange between the partners made the daily Sobriety Contract a caring behavior rather than a "checking-up" procedure. Stephen said there was substantially less stress in the home because Ellen did not bring up his past drinking and did not call him a liar when he reported he was not drinking. Stephen's AA involvement provided him with a support network that did not include friends with whom he drank. Ellen reported she occasionally attended an Al-Anon group for wives of alcoholics, which gave her a supportive forum to discuss her marriage.

Communication skills training focused on slowing down the partners' verbal exchanges, with an emphasis on focusing on a single issue at a time. The partners were trained to make positive specific requests and to use "I" statements as a way to own their feelings rather than attributing how they feel to their spouse.

Later sessions addressed identified relationship problems. Assignments such as Catch Your Partner Doing Something Nice and shared rewarding activities served to increase positive verbal exchanges and mutual caring, along with reestablishing a long-term commitment to the relationship. Toward the end of therapy, the partners reported that BCT helped them learn to "enjoy each other again." They noted that their sex life had improved dramatically and, with a referral, they had sought the services of a credit counselor to assist them with some of their financial problems.

After completion of primary treatment, the couple entered the aftercare phase of treatment, during which the partners were seen once every other month for a year to stabilize Stephen's sobriety and the couple's relationship satisfaction. During this period, Stephen reported he had remained sober and continued to take disulfiram. Both partners reported that they made a point of doing something together that was mutually rewarding at least once per week. Stephen was attending AA meetings three times weekly and was generally "working the steps" of AA. Although the partners continued to have money problems, Ellen received a work promotion, which helped to alleviate some of the financial stress.

This case example highlights some important issues. First, with some coaching from a therapist, Ellen confronted her husband about his alcohol use and encouraged him to get an evaluation. The physician's evaluation increased his motivation to enter into formal treatment. The interrelatedness of Stephen's alcohol use and the relationship difficulties suggested that a couple-based treatment, addressing both sets of problems concurrently, would be helpful. Lastly, the couple continued to participate in aftercare treatment effectively to stabilize their treatment gains.

CONCLUSION

As is evidenced by the breadth of interventions described in this chapter, there is no shortage of family-based treatment methods for therapists treating substance users. Although family treatment was, at one time, frowned upon by the treatment community, it is now an integral part of all phases of the treatment process, from motivating reluctant substance users, through primary treatment, to helping maintaining long-term sobriety after treatment. With the exception of somewhat unusual circumstances, such as reluctance by family members to be involved, many would consider failure to involve family members in at least some aspects of the treatment process to represent substandard care.

Given the popularity of family treatment in the substance abuse treatment community, it may come as a surprise that there remain significant gaps in the research literature on the effectiveness of the various treatment interventions used. For example, although systematic reviews have concluded that family therapy is effective in promoting positive outcomes for substance-abusing patients (e.g., O'Farrell & Fals-Stewart, in press; Stanton & Shadish, 1997), very few dismantling studies have been conducted to determine the active ingredients of the interventions described. It is likely that, unless a treatment provider is in a research setting using a detailed treatment manual, he or she is likely to draw techniques from all of the methods described here. It would be helpful if decisions as to which techniques to use were informed by research establishing which techniques produce important behavior change.

In addition, the findings from other studies indicate that family-based methods that have been shown to be particularly effective are not widely used in community-based treatment programs. For example, BCT appears to be a very effective treatment for married or cohabiting substance-abusing patients, but is rarely used by substance abuse treatment providers in nonresearch settings (Fals-Stewart & Birchler, 2001). As another example, the Johnson Institute Intervention is very popular and proponents often state that the approach is very effective, but systematic research has demonstrated that methods such as CRAFT are far more effective (Miller et al., 1999).

But the responsibility of dissemination of effective family-based treatment methods is a shared one between researchers and primary treatment providers. Investigators need to examine family treatment techniques that providers can adopt, given the economic and system constraints faced by community programs. For example, the involvement of managed care in substance abuse treatment has resulted in the more routine use of brief interventions. Thus, family-based treatment methods that require multiple therapy sessions over the course of several months are not likely to be adopted, regardless of their effectiveness. Conversely, it is the responsibility of providers and treatment programs to entertain using family-based treatment methods that may be less familiar (e.g., behavioral interventions), but nonetheless more effective, than traditional approaches. This would require challenging preconceived notions about what long-standing clinical wisdom may dictate as effective; although difficult, the beneficiaries are likely to be the substance users and their families.

ACKNOWLEDGMENT

Preparation of this chapter was supported by grants from the National Institute on Drug Abuse (Nos. DA12189, DA14402, and DA015937).

REFERENCES

Akers, R. L., Krohn, M. D., Lanza Kaduce, L., & Radosevich, M. (1979). Social learning and deviant behavior: A specific test of a general theory. *American Sociology Review, 44*, 636–655.

Al-Anon Family Groups. (1981). *This is Al-Anon.* New York: Al-Author.

Azrin, N. H. (1976). Improvements in the community-reinforcement approach to alcoholism. *Behaviour Research and Therapy, 14*, 339–348.

Azrin, N. H., Donohue, B., Besalel, V. A., Kogan, E. S., & Acierno, R. (1994). Youth drug abuse treatment: A controlled outcome study. *Journal of Child and Adolescent Substance Abuse, 3*, 1–16.

Barber, J. G., & Crisp, B. R. (1995). The "pressure to change" approach to working with the partners of heavy drinkers. *Addiction, 90*, 269–276.

Barber, J. G., & Gilbertson, R. (1998). Evaluation of a self-help manual for the female partners of heavy drinkers. *Research in Social Work Practice, 8*, 141–151.

Coleman, S. B., & Davis, D. T. (1978). Family therapy and drug abuse: A national survey. *Family Process, 17*, 21–29.

Donovan, D. M. (1998). Continuing care: Promoting the maintenance of change. In W. R. Miller & N. Heather (Eds.), *Treating addictive behaviors* (2nd ed., pp. 317–336). New York: Plenum Press.

Faber, E., & Keating-O'Connor, B. (1991). Planned family intervention: Johnson Institute method. *Journal of Chemical Dependency Treatment, 4*, 61–71.

Fals-Stewart, W., & Birchler, G. R. (2001). A national survey of the use of couples therapy in substance abuse treatment. *Journal of Substance Abuse Treatment, 20*, 277–283.

Galanter, M. (1999). *Network therapy for alcohol and drug abuse.* New York: Guilford Press.

Garrett, J., Landau-Stanton, J., Stanton, M. D., Stellato-Kabat, J., & Stellato-Kabat, D. (1977). ARISE: A method for engaging reluctant alcohol- and drug-dependent individuals in treatment. *Journal of Substance Abuse Treatment, 14,* 235–248.

Gondoli, D. M., & Jacob, T. (1990). Family treatment of alcoholism. In R. R. Watson (Ed.), *Drug and alcohol abuse prevention* (pp. 245–262). Totowa, NJ: Humana Press.

Haley, J. (1976). *Problem-solving therapy.* San Francisco: Jossey-Bass.

Hasin, D. S. (1994). Treatment/self-help for alcohol-related problems: Relationship to social pressure and alcohol dependence. *Journal of Studies on Alcohol, 55,* 660–666.

Henggeler, S. W., Borduin, C. M., Melton, G. B., Mann, B. J., Smith, L. A., Hall, J. A., Cone, L., & Fucci, B. R. (1991). Effects of multisystemic therapy on drug use and abuse in serious juvenile offenders: A progress report from two outcome studies. *Family Dynamics of Addiction Quarterly, 1,* 40–51.

Jellinek, E. M. (1960). *The disease concept of alcoholism.* New Haven, CT: Hillhouse Press.

Kaufman, E. (1985). Family therapy in the treatment of alcoholism. In E. T. Bratter & G. G. Forrest (Eds.), *Alcoholism and substance abuse: Strategies for clinical interventions* (pp. 376–397). New York: Free Press.

Kaufman, E. (1994). Family therapy: Other drugs. In M. Galanter & H. D. Kleber (Eds.), *The American Psychiatric Association textbook of substance abuse treatment* (pp. 331–348). Washington, DC: American Psychiatric Association Press.

Kaufman, E., & Kaufman, P. (1992). *Family therapy of drug and alcohol abuse* (2nd ed.). Needham Heights, MA: Allyn & Bacon.

Keller, M. (1974). Trends in treatment of alcoholism. In *Second special report to the U.S. Congress on alcohol and health* (pp. 145–167). Washington, DC: Department of Health, Education, and Welfare.

Krampen, G. (1989). Motivation in the treatment of alcoholism. *Addictive Behaviors, 14,* 197–200.

Laundergan, J. C., & Williams, T. (1993). The Hazelden residential family program: A combined systems and disease model approach. In T. J. O'Farrell (Ed.), *Treating alcohol problems: Marital and family interventions* (pp. 145–169). New York: Guilford Press.

Liepman, M. R. (1993). Using family influence to motivate alcoholics to enter treatment: The Johnson Institute Intervention approach. In T. J. O'Farrell (Ed.), *Treating alcohol problems: Marital and family interventions* (pp. 54–77). New York: Guilford Press.

Marlatt, G. A., & Gordon, J. R. (Eds.). (1985). *Relapse prevention.* New York: Guilford Press.

McCrady, B. S. (1986). The family in the change process. In W. R. Miller & N. H. Heather (Eds.), *Treating addictive behaviors: Process of change* (pp. 305–318). New York: Plenum Press.

McCrady, B. S. (1989). Extending relapse prevention models to couples. *Addictive Behaviors, 14,* 69–74.

McCrady, B. S. (1993). Relapse prevention: A couples-therapy perspective. In T. J. O'Farrell (Ed.), *Treating alcohol problems: Marital and family interventions* (pp. 327–350). New York: Guilford Press.

Meyers, R. J., Smith, J. E., & Miller, E. J. (1998). Working through the concerned significant other. In W. R. Miller & N. Heather (Eds.), *Treating addictive behaviors* (2nd ed., pp. 149–161). New York: Plenum Press.

Miller, P. M., Meyers, R. J., & Tonigan, J. S. (1999). Engaging the unmotivated in treatment for alcohol problems: A comparison of three strategies for intervention through family members. *Journal of Consulting and Clinical Psychology, 67*, 688–697.

Minuchin, S. (1974). *Families and family therapy.* Cambridge, MA: Harvard University Press.

Moos, R. H., Finney, J. W., & Cronkite, R. C. (1990). *Alcoholism treatment: Context, process, and outcome.* New York: Oxford University Press.

O'Farrell, T. J. (1993a). Couples relapse prevention sessions after a behavioral marital therapy couples group program. In T. J. O'Farrell (Ed.), *Treating alcohol problems: Marital and family interventions* (pp. 305–326). New York: Guilford Press.

O'Farrell, T. J. (Ed.). (1993b). *Treating alcohol problems: Marital and family interventions.* New York: Guilford Press.

O'Farrell, T. J. (1995). Marital and family therapy. In R. Hester & W. Miller (Eds.), *Handbook of alcoholism treatment approaches* (2nd ed., pp. 195–220). Boston: Allyn & Bacon.

O'Farrell, T. J., Choquette, K. A., & Cutter, H. S. (1998). Couples relapse prevention sessions after behavioral marital therapy for male alcoholics: Outcomes during the three years after starting treatment. *Journal of Studies on Alcohol, 59*, 357–370.

O'Farrell, T. J., & Fals-Stewart, W. (in press). Family-involved alcoholism treatment: An update. In M. Galanter (Ed.), *Recent developments in alcoholism: Vol. 15. Services research in the era of managed care.* New York: Plenum Press.

Ossip-Klein, D. J., & Rychtarik, R. G. (1993). Behavioral contracts between alcoholics and family members: Improving aftercare participation and maintaining sobriety after inpatient alcoholism treatment. In T. J. O'Farrell (Ed.), *Treating alcohol problems: Marital and family interventions* (pp. 281–304). New York: Guilford Press.

Schaef, A. (1986). *Codependence misunderstood/mistreated.* New York: Harper & Row.

Stanton, M. D. (1997). The role of family and significant others in the engagement and retention of drug-dependent individuals. In L. S. Onken, J. D. Blaine, & F. J. Boren (Eds.), *Beyond the therapeutic alliance: Keeping the drug dependent individual in treatment* (pp. 157–180). Rockville, MD: National Institute on Drug Abuse.

Stanton, M. D., & Heath, A. W. (1997). Family and marital treatment. In J. H. Lowinson, P. Ruiz, R. B. Millman, & J. G. Langrod (Eds.), *Substance abuse: A comprehensive textbook* (3rd ed., pp. 448–454). Baltimore: Williams & Wilkins.

Stanton, M. D., & Shadish, W. R. (1997). Outcome, attrition, and family/couples treatment for drug abuse: A meta-analysis and a review of controlled, comparative studies. *Psychological Bulletin, 122*, 170–191.

Stanton, M. D., Todd, T. C., & Associates. (1982). *The family therapy of drug abuse and addiction.* New York: Guilford Press.

Steinglass, P., Bennett, L., Wolin, S., & Reiss, D. (1987). *The alcoholic family.* New York: Basic Books.

Szapocznik, J., Kurtines, W. M., Foote, F. H., Perez-Vidal, A., & Hervis, O. (1983). Conjoint versus one-person family therapy: Some evidence for the effectiveness of conducting family therapy through one person. *Journal of Consulting and Clinical Psychology, 51,* 889–899.

Szapocznik, J., Perez-Vidal, A., Brickman, A. L., Foote, F. H., Santisteban, D., Hervis, O., & Kurtines, W. M. (1988). Engaging adolescent drug abusers and their families in treatment: A strategic structural systems approach. *Journal of Consulting and Clinical Psychology, 56,* 552–557.

Thomas, E. J. (1994). The spouse as a positive rehabilitative influence in reaching the uncooperative alcohol abuser. In D. K. Granvold (Ed.), *Cognitive and behavioral treatment: Methods and applications* (pp. 159–173). Pacific Grove, CA: Brooks/Cole.

Thomas, E. J., & Ager, R. D. (1993). Unilateral family therapy with spouses of uncooperative alcohol abusers. In T. J. O'Farrell (Ed.), *Treating alcohol problems: Marital and family interventions* (pp. 3–33). New York: Guilford Press.

7

Cognitive-Behavioral Theories of Substance Abuse

Frederick Rotgers

Cognitive-behavioral (CB) theories of treatment for psychoactive substance use disorders (PSUDs) are based on principles of learning and behavior change in both animals and humans that have been delineated by experimental psychologists (Eysenck, 1982). They are a part of the larger group of behavior change techniques that fall under the rubric of "behavior therapy." This chapter reviews the current status of CB theory of substance abuse treatment, beginning with a delineation of basic assumptions, followed by a brief outline of the processes presumed to operate in treatment of PSUDs and behavior change efforts in general. This review is followed by a consideration of the etiology, maintenance, and individual client characteristics in treating PSUDs within a CB framework. Discussion then proceeds to the tasks cognitive behaviorally oriented clinicians attempt to accomplish in treatment and what CB theory has to say about the issue of treatment goal selection. The chapter concludes with a review of the advantages and disadvantages of CB theories of PSUDs.

The author of Chapter 8 and I have made the decision to exclude substantive consideration of operant and contingency management approaches from these two chapters on CB technique. Operant and contingency management approaches are clearly part of the overall behavior therapy approach to PSUDs, and in order to be most effective they are typically used in conjunction with each other. Due to the significant increase in the use of operant and contingency management approaches and the burgeoning research literature supporting the efficacy of these approaches it was our assessment that operant and contingency management approaches deserved extensive consideration in their own right. Chapters 9 and 10 in this volume present that discussion of operant and contingency management theory and technique. This is a somewhat artificial separation of CB from these other behavioral approaches. Therefore, we want to emphasize that, in practice, CB approaches are often used in conjunction with operant approaches.

Basic Assumptions

CB theories are based on psychological learning principles as delineated in animal and human experiments during the course of the last 75 years. The advent of the "cognitive revolution" in psychology in the 1970s (Baars, 1986) led to the addition of a number of components to theories of the development and treatment of PSUDs. The microtheories of behavior change that can be included under the rubric of CB differ from each other somewhat in the aspects of the person–environment interactions on which they focus. Nonetheless, regardless of the particular microtheory of behavior and behavior change on which a set of CB techniques is based, all share seven basic assumptions that characterize a CB approach to therapeutic change. These assumptions are outlined in Table 7.1.

First and most fundamental to these assumptions is the conviction that despite some evidence for biological or genetic components to human behavior, human behavior is largely learned. Many behavioral theorists (Bandura, 1977; Eysenck, 1982) assume that biological factors form a substrate on which a person's experiences build in producing individual patterns of behavior. Learning is thus the result of interactions between the person and the environment. While the process of learning may vary depending on the particular behavior at issue, biological and genetic factors are presumed by most CB theorists to take a backseat in the formation and change of behavior. CB theorists

---

TABLE 7.1. Basic Assumptions of Cognitive-Behavioral Theories of Psychoactive Substance Use Disorders and Their Treatment

1. Human behavior is largely learned rather than being predominantly determined by genetic factors.

2. The same learning processes that create problem behaviors can be used to change them.

3. Behavior is largely determined by contextual and environmental factors.

4. Covert behaviors such as thoughts and feelings are subject to change through the application of learning principles.

5. Actually engaging in new behaviors in the contexts in which they are to be performed is a critical part of behavior change.

6. Each client is unique and must be assessed as an individual in a particular context.

7. The cornerstone of adequate treatment is a thorough CB assessment.

tend to believe that biological and genetic factors are largely immutable given our current level of knowledge, and that change efforts are better focused on a higher-order level: that of behavior itself. Often the behavior focused on is the behavior that would help the person cope with the biological factors that may be maintaining substance use (e.g., withdrawal symptoms).

A corollary to the first assumption is that the same processes by which behavior develops can be harnessed in helping a person to change unwanted or undesirable behavior (Krasner, 1982). A sophisticated technology has been developed, and is described in more detail in the companion chapter to this one (Morgan, Chapter 8, this volume), based on the notion that any behavior shaped by learning can be reshaped, reduced, or even eliminated by the same process.

A third assumption is that contextual and environmental factors are significant in the initiation, maintenance, and change of behavior. Consistent with the focus of CB theories on person–environment interactions, many CB techniques focus explicitly on altering aspects of this interaction as a means of changing behavior. The degree to which importance is placed on changing environment versus changing individual reactions to the environment varies from microtheory to microtheory. Techniques such as the community reinforcement approach of Azrin and Sisson (Azrin, Sisson, Meyers, & Godley, 1982), based explicitly on operant learning theory, rely heavily on environmental changes to promote changes in behavior (see Chapters 9 and 10, this volume, for a more detailed discussion of such approaches). In contrast, more cognitive theories, such as those of Ellis (Ellis, McInerney, DiGiuseppe, & Yeager, 1988) and Beck (Beck, Wright, Newman, & Liese, 1993), place a greater emphasis on changing individual reactions to the environment. All, however, recognize the importance of context and environment in both the origins and treatment of PSUDs.

The fourth assumption common to CB approaches is that all behaviors that appear to be internal or covert (e.g., thoughts, feelings, and physiological changes) are changeable through the application of learning theory principles. This assumption has been borne out in numerous studies of the changes in internal processes that occur in response to treatment of a variety of disorders other than PSUDs. Specifically, there is substantial evidence from research on anxiety disorders and depression, among other disorders, that the application of learning theory-based approaches brings about changes in internal processes in addition to changes in overt observable behavior.

The fifth basic assumption is that techniques should emphasize actually engaging in new behaviors in the contexts that are problematic for clients. Whereas the practice of new skills and behaviors in the office setting is helpful as a first step in changing behavior, actual confrontation of problem situations in the real world is considered to be a more effective way of ensuring long-term behavior change.

Sixth, CB therapists assume that although general principles of behavior change can be applied to any client's circumstance, each client presents a unique case that requires a thorough understanding within a CB framework in order for treatment to be successful. Approaching each client uniquely means that CB therapists attempt to delineate the particular configuration of forces that produce and maintain the target behavior. Thus, while a cognitive behaviorist may believe that there are certain common errors in thinking and reasoning that produce or maintain substance use, each individual is still presumed to suffer from a combination of errors that is distinct.

The previous assumption leads logically into the seventh assumption: that treatment within a CB context must be preceded by a thorough and rigorous assessment of the client's behavior (Donovan, 1988). Without a thorough initial assessment focusing on how specific learning processes operate in a particular client's case, therapy and consequent behavior change are bound to fail.

In addition to adherence to these basic assumptions about the nature of PSUDs and the process of treatment and behavior change, cognitive behavioral theorists also place a heavy emphasis on empirical validation of the efficacy of their techniques. Although behavior therapy has often been equated with a rigid, mechanistic, and authoritarian approach to behavior change, nothing could be further from the truth in practice. Behavior therapists, and those who adhere to a cognitive behavioral theory of substance abuse treatment, by and large adopt an approach to the therapeutic enterprise that insists on rigorous, but humanistically based, application of well-validated principles to help people change unwanted behavior that is standing in the way of a more fulfilling life.

With the basic assumptions of CB theory as background, let us now turn to a consideration of the processes CB theorists view as central to the initiation, maintenance, and change of PSUDs. The discussion that follows is brief and presents only a bare outline of each process. (For more specific information about how these processes are applied to form a detailed theory of the development of PSUDs, see Abrams & Niaura, 1987.) Although focused on alcohol and alcoholism, this chapter provides a CB framework that is also applicable to other PSUDs.

BASIC COGNITIVE-BEHAVIORAL PROCESSES AND MODELS OF PSYCHOACTIVE SUBSTANCE USE DISORDERS

There are three basic learning theory processes that contribute to the initiation, maintenance, and change of behavior: classical conditioning, operant conditioning, and psychological modeling. These three processes form the core of most behavioral theories of substance abuse treatment. In addition, since the cognitive revolution in psychology, increasing emphasis has been placed by some theorists (notably those who adopt Bandura's, 1977, social learning models and followers of Ellis et al.'s, 1988, and Beck et al.'s, 1993, cognitive approaches) on the role of cognitive processes in the initiation and maintenance of behavior. In the sections that follow, I outline classical conditioning and modeling formulations of various aspects of PSUDs (leaving out operant conditioning, which is addressed in Chapters 9 and 10). I then discuss cognitive factors in substance abuse and treatment as presented in SLT and CB theories. The focus in the final sections is on how basic learning and cognitive processes are presumed to operate in substance abuse and can be brought to bear in changing substance use behavior.

Classical Conditioning

Classical conditioning is a basic learning process that was first intensively studied experimentally and systematically by the Russian physiologist Ivan Pavlov (1927) and the American psychologist J. B. Watson (1919) around the turn of the century. As one example of a classical conditioning paradigm, consider a person who drinks in a bar. The conditioned stimulus (CS), alcohol, is paired with the unconditioned stimulus (UCS), social interaction, until the alcohol itself elicits what the UCS formerly produced: feelings of warmth, satisfaction, and companionship. Of course, being with others might normally produce such feelings, but over time the alcohol on its own produces this conditioned response (CR). Whether a cue will elicit a CR depends, among other factors, on the frequency with which the UCS and the CS have been paired, the intensity of the CS when it is presented, and the physiological and psychological state of the organism at the time the CS is presented. Thus, for a hungry person, the mere sight of a picture of a Big Mac, without any of the associated cues of smell and taste, may elicit a salivation response or a subjective feeling of desire or craving to go out and buy lunch.

Classical conditioning has been most often invoked as the primary process by which environmental cues come to elicit urges or cravings to use psychoactive substances. While working at the U.S. Public Health Service Hospital in Lexington, Kentucky, in the 1960s, Wikler discovered that some of the chronic heroin users being treated there experienced what appeared to be withdrawal symptoms from the mere sight of the paraphernalia associated with heroin use. In a series of studies, Wikler and others (outlined in Wikler, 1965, 1973) provided addicts with paraphernalia and an opportunity to engage in the ritual of preparing and injecting what they thought to be heroin, but what was in reality an inert substance. In many of the subjects, the sight of the paraphernalia elicited physiological and subjective signs of withdrawal, which Wikler began to view as conditioned withdrawal phenomena. Moreover, when presented with the opportunity to "use" what they thought was heroin, these individuals often experienced a "high" even when the substance they injected was merely an inert solution that resembled heroin in appearance.

According to a classical conditioning model, in Wikler's studies the UCS was heroin and the UCR was the withdrawal symptoms and subsequent high that the users experienced after injecting heroin. The CS was the paraphernalia associated with heroin preparation and use and the CR was the pseudowithdrawal and pseudohigh experienced by the experimental subjects when preparing and injecting an inert solution. Based on findings such as these, classical conditioning theorists postulate that substance users actually condition many stimuli in the environment to the rituals, paraphernalia, and use of their drug of choice by repeatedly using the drug in specific settings, with specific people, and according to a specific ritual. The types and variety of cues that become CSs for substance users are vast, and the specific cues are unique to each individual's experience and substance use pattern.

Classical conditioning theory has formed the basis for at least four prominent procedures in the treatment of PSUDs: cue exposure treatments (e.g., Childress et al., 1993; McLellan, Childress, Ehrman, & O'Brien, 1986), stimulus control techniques (e.g., Bickel & Kelly, 1988), relaxation training (e.g., Monti, Cooney, Kadden, Rohsenow, & Abrams, 2002), and covert sensitization and other aversion therapy techniques (Rimmele, Miller, & Dougher, 1989). In addition, they form part of the theoretical basis for teaching drinking refusal skills (Monti et al., 2002). Other than aversion therapy, all these procedures attempt, at least in part, to break the conditioned connection between particular aspects of the client's environment and the conditioned withdrawal or cravings presumed to form the motivational basis for substance seeking and subsequent use. Aversion therapy and its variant covert sensitization apply classical conditioning theory in a different fashion by attempting to condition a new, aversive response to substance use and the cues associated with it.

Modeling

Modeling (Bandura, 1977) is a second basic learning process that has been used in developing CB theories of substance abuse treatment. Of the three basic learning processes (the others being classical conditioning and operant conditioning), modeling is the one that appears to be most efficient and most rapid in producing new learning. Modeling involves, as its name implies, observation of another's behavior and then performance of that behavior given appropriate reinforcement contingencies. Modeling is an efficient way to learn new behaviors because humans can learn many complex behaviors with very few observations. In fact, many complicated behaviors can be learned and accurately performed after only a single observation.

The modern theory of modeling began with the work of Albert Bandura (1977), also one of the founders of SLT. He and his coworkers mapped out the parameters of modeling as a learning process. Modeling involves two subprocesses: observational learning and performance. Learning can occur by observation, and the newly learned behavior can be reproduced quite accurately without any prior practice. Bandura postulates that a process of cognitive mapping occurs at this stage in which the individual stores aspects of the behavior that are later reproduced from this cognitive map. The adequacy with which this cognitive representation of the modeled behavior occurs depends on, among other factors, how well the observer attended to the model's behavior and how the behavior was encoded (e.g., verbal, visual, tactile, etc.). The more modalities the learner uses to encode the behavior, the more efficiently the behavior is learned. Thus, when sensory, emotional, cognitive, and motor modalities are all engaged in encoding newly modeled behavior, that behavior is most efficiently stored and retrieved.

Whether behavior learned by observation will actually be performed depends on factors other than the cognitive map. The actual performance of the behavior depends on characteristics of the model (e.g., the degree to which the observer holds the model in esteem and as a person to be imitated), whether the model is seen as being reinforced or punished for engaging in the behavior, whether the observer has an incentive to perform the modeled behavior, and whether the observer expects to be reinforced in a similar fashion to the model if the behavior is performed.

Modeling processes have been strongly implicated in the development of PSUDs in adolescence. Adolescents who observe substance-using peers with whom they wish to relate, or the behavior of persons whom they view as powerful or popular and who use alcohol or drugs, may both learn and perform those behaviors quite rapidly. Modeling also influences the maintenance of PSUDs in that people will often engage in behaviors that members of their peer group engage in as a means of ensuring inclusion in the group.

The efficiency of modeling as a learning process (it can occur in only a few trials, without the necessity of repeated experiences, as is the case in both classical and operant learning) has led to its utilization as a major process in CB treatment of PSUDs. Persons with PSUDs often lack skills that would enable them to cope with situations that evoke substance use. Persons who lack assertiveness or refusal skills or who are prone to inappropriate thought processes that lead to substance use can be taught new skills and thought processes by observing skilled others modeling those processes and behaviors. Thus, modeling theory provides the theoretical basis for social skills approaches to the treatment of PSUDs, as well as forming a component of the teaching of other intrapersonal skills such as relaxation, coping self-statements, and anger management. Almost any new behavior that does not rely directly on repeated pairings of environmental stimuli with client responses can be taught or its teaching enhanced by inclusion of modeling processes.

Cognitive Mediation of Behavior

Cognitive mediation of behavior is another basic process that CB theorists have integrated into their thinking about PSUDs, particularly since the 1970s. Several theoretical accounts of PSUDs heavily emphasize the roles of various cognitive processes in the initiation, maintenance, and change of substance use behavior (e.g., Abrams & Niaura, 1987; Goldman, Brown, & Christiansen, 1987; Sher, 1987). These cognitive theories vary in the amount of emphasis they place on cognitive mediators, but all rely heavily on the three basic learning processes to promote behavior change in treatment.

SLT represents an extension of the theories of classical conditioning, operant conditioning, and modeling as previously discussed. In addition, SLT assumes that certain cognitive factors mediate these basic learning processes. Primarily associated with the work of Bandura (1977), SLT is a comprehensive theory of the development, maintenance, and change of learned behavior. While firmly rooted in the animal experimental literature, SLT research has focused largely on humans. In a nutshell, SLT postulates that human behavior develops by a combination of classical conditioning, operant conditioning, and modeling, which not only produce overt behaviors but lead to the development of patterns of thought and emotion that themselves guide and shape behavior.

A central concept in SLT is *reciprocal determinism*, the belief that people both influence and are influenced by their environments. This implies that behavior change can be brought about by changing a person's environment, but it also implies that behavior change can be engineered by the person him- or herself through a planned process of self-control or self-initiated changes in his or her environment. This "self" control is a central feature of SLT-based approaches to treatment of PSUDs.

In addition to postulating a reciprocally determined relationship between environment and behavior, SLT emphasizes the role of cognition in the control and performance of behavior. A person's thoughts, feelings, and expectations with regard to whether a particular behavior will be reinforced, his or her confidence about the adequacy with which the behavior can be performed, and the level of skill that person can bring to bear to cope with problematic situations—all these influence the coping strategies and behaviors he/she will use in navigating through life. The interaction of expectations and skill levels is encapsulated in the notion of self-efficacy, a central concept of SLT. *Self-efficacy* refers to the person's expectations that he or she will be able to perform a coping response in a given situation, coupled with the expectation that performance of that response will be reinforced. The extent to which a person lacks requisite coping skills, or views his or her ability to execute those skills as being deficient, contributes to the person's self-efficacy expectations for coping in a given situation. According to SLT, self-efficacy expectations are primary cognitive mediators that determine whether or not a person will engage in a particular coping response. When self-efficacy is high, the person will be more likely to enact that skill in an attempt to cope with life. If, on the other hand, self-efficacy is low with regard to a particular skill, the person will likely choose some other skill or coping strategy with which he or she feels more comfortable.

SLT views PSUDs as basically a failure of coping (Abrams & Niaura,

1987). This failure may be due to any combination of inappropriate conditioning, reinforcement contingencies, modeling of inappropriate behaviors, failure to model appropriate coping skills, and reduced self-efficacy with regard to behaviors that not only enhance coping but are also widely reinforced. Failure to perform skills one already knows may also be the result of reduced self-efficacy or outcome expectations or may be due to physiological, emotional, or other cognitive factors that interfere with effective skill performance.

Following logically from this view of PSUDs, SLT-based approaches to treatment of PSUDs emphasize skills training and practice. In addition, SLT approaches seek not only to teach skills for coping with known stresses or problems but to enhance the possibility of future avoidance of substance use by helping the client anticipate situations in which he or she either lacks appropriate coping skills or has low self-efficacy with regard to performance of those skills. This process, coupled with teaching clients to address the cognitive aspects of relapse (e.g., how to cope with the abstinence violation effect that results from a slip back to use after a period of abstinence) forms the core of relapse prevention approaches to PSUDs (Marlatt & Gordon, 1985). Treatments within this framework are initiated following a thorough functional analysis of substance use behavior to determine whether substance use is maintained because the person lacks other coping skills, because the person has adequate coping skills but low self-efficacy expectations with regard to using those skills, or because the person expects that using the available coping skills will be ineffective. The client is also assessed with regard to physiological or emotional factors that may be interfering with skill performance (e.g., high levels of anxiety, depression, or anger) or which may themselves drive substance use. Assessment of skills and expectations continues throughout treatment in order to measure progress toward adequate, substance-free coping.

Treatments that have been developed within an SLT framework include social and communication skills training, assertiveness training, anger and stress management training, self-control training, and relapse prevention training following a model developed by Marlatt (Marlatt & Gordon, 1985). Marital and family approaches to treatment have also been developed from an SLT perspective (see McCrady, Epstein, & Sell, Chapter 5, this volume).

Two other cognitive theories of treatment bear mention. These have grown primarily out of the work of two theorists: Ellis, the founder of rational–emotive therapy (RET), and Beck, the founder of cognitive therapy (CT). Although differing somewhat in their details, both of these cognitive theories view thought (cognition) as a primary causal factor in emotion and substance use, and regard abuse primarily as an effort to cope with negative emotional states that arise as a result of illogical or distorted thinking.

Ellis's (Ellis et al., 1988) RET approach is an excellent example of how a cognitive framework addresses the role of cognition (thoughts) in the development of emotional disturbance and the consequent development of PSUDs in some people as a means of coping with negative emotions. Ellis has developed what he calls the A–B–C model of emotion. According to the A–B–C model of emotion, the events or situations a person encounters (A) do not, in and of themselves, create negative emotions. Rather the person's assessment or interpretation (B) of the meaning of events based on his or her beliefs is what creates the negative emotion (C). In order for change in emotions to occur, the client must begin to identify and challenge the thoughts occurring at B through a process of rational disputation. Ellis has identified a variety of irrational beliefs that, coupled with what he views as the addict's inability to tolerate frustration or other negative emotions, are believed to set the stage for use of drugs or alcohol as a means of coping with negative emotions. According to Ellis, a further factor that triggers alcohol or drug use to cope with emotions is poor ability to tolerate negative affect. This results in a belief that Ellis calls "I-can't-stand-it-itis." This belief prompts people suffering from PSUDs to react impulsively in order to alleviate negative emotions immediately. Ellis refers to this tendency as low frustration tolerance and believes that this additional set of beliefs must be addressed for substance abuse to be successfully treated.

Beck (Beck, Rush, Shaw, & Emery, 1979; Beck et al., 1993) has also articulated a complex theory of negative emotion based on an inventory of illogical or irrational reasoning processes that he terms "core beliefs." These beliefs are commonly held, but irrational, ideas about the nature of the world or what a person needs in order to lead a contented life. When the person faces a problematic situation or other activating cues, these core beliefs are activated as a way of construing the meaning of the experience and of generating coping responses. Because these core beliefs are maladaptive or illogical, the coping responses they trigger are often illogical or maladaptive. Coupled with these core beliefs are highly stereotyped "automatic" thoughts, which are similar to the "B" component of Ellis's A–B–C model of emotion. The occurrence of these automatic thoughts is presumed to activate urges or cravings to use drugs or alcohol to alleviate negative emotions produced by the automatic thoughts. Action on urges or cravings in substance abusers is presumably triggered by additional thoughts or beliefs, which Beck terms "facilitating beliefs." Facilitating beliefs are, in Beck's model, the proximate cause of drug- and alcohol-seeking behavior in an addicted person faced with problematic situations or emotions.

Despite their emphasis on cognitive processes, cognitive therapies rely heavily on techniques based on SLT to facilitate the changes in cognition that are viewed as being crucial to the treatment of PSUDs. Cognitive theorists do, however, believe that lasting behavior change is difficult to achieve without changing the underlying faulty patterns of thinking that lie at the root of most emotional upsets and thereby trigger substance use.

Techniques for treating PSUDs that derive wholly or in part from cognitive theories are anger management training, rational disputation of positive thoughts about alcohol/drug use, and rational disputation of thoughts linking substance use to alleviation of negative emotional states. Techniques based on cognitive theory tend to blend quite nicely with SLT-based techniques. Current research aimed at enhancing aspects of techniques based on other behavioral theories (e.g., cue–exposure based on classical conditioning theory) is beginning to incorporate explicit cognitive strategies into treatment. With its flexibility and inclusiveness, SLT has emerged in the last two decades as the predominant CB theory of addictions origin and treatment.

With this brief overview of CB theories of substance abuse treatment in mind, let us now turn to a discussion of critical issues in treating substance abusers as viewed through the lens of CB theory. These issues are discussed from the perspective of SLT because that theory provides the most comprehensive behavior theoretical framework currently available.

CRITICAL ISSUES IN SUBSTANCE ABUSE TREATMENT

Etiology and Maintenance of Substance Use

CB theories view PSUDs as resulting from a combination of factors presumed to interact in different ways to produce PSUDs depending on each individual's unique characteristics and environment. Although explicitly endorsing a "biopsychosocial" perspective from which to view the origins of PSUDs, CB theories tend to minimize the causal role of genetic factors while placing a heavier emphasis on the interacting influences of an individual's environment, innate biological makeup or temperament, and learning processes. These factors are presumed to interact with each other in individual-specific fashion to produce PSUDs.

CB theories view the initiation of substance use as primarily due to a combination of environmental factors (particularly substance availability and peer group norms) and individual physiological responses to initial use, resulting in substance use being either reinforcing or punishing for the individual. Whether substance use will be initiated and continued depends on the availability of substances in a person's environment, peer group behavior and norms with respect to substance use, the degree of importance of the peer group in the individual's life, and whether or not initial use of the substance is pleasurable. Parental attitudes and behaviors also play a role, with parental behavior being more likely to be modeled than parental dictates, especially if other factors (e.g., substance availability or peer group norms) favor substance use. The combined effect of these factors is the development of drinking and drug use outcome expectancies that appear to play an important role in the initiation and maintenance of early drinking (Christiansen, Smith, Roehling, & Goldman, 1989).

For persons who develop PSUDs, CB theories postulate that the pharmacological and social reinforcements attendant on initial use increase the probability of substance use behavior. With increased use, the person begins to recognize the role that drugs or alcohol can play in reducing negative emotions and may fail to learn alternative coping responses. In a somewhat different fashion, persons who have failed to learn adequate coping skills prior to the onset of substance use may begin to use drugs or alcohol as a means of compensating for the lack of those skills. Finally, some substance users may, by virtue of temperamental factors such as sensation seeking and impulsivity, use alcohol or drugs initially for their excitement-producing properties rather than as a means of coping.

The processes presumed to operate in the development of PSUDs at the earliest, or less severe, stages are largely modeling, operant conditioning (reinforcement of substance use), and cognitive mediators such as expectancies that substance use will result in highly positive outcomes. With repeated substance use and at more severe stages of dependence, classical conditioning factors begin to play a more prominent role in the development of PSUDs, with both conditioned craving and withdrawal playing an important part in producing severe dependence in some individuals. There is also evidence that tolerance is, at least to some extent, a learned phenomenon (Vogel-Sprott, 1992). At severe levels of dependence, use is often driven by the reinforcing value of avoiding withdrawal (negative reinforcement) rather than the pleasurable effects of use. It is clear that at more severe levels of dependence, the person's body has adapted to the continuing presence of alcohol or drugs, and that these physiological changes play an important role in shifting the reinforcing contingencies of substance use. At this latter stage, CB theories of treatment shift the focus of treatment somewhat toward coping with the effects of these physiological changes, particularly withdrawal symptoms that may trigger a return to use following brief abstinence. Nonetheless, the basic processes by which treatment proceeds remain the same and involve implementation of learning strategies to cope with the long-term effects of substance use.

As substance use begins to assume a greater role in the individual's life, the negative consequences of use may also increase. These consequences are often unique to the individual and may require active coping responses. Coping skill deficits become important again as the individual may be unable to cope with the problems associated with substance use itself (e.g., family, work, or legal problems) and increase their use in an effort to cope with increasingly frequent negative emotions. The immediate reinforcing value of substance use assumes a prominent role in maintaining the habit, despite the negative consequences, because substance use produces immediate reinforcement whereas the punishment of negative consequences might be greatly delayed.

As the severity of an individual's PSUD increases, several things may happen. Often substance use itself becomes stereotyped and limited to certain situations. These settings and the associated stimuli may become conditioned to substance use and come to elicit physiological or psychological responses that further prompt it. With increasingly complex problems to face, the individual's coping skills may be overwhelmed and his or her substance use increased as a means of alleviating the negative emotions that stem from failure to cope adequately.

Associations with peer groups whose members are themselves substance users may exert pressure on the individual to maintain substance use as a means of interaction with peers or of retaining the reinforcement of group membership. Peers may also reinforce unrealistically positive expectancies for drug or alcohol by their own behavior under the influence.

Consistent with natural history studies of the development of PSUDs, CB theories suggest that although the nature and quality of reinforcement for substance use may change over the course of a particular individual's substance use history, principles of classical conditioning, operant conditioning, modeling, and cognitive mediation of behavior still operate in maintaining substance use behavior. In the many cases now being documented in which persons suffering from PSUDs stop using drugs or alcohol on their own without any treatment, a combination of shifting reinforcement contingencies and cognitive changes appears to explain the change in behavior (Sobell, Sobell, Toneatto, & Leo, 1993).

Homogeneity/Heterogeneity of Persons with Psychoactive Substance Use Disorders

CB theories are entirely consistent with current views of substance use as falling along a continuum ranging from no use at all to severely dependent use (Institute of Medicine, 1990). CB theories view each individual as forming a unique constellation of biological bases, learning history, and current environment. In spite of the uniqueness of every individual's substance use history, CB theories believe that there are also commonalities among substance users and abusers. Nonetheless, CB theories tend to minimize the importance of global subtyping or labeling of individuals in treatment. Although guided by empirical evidence that suggests differences in treatment outcomes and the advisability of various treatment goals among persons with PSUDs who have particular genetic backgrounds, personality makeups, and environments, CB theorists tend to use these data as guidelines rather than as strict determinants of treatment.

In essence, although CB theorists recognize groups of PSUDs that result from personality disorders, depression, or anxiety, a thorough assessment and treatment must still be based on an individualized CB analysis rather than on assumptions about group membership. CB theories of treatment emphasize the matching of treatment procedures and goals to patient needs to a greater extent than do other theories of treatment. Although the therapist's armamentarium of techniques is relatively constant, the application of those techniques is based on analyses of a particular client's skill assets and deficits.

Role of Genetics/Biological Factors in Psychoactive Substance Use Disorders

It would be foolish to deny that human beings are to some extent the product of their biology. All behavior at the levels at which therapy takes place (e.g., the overtly or subjectively observable) ultimately has a biological substrate. All learning, at bottom, involves changes at the neuronal level, if not change at the molecular level. The role of genetics in human behavior is not clearly specified, and at the present time the genetic substrate of human behavior is immutable by available methods. Thus, while biological and genetic factors are viewed as risk factors that must be taken into account in one's analysis of a particular individual's substance use patterns and addressed in the selection of treatment goals, they do not play a significant role in treatment itself.

CB theorists believe that changes in behavior require something more than changes in a person's biological or neurochemical functioning. This belief rests on the assumption that environmental contingencies play a key role in the cause and control of behavior, as well as on the notion that skill assets and deficits are important contributors to the development, maintenance, and change of PSUDs.

CB theories of change emphasize helping the client to learn coping skills that will be more effective in managing day-to-day life without using drugs or alcohol. While not rejecting the potential role of pharmacotherapeutic interventions, CB theorists point out that although some effective pharmacotherapeutic measures exist for helping some persons with PSUDs (e.g., disulfiram [Antabuse] for alcoholics [Volpicelli, Alterman, Hayashida & O'Brien, 1992] and opiate addicts), these approaches have not yet made a wide impact on the treatment of PSUDs. The reason for this relatively minimal impact to date is most likely due to difficulties in persuading persons with PSUDs to take these medications reliably, and to a lack of knowledge as to which clients will best respond to pharmacological interventions. This sort of client–treatment matching is an issue that CB treatment techniques are uniquely equipped to address.

Tasks of Treatment

CB theories typically view treatment as needing to accomplish several tasks in order to be successful. As with all psychosocial treatment approaches, the first task in treatment, if necessary, is to detoxify the client from hazardous or potentially life-threatening levels of substance use, preferably to a level of temporary abstinence, although CB theories do not usually make total abstinence a precondition for treatment, or even a necessary treatment goal for some clients.

Once detoxification has been accomplished, the therapist must conduct, in collaboration with the client, a thorough functional analysis of substance use behavior and its triggering and maintaining factors. This analysis should focus on both skill deficits and on the client's environment, with a particular emphasis on identifying those person-specific (e.g., emotional states and thoughts) and environmental factors that are associated with, or perhaps trigger, substance use. These high-risk situations, which may be both internal and external, need to be addressed in order for treatment to succeed and treatment gains to be maintained. Without this thorough assessment, treatment cannot proceed and is likely to fail.

Following a functional analysis, work then proceeds on teaching the client a specifically tailored menu of techniques and strategies aimed at intervening in the problems identified in the assessment. In CB treatments, assessment and treatment are closely linked, and assessment is reiterated throughout the process of treatment in order to gauge progress and identify continuing problem areas and behaviors. The fact that problems may continue to emerge during treatment reinforces the importance of ongoing assessment.

The final task of CB treatments is to assist the client in identifying and planning strategies for coping with high-risk situations that may occur in the future. This task is designed to provide the client with the tools necessary to prevent relapse to substance use—the core of CB notions of relapse prevention. Clients are also taught how to cope with slips or relapses, should they occur, in ways that will shorten the length and intensity of any future return to substance use.

The three core tasks of treatment from a CB perspective—functional analysis, skills training, and relapse prevention—are accomplished both by individual work with the client and by helping the client make active attempts to change environmental factors that may be triggering or maintaining substance use. Thus, clients may be encouraged to make significant lifestyle changes, or changes in their daily routine or interactions with family and friends, that the functional analysis suggests might enhance the client's ability to cope without the use of drugs or alcohol. Although not always explicitly addressed, the key role of the environment in PSUDs is always a factor in guiding treatment.

Treatment Goals

Because they place heavy emphasis on matching treatments to specific client characteristics and needs, CB approaches to the treatment of PSUDs, imply flexibility in the selection of treatment goals. Unlike other theoretical positions that insist on abstinence as the only legitimate goal of treatment and that often make abstinence a prerequisite for treatment entry, CB theories allow for a more flexible and incremental approach to substance use reduction that is often more attractive to clients who might otherwise avoid treatment.

Although individual therapists may vary in the degree to which they insist on an abstinence goal for their clients, there is a substantial body of literature suggesting that many persons with PSUDs, particularly those with less severe dependence, can and do become moderate users, often without any treatment at all (Booth, Dale, Slade, & Dewey, 1992; Duckert, Amundsen, & Johnsen, 1992; Sobell et al., 1993). In fact, many who have been treated for PSUDs in abstinence-oriented programs become moderate users, and many who set out to achieve only a reduction in substance use ultimately become abstinent. There appear to be cognitive variables that have an impact upon the decision to change substance use behavior. There are now data to suggest that a particular individual's stage of readiness to change (Prochaska, DiClemente, & Norcross, 1992) strongly influences the process of treatment participation and commitment.

Being guided by the scientific literature, CB oriented therapists will typically work with a client incrementally toward abstinence and its maintenance, if that is what the client insists on, and if the client's level of substance use at treatment entry does not carry with it the risk of immediate catastrophic consequences (e.g., liver failure, legal contingencies) if some level of use continues. The process of goal determination is one of negotiation rather than therapist insistence, consistent with the notion that the more committed the client is to the particular treatment goal, the greater the likelihood of reaching it.

Recently, another approach to treatment goals has emerged that has been termed "harm reduction" (Marlatt & Tapert, 1993). The harm reduction approach attempts to reflect the realities of treating persons with PSUDs in recognizing that complete lifelong abstinence is often extremely difficult to accomplish, even though that may be the healthiest goal for a particular client, even when a client is committed to abstinence. When immediate cessation of substance use is not likely to or does not occur (due, perhaps, to the severity of the individual's PSUD), taking a harm reduction approach leads to working in an incremental fashion, in smaller steps, toward an ultimate goal of abstinence. The ultimate aim of harm reduction is to enhance health by minimizing or reducing the impact of behaviors or other factors that threaten health. From this perspective, any change in the environment or client behavior that leads to reduced substance use is one that should be promoted.

EMPIRICAL RESEARCH AND COGNITIVE-BEHAVIORAL THEORY

Of all the approaches presented in this book, with the exception of motivational and pharmacotherapeutic approaches, cognitive-behaviorally based approaches are the most closely linked with existing scientific knowledge of PSUDs. Empirical validation of treatment techniques has been an integral part of the CB theory of treatment from the beginnings of the behavior therapy movement in the early 1950s. CB therapists view each client and his or her treatment as, in a sense, a minilaboratory within which the therapist and client collaborate to assess client needs and apply and evaluate the effect of various treatment technologies.

Not only are CB treatments open to scientific scrutiny, they insist on it. Without well-designed experimental studies of treatment outcomes, CB theorists believe that no progress can be made toward resolving the most difficult issue when treating PSUDs: what treatments work best under what conditions with what clients. This is the crux of the patient–treatment matching research that has been conducted under the auspices of the National Institute of Alcohol Abuse and Alcoholism (Donovan & Mattson, 1994). The behavior therapy movement, from which CB theories of treating PSUDs are derived, insists on empirical validation of the techniques used to treat clients as a cornerstone of ethical professional practice. To apply scientifically untested or untestable techniques routinely, solely on the basis of single case histories or client testimonials, is considered by most CB therapists to be unethical practice, especially when empirically validated techniques exist and could be more widely used were practitioners aware of them.

ADVANTAGES AND DISADVANTAGES OF COGNITIVE-BEHAVIORAL APPROACHES

Advantages of Cognitive-Behavioral Approaches

Approaches to treating PSUDs based on CB theory have a number of advantages over other currently available approaches to treatment. This can be seen by the extent to which concepts that were originally developed by CB theorists (e.g., Marlatt's [Marlatt & Gordon, 1985; Marlatt & Tapert, 1993] relapse prevention concept) have begun to be incorporated, although often in altered form, into the practice of therapists trained in other approaches (Morgenstern & McCrady, 1992; Rotgers & Morgenstern, 1994). There are seven clear advantages to adopting a CB view of PSUDs and their treatment. These are outlined briefly in Table 7.2.

FLEXIBILITY IN TAILORING TREATMENT TO CLIENT NEEDS

Because CB approaches eschew global labeling and place a heavy emphasis on individualized assessment, they are ideally suited to matching treatments to client needs. This flexibility extends to treatment goal selection as well as to se-

**TABLE 7.2. Advantages of Cognitive-Behavioral Theories
of Psychoactive Substance Use Disorders and Their Treatment**

1. Flexibility in meeting specific client needs.
2. Readily accepted by clients due to high level of client involvement in treatment planning and goal selection.
3. Soundly grounded in established psychological theory.
4. Emphasis on linking scientific knowledge to treatment practice.
5. Clear guidelines for assessing treatment progress.
6. Empowerment of clients in making their own behavior change.
7. Strong empirical and scientific evidence of efficacy.

lection of the particular interventions to be used with a given client. CB theory allows for specific matching of client problems, goals, and readiness for change, as well as selection of treatment interventions.

READY ACCEPTANCE BY CLIENTS THROUGH AVOIDANCE
OF LABELING AND GOAL IMPOSITION

CB treatments for PSUDs are readily accepted by clients. This is because therapists operating within this perspective adopt a collaborative rather than a confrontational stance with clients and avoid labeling them with terms that in our society carry pejorative connotations. Likewise, CB approaches are explicitly carried out in a collaborative fashion in which client input is given a high level of attention and consideration. Clients are not forced to accept a unitary explanation of their behavior as a precondition for behavior change efforts. CB theory allows for a high degree of individualization of treatment, in contrast to other approaches that attempt to apply a similar formula for recovery to all clients.

Within traditional approaches, if a client rejects that approach's conception of PSUDs and what is necessary to bring about change, treatment is likely to fail. The therapist is then often left with only two alternatives if he or she wishes to remain within the constraints of the approach: to continue to attempt to convince the client of the validity of the approach or to terminate treatment. If the therapist adopts the first approach, the results are often countertherapeutic due to the elicitation of strong reactance on the part of the client against the therapist's views. This is likely to lead to treatment dropout and may become a barrier to that client seeking treatment elsewhere.

SOUND BASIS IN PSYCHOLOGICAL THEORY

Unlike other widely used approaches, CB approaches have a clear, coherent, well-tested theoretical basis that is rooted in scientific psychology. Having a clear, coherent theory of behavior change has been cited as a factor in treatment success in substance abuse treatment (Onken, 1991).

EMPHASIS ON LINKING SCIENCE TO TREATMENT

A corollary to this sound basis in psychological science is a strong emphasis on linking science to treatment. Scientific evaluation and knowledge are important both at the individual client–therapist level and at the systemic or treatment system level. In the client–therapist relationship, the emphasis on continuous testing of assessment hypotheses and technique success is integral to the achievement of behavior change. At the systemic level, scientific evaluation of techniques derived from CB theory plays an integral role in ensuring that consumers of CB treatments get the best available treatment and in providing the scientific knowledge that can lead to development of more efficient and more effective treatments in the future.

CLEAR GUIDELINES FOR ASSESSING TREATMENT PROGRESS

By focusing on continued assessment of the factors contributing to a particular client's substance use, as well as the degree to which clients are learning and implementing new coping skills and lifestyle changes, CB approaches provide clear milestones for evaluating individual treatment progress or the lack thereof. Knowing whether and how well a client is progressing is essential both to altering treatment strategies that may be ineffective and to determining when it is appropriate to terminate treatment with a particular client. Because client and therapist mutually agree upon treatment goals at the beginning of treatment, progress toward termination is more easily assessed. This allows the length of treatment to be tailored explicitly to client needs on the basis of definable criteria.

EMPOWERMENT OF CLIENTS AS EFFECTIVE AGENTS
IN CHANGING THEIR OWN BEHAVIOR

In contrast to traditional approaches that emphasize, in somewhat paradoxical (and often puzzling-to-clients) fashion, clients' powerlessness over their own addiction, CB approaches explicitly attempt to enhance clients' sense of personal efficacy and problem-solving ability. By teaching clients not only that they can be effective problem solvers without using alcohol or drugs to cope but that they can learn new skills necessary to solve new, unforeseen problems in the future, CB techniques accomplish two major tasks: they destigmatize addiction and help enhance self-efficacy and self-esteem. In a related way, they may also reduce the need for future treatment by teaching clients the requisite skills to analyze and solve problems themselves. In this, CB approaches are consistent with the adage, "When you give a man a fish, you feed him for a day, but when you teach him to fish, you feed him for a lifetime."

EMPIRICAL EVIDENCE OF EFFICACY

In contrast to the bulk of treatment approaches currently employed in practice, approaches based on CB theory have garnered substantial scientific evidence of efficacy in controlled clinical trials (Holder, Longabaugh, Miller, & Rubonis, 1991). In addition, there is evidence that CB approaches may be more effective than other approaches with a group of clients that have generally poor prognosis: those that suffer from antisocial personality disorder (Kadden, Cooney, Getter, & Litt, 1989). Given evidence that a very high percentage of clients with PSUDs also suffer from antisocial personality disorder (Regier et al., 1990; Ross, Glaser, & Germanson, 1988), the finding of relative efficacy of CB techniques with this group is a strong reason to consider them.

Disadvantages of Cognitive-Behavioral Approaches

Despite the numerous advantages just presented, CB approaches as they currently exist have several disadvantages. These disadvantages have more to do with the current state of scientific knowledge than with any inherent difficulties with CB approaches. As scientific knowledge accumulates, it is likely that these disadvantages will disappear. As it now stands, these disadvantages could more reasonably be termed "limitations" of the approach.

First, while there is evidence of differential effectiveness for CB approaches, the exact reason for this is unclear. For example, the extent to which clients actually use the skills they are taught in treatment and the relationship of skill use to relapse or maintenance of change are unclear.

Second, there is a distinct, and surprising lack of empirical support for the advantage of adding relapse prevention procedures to treatment as a means of enhancing long-term outcomes. Although some data suggest that those who learn relapse prevention techniques are able to curtail the length and severity of their relapses, the overall advantage predicted to accrue to clients as a result of the introduction of relapse prevention technologies has not been strongly validated empirically (Wilson, 1992).

Third, and unrelated to the scientific basis of CB techniques, is the fact that few treatment providers are well trained in these techniques, and that some aspects of CB practice are rejected out of hand by some therapists working from a more traditional perspective. Specifically, some who hold a more traditional perspective reject the possibility of moderated use as a treatment goal, in spite of evidence that moderated use can be common under certain conditions (Miller, Walters, & Bennett, 2001).

The lack of emphasis on a spiritual aspect to PSUDs is also disturbing to some practitioners, particularly ones who have themselves benefited from more traditional, 12-step-based approaches to treatment, predominantly a reflection of the Alcoholics Anonymous philosophy. Although a CB approach is not inherently antithetical to a spiritual notion of PSUDs, the notion of powerlessness often associated with spirituality in addictions treatment is. For those who rely more strongly on personal belief rather than on scientific evidence to guide their practice, this may be an unbreachable barrier to the use of CB techniques in practice. For patients who reject the spiritual aspects of Alcoholics Anonymous, there are a number of alternative self-help approaches, such as Rational Recovery, that are more directly based on CB approaches to recovery (McCrady & Delaney, 1995; Trimpey, 1992).

CONCLUSION

In the last quarter century, CB theories have been among the most productive in advancing empirically validated knowledge of the origins and treatment of PSUDs. The notion of solidly basing treatment on knowledge of the psychological processes of human behavior has led to the development of a variety of new, demonstrably effective, treatment technologies. Marital/family and motivational approaches (discussed elsewhere in this volume) are based largely on the work of CB theorists, although substantial progress beyond basic CB theory characterizes those approaches as well.

Although CB based treatments still do not reliably and predictably produce the sorts of treatment outcomes all therapists desire (i.e., long-lasting, positive behavior change), they do offer some of the most promising approaches currently available to therapists treating PSUDS. They also hold the promise, based on the strong emphasis by CB oriented therapists on scientific study of both the efficacy and process of behavior change in addictions, of advancing our knowledge of how best to treat these difficult and socially costly problems.

REFERENCES

Abrams, D. B., & Niaura, R. S. (1987). Social learning theory. In H. T. Blane & K. E. Leonard (Eds.), *Psychological theories of drinking and alcoholism* (pp. 131–178). New York: Guilford Press.

Azrin, N. H., Sisson, R. W., Meyers, R., & Godley, M. (1982). Alcoholism treatment by disulfiram and community reinforcement therapy. *Journal of Behavior Therapy and Experimental Psychiatry, 13*, 105–112.

Baars, B. J. (1986). *The cognitive revolution in psychology.* New York: Guilford Press.

Bandura, A. (1977). *Social learning theory.* Englewood Cliffs, NJ: Prentice-Hall.

Beck, A. T., Rush, A. J., Shaw, B. F., & Emery, G. (1979). *Cognitive therapy of depression.* New York: Guilford Press.

Beck, A. T., Wright, E. D., Newman, C. F., & Liese, B. S. (1993). *Cognitive therapy of substance abuse.* New York: Guilford Press.

Bickel, W. K., & Kelly, T. H. (1988). The relationship of stimulus control to the treatment of substance abuse. In B. A. Ray (Ed.), *Learning factors in substance abuse* (NIDA Research Monograph 84, pp. 122–140). Washington, DC: U.S. Government Printing Office.

Booth, P. B., Dale, B., Slade, P. D., & Dewey, M. E. (1992). A follow-up study of problem drinkers offered a goal choice option. *Journal of Studies on Alcohol, 53,* 594–600.

Childress, A. R., Hole, A. V., Ehrman, R. N., Robbins, S. J., McLellan, A. T., & O'Brien, C. P. (1993). Cue reactivity and cue reactivity interventions in drug dependence. In L. S. Onken, J. D. Blame, & J. J. Boren (Eds.), *Behavioral treatments for drug abuse and dependence* (NIDA Research Monograph 137, pp. 73–96). Washington, DC: U.S. Government Printing Office.

Christiansen, B. A., Smith, G. T., Roehling, P. V., & Goldman, M. S. (1989). Using alcohol expectancies to predict adolescent drinking behavior after one year. *Journal of Consulting and Clinical Psychology, 57,* 93–99.

Donovan, D. M. (1988). Assessment of addictive behaviors: Implications of an emerging biopsychosocial model. In D. M. Donovan & G. A. Marlatt (Eds.), *Assessment of addictive behaviors* (pp. 5–14). New York: Guilford Press.

Donovan, D. M., & Mattson, M. E. (Eds.). (1994, December). Alcoholism treatment matching research: Methodological and clinical approaches. *Journal of Studies on Alcohol* (Suppl. No. 12), 5–14.

Duckert, E., Amundsen, A., & Johnsen, J. (1992). What happens to drinking after therapeutic intervention? *British Journal of Addiction, 87,* 1457–1467.

Ellis, A., McInerney, J. F., DiGiuseppe, R., & Yeager, R. J. (1988). *Rational–emotive therapy with alcoholics and substance abusers.* New York: Pergamon Press.

Eysenck, H. J. (1982). Neobehavioristic (S–R) theory. In G. T. Wilson & C. M. Franks (Eds.), *Contemporary behavior therapy: Conceptual and empirical foundations* (pp. 205–276). New York: Guilford Press.

Goldman, M. S., Brown, S. A., & Christiansen, B. A. (1987). Expectancy theory: Thinking about drinking. In H. T. Blane & K. E. Leonard (Eds.), *Psychological theories of drinking and alcoholism.* New York: Guilford Press.

Holder, H. D., Longabaugh, R., Miller, W. R., & Rubonis, A. V. (1991). The cost effectiveness of treatment for alcoholism: A first approximation. *Journal of Studies on Alcohol, 52,* 517–540.

Institute of Medicine. (1990). *Broadening the base of treatment for alcohol problems: Report of a study by a committee of the Institute of Medicine, Division of Health and Behavioral Medicine.* Washington, DC: National Academy Press.

Kadden, R. M., Cooney, N. L., Getter, H., & Litt, M. D. (1989). Matching alcoholics to coping skills or interactive therapies: Posttreatment results. *Journal of Consulting and Clinical Psychology, 57,* 698–704.

Krasner, L. (1982). Behavior therapy: On roots, contexts and growth. In G. T. Wilson & C. M. Franks (Eds.), *Contemporary behavior therapy: Conceptual and empirical foundations* (pp. 11–64). New York: Guilford Press.

Marlatt, G. A., & Gordon, J. R. (Eds.). (1985). *Relapse prevention: Maintenance strategies in the treatment of addictive behaviors.* New York: Guilford Press.

Marlatt, G. A., & Tapert, S. F. (1993). Harm reduction: Reducing the risks of addictive behaviors. In J. S. Baer, G. A. Marlatt, & R. J. McMahon (Eds.), *Addictive behaviors across the life span: Prevention, treatment and policy issues.* Newbury Park, CA: Sage.

McCrady, B. S., & Delaney, S. I. *(1995).* Self-help groups. In R. K. Hester & W. R. Miller (Eds.), *Handbook of alcoholism treatment approaches: Effective alternatives* (2nd ed., pp. 160–175). Needham Heights, MA: Allyn & Bacon.

McLellan, A. T., Childress, A. R., Ehrman, R. N., & O'Brien, C. P. (1986). Extinguishing conditioned responses during treatment for opiate dependence: Turning laboratory findings into clinical procedure. *Journal of Substance Abuse Treatment, 3,* 33–40.

Miller, W. R., Walters, S. T., & Bennett, M. E. (2001). How effective is alcohol treatment in the United States? *Journal of Studies on Alcohol, 62,* 211–220.

Monti, P. M., Kadden, R. M., Rohsenow, D. J., Cooney, N. L., & Abrams, D. B. (1989). *Treating alcohol dependence: A coping skills training guide* (2nd ed.). New York: Guilford Press.

Morgenstern, J., & McCrady, B. S. (1992). Curative factors in alcohol and drug treatment: Behavioral and disease model perspectives. *British Journal of Addiction, 87,* 901–912.

Onken, L. S. (1991). Using psychotherapy effectively in drug abuse treatment. In R. W. Pickens, C. G. Leukefeld, & C. R. Schuster (Eds.), *Improving drug abuse treatment* (pp. 267–278). Washington, DC: U.S. Government Printing Office.

Pavlov, I. P. (1927). *Lectures on conditioned reflexes.* New York: International Publishers.

Prochaska, J. O., DiClemente, C. C., & Norcross, J. C. (1992). In search of how people change: Applications to addictive behaviors. *American Psychologist, 47,* 1102–1114.

Regier, D. A., Farmer, M. E., Rae, D. S., Locke, B. Z., Keith, S. J., Judd, L. L., & Goodwin, F. K. (1990). Comorbidity of mental disorders with alcohol and other drug abuse: Results from the Epidemiologic Catchment Area (ECA) study. *Journal of the American Medical Association, 264,* 2511–2518.

Rimmele, C. T., Miller, W. R., & Dougher, M. J. (1989). Aversion therapies. In R. K. Hester & W. R. Miller (Eds.), *Handbook of alcoholism treatment approaches: Effective alternatives* (pp. 134–147). New York: Pergamon Press.

Ross, H. E., Glaser, F. B., & Germanson, T. (1988). The prevalence of psychiatric disorders in patients with alcohol and other drug problems. *Archives of General Psychiatry, 45,* 1023–1031.

Rotgers, F., & Morgenstern, J. (1994). *Processes comprising successful substance abuse treatment: A survey of counselors.* Unpublished manuscript, Rutgers University, Center of Alcohol Studies, Piscataway, NJ.

Sher, K. J. (1987). Stress response dampening. In H. T. Blane & K. E. Leonard

(Eds.), *Psychological theories of drinking and alcoholism* (pp. 227–271). New York: Guilford Press.

Sobell, L. C., Sobell, M. B., Toneatto, T., & Leo, G. I. (1993). What triggers the resolution of alcohol problems without treatment? *Alcoholism: Clinical and Experimental Research, 17,* 217–224.

Trimpey, J. (1992). *The small book: A revolutionary alternative for overcoming alcohol and drug dependence* (3rd ed.). New York: Delacorte Press.

Vogel-Sprott, M. (1992). *Alcohol tolerance and social drinking: Learning the consequences.* New York: Guilford Press.

Volpicelli, J. R., Alterman, A. I., Hayashida, M., & O'Brien, C. P. (1992). Naltrexone in treating alcohol dependence. *Archives of General Psychiatry, 49,* 876–880.

Watson, J. B. (1919). *Psychology from the standpoint of a behaviorist.* Philadelphia: Lippincott.

Wikler, A. (1965). Conditioning factors in opiate addiction and relapse. In D. L. Wilner & G. G. Kassenbaum (Eds.), *Narcotics* (pp. 85–100). New York: McGraw-Hill

Wikler, A. (1973). Dynamics of drug dependence: Implications of a conditioning theory for research and treatment. *Archives of General Psychiatry, 28,* 611–616.

Wilson, P. H. (1992). Relapse prevention: Conceptual and methodological issues. In P. H. Wilson (Ed.), *Principles and practice of relapse prevention* (pp. 1–22). New York: Guilford Press.

8

Behavioral Treatment Techniques for Psychoactive Substance Use Disorders

Thomas J. Morgan

Basic Tasks of All Behavioral Interventions

Whether working with substance abuse patients or with a general psychiatric population, there are several essential tasks the behavioral clinician must accomplish during treatment. These tasks include (1) developing a collaborative therapeutic relationship, (2) enhancing patient motivation to make changes, (3) using a functional analysis to make a thorough assessment of the patient's presenting problem, (4) developing and implementing treatment goals, and (5) evaluating patients' treatment progress and terminating service.

Developing a Therapeutic Relationship

The importance of a positive therapeutic relationship with patients has long been emphasized. Since Rogers (1957) first defined unconditional positive regard, accurate empathy, genuineness, and therapist congruence as necessary conditions for positive change, the scientific and treatment communities have been interested in the therapeutic relationship and its contribution to successful treatment. In the substance abuse field, Valle (1981) has shown that the level of a counselor's empathy and general interpersonal skills predicts long-term outcomes for alcoholics. Additionally, there is some evidence that alcoholic patients have poorer treatment outcomes when clinicians use a confrontational style (Lieberman, Yalom, & Miles, 1973; MacDonough, 1976; Miller, Benefield, & Tonigan, 1993). Finally, in Project MATCH, higher therapeutic alliance ratings were predictive of increased treatment participation and improved drinking outcomes among outpatient clients (Connors, Carroll, DiClemente, Longabaugh, & Donovan, 1997).

In developing a positive collaborative relationship with a patient, the clinician should spend time focusing on aspects of the therapeutic relationship. One important aspect includes exploring patient expectations about treatment. Time is needed to discuss previous experiences with treatment and to understand patient expectations about how treatment should proceed. Clinicians should explain to the patient what to expect in the current treatment, such as how long it might last, how sessions are structured, and issues concerning confidentiality.

Another important aspect of the collaborative relationship is having a sense of empathy for the patient's experiences. McCrady (2001) has suggested several actions therapists can take to enhance empathy for their substance–abusing patients. These activities include attempting to change an addictive behavior or deeply held habit of one's own, attending self-help meetings, and listening carefully to the client. Also, in developing a good therapeutic alliance, a clinician can ask questions that reflect an interest in the patient and his or her life outside of substance use. For example, one way to enhance rapport is to ask about a patient's family, work, hobbies, or family pet in addition to substance abuse history.

Enhancing Motivation to Change

For nearly two decades, motivational aspects of substance abuse treatment have been the focus of much discussion. Miller (1985), for instance, has written an excellent article that reviews the concepts of "denial" and motivation in alcoholism treatment. Miller and Rollnick (2002) have written a superb text that describes the "how-to" of motivational interviewing with substance abuse clients. Today, motivational interviewing is a popular and effective intervention as an add-on component to standard treatment, as well as a stand-alone treatment in itself. In a meta-analytic study of controlled alcohol treatment studies, Miller and Wilbourne (2002) reported strong evidence for the effectiveness of motivationally based interventions. Additionally, results from Project MATCH highlight the effectiveness of motivational enhancement as a stand-alone treatment (Project MATCH Research Group, 1998). Readers are directed to Chapters 11 and 12 in this text for a more detailed presentation of the theoretical and clinical aspects of motivation within the addictions field.

Assessment via Functional Analysis

The prelude to good behavioral treatment is a thorough assessment and understanding of the patient. In a behavioral assessment, a patient's substance use is examined in terms of factors that initiate and maintain the substance use.

One area to assess is the unique precursors or triggers to a patient's substance use. This assessment includes evaluating interpersonal situations, emotional states, and environmental situations that are associated with a patient's drinking or drug use. Each patient is different, so it is important to identify the individualized "triggers" of substance use, as this will be invaluable in identifying and coping with later high-risk situations.

The clinician also needs to assess the consequences of the patient's substance use, both immediate and long term, as well as the positive and negative reinforcers associated with the substance use. In identifying consequences, it is important to inquire about different areas of a patient's life that are often affected by substance use:

- *Relationship problems.* Arguments with family and/or friends about substance use; separations, breakups, or divorce due to substance use; family and/or friends becoming annoyed or criticizing the patient's alcohol/drug use.
- *Work problems.* Coming in late or missing work due to intoxication or hangover; being intoxicated or high while at work; being warned at work and/or being fired due to substance use.
- *Legal problems.* Being arrested, placed on probation, and/or incarcerated for alcohol- or drug-related offenses such as driving while intoxicated (DWI); being disorderly; possessing controlled dangerous substances (CDS); or possessing with intent to distribute. Additionally, dependence on alcohol and/or drugs may lead to other illegal activities such as burglary, larceny, or prostitution, and resultant criminal charges.
- *Medical/physical problems.* Having a history of alcohol-related traumas and liver or pancreatic problems, being hospitalized for alcohol- or drug-related illnesses, or having been advised by a physician to cut down on or quit drinking or drug use; having blackouts, hangovers, or withdrawal symptoms such as nausea, shakes, convulsions, or seizures after using substances.
- *Financial problems.* Experiencing heavy debt due to substance use; not paying bills in order to have money to buy alcohol and/or drugs.
- *Intrapersonal problems.* Experiencing feelings of guilt, shame, and regret about substance use; feeling depressed, paranoid, and/or anxious as a result of using substances.

Whenever possible, it is important to gather collateral information about the patient's substance use and its effects on other people. Gaining a perspective on the patient's substance use from his or her spouse/partner, an employer, a probation officer, and/or physician can be extremely helpful. Before talking to collaterals, however, you must discuss with the patient the importance of getting collateral information and obtain appropriate releases.

Finally, a clinician should assess a patient's cognitions regarding the antecedents or triggers to his or her substance use, as well as the patient's expectancies about the effects the substance use will have for him or her. For example, a patient believes that after a particularly long and stressful day at work, "I deserve to have a beer and relax." This cognition may highlight the patient's interpretation of personal stress and discomfort as intolerable and his or her sense of entitlement to a stress-free life. It also emphasizes the patient's expectation that alcohol will have a soothing, calming effect. (For those readers interested in more detailed accounts of substance abuse assessment, see Donovan, 1999, and Miller, Westerberg, & Waldron, 1995.)

Developing and Implementing Treatment Goals.

Developing individualized treatment plans has been one hallmark of behavioral treatment. However, within addictions treatment, the traditional disease model has historically prescribed a generic treatment plan for all. From this traditional perspective, treatment would typically include confrontation of patient denial, education about the disease concept of addiction, and facilitation of the patient into a 12-step program such as Alcoholics Anonymous (AA) or Narcotics Anonymous (NA). The goal for all patients would be lifetime abstinence from alcohol and drugs.

Providing options for substance abusers, specifically alcohol abusers, is consistent with the behavioral tenant of individualized treatment plans. The possibility of moderated drinking by alcoholic patients was first reported by Davies (1962) and later suggested by Sobell and Sobell (1976), Miller and Caddy (1977), and Polich, Armor, and Braiker (1981). It was the Sobells' study that received so much attention and ignited so much controversy from traditional treatment providers. (For a more detailed account of the controlled drinking controversy, see excellent reviews by Nathan & Niaura, 1985 and by Marlatt, Larimar, Baer, & Quigley, 1993.) More recently, there has been a consistent and growing literature that supports moderated drinking for *some* problem drinkers. For instance, in their review of multisite treatment trials, Miller, Walters, and Bennett (2001) found that 10% of alcohol-dependent patients who underwent treatment were able to sustain moderate, asymptomatic drinking for at least 1 year. However, despite this evidence, it still is clear that most alcohol-dependent individuals are not appropriate candidates for moderation-based drinking goals. (For a cogent review of the literature on controlled drinking, see Rosenberg, 1993.)

From the behavioral perspective, it is important that treatment goals are collaboratively determined. Studies have emphasized the importance of patient choice in determining treatment goals. Regardless of the goal preferences of treatment providers, studies have shown that patients will ultimately decide on substance use goals that suit them. This includes alcohol-dependent patients who moderate their drinking when treated in an abstinence-based program (McCabe,

1986; Nordstrom & Berglund, 1987; Sanchez-Craig, Annis, Bornet, & MacDonald, 1984; Vaillant & Milkofsky, 1982), as well as patients who abstain from drinking even after they have been treated in a moderation-based program (Miller, Leckman, Delaney, & Tinkcom, 1992; Rychtarik, Foy, Scott, Lokey, & Prue, 1987). Also, allowing patients to self-select their own goal is an important factor in developing motivation, commitment, and engagement in treatment (Marlatt et al., 1993; Ogborne, 1987; Sobell, Toneatto, & Sobell, 1992). Finally, goal choice has become more popular as studies have suggested that successful outcomes are more likely if the treatment goals are consistent with the patient's goal preference (Booth, Dale, & Ansari, 1984; Orford & Keddie, 1986). (For further information on goal setting, see Kadden & Skerker, 1999.)

Evaluating Treatment Progress and Terminating Treatment

As treatment progresses, the therapist needs to continually evaluate the progress of the work or, if there is a lack of progress, immediately address this issue in treatment. By regularly assessing progress, both therapist and patient can see concrete positive changes and the patient can be reinforced for making these changes. When progress is not being made, the therapist and patient can identify and discuss obstacles to reaching treatment goals. It may be true that the goals of treatment are unrealistic, that the patient has become ambivalent with respect to them, or that the assessment of the problems/circumstances in the patient's life is not accurate. It is often helpful to consult with colleagues and supervisors when one's work with a case becomes "stuck."

Ideally, termination of treatment from a behavioral perspective is mutually determined. Treatment ends when goals have been reached or there is an acknowledgment that treatment might follow a different direction (e.g., referral to another practitioner or a higher level of care). In terminating treatment, the patient and the clinician should review the course of treatment and acknowledge and reinforce behavior changes. Also during termination there should be a discussion of "warning signs" that will signal the patient to consider returning to therapy or renew a process of self-change.

SPECIFIC BEHAVIORAL TREATMENT TECHNIQUES AND INTERVENTIONS

In should be noted that the following description of behavioral treatment techniques is relevant for both alcohol- and drug-abusing patients. Due to space constraints I will primarily describe the use of behavioral techniques with alcohol-abusing patients. (For a detailed description of behavioral treatment with drug abuse populations, see Onken, Blaine, & Boren, 1993, and Sobell et al., 1992.)

Classical conditioning theory assumes that substance users become conditioned to certain stimuli in the environment through repeated pairing of substances with specific settings, people, and rituals. These cues, or "triggers" (conditioned stimuli), are quite diverse and are unique to each individual. The assumption is that if certain conditioned stimuli have come to be associated with substance use, then these cues can be unlearned or extinguished. The following section provides a summary of the most well known treatments for substance abuse disorders following the classical conditioning paradigm.

Aversion Treatments

One of the first behavioral treatments for substance use disorders, specifically alcohol dependence, was aversion therapy. This treatment paired an aversive experience with the stimuli ("triggers") of drinking so that the patient would develop a negative reaction to alcohol and thus lose the urge to drink. Over the years, electrical aversion, chemical aversion, and covert sensitization were used in an attempt to condition an aversive response to alcohol. Since electrical and chemical aversion have shown inconsistent empirical support and are no longer considered a serious treatment for alcohol disorders, I will limit my discussion here to covert sensitization techniques.

COVERT SENSITIZATION

In covert sensitization, the aversive conditioning to alcohol or drugs occurs through the patient's verbal and imaginal modalities. This treatment protocol continues to follow the learning principles of counterconditioning but is not as invasive or painful as electrical and chemical aversion treatments. In addition, medical supervision and special equipment are not needed, so the protocol can be carried out on an outpatient basis.

In covert sensitization, specific information is gathered regarding usual antecedents or cues to the patient's alcohol and/or drug use as well as information regarding negative or feared consequences. This information is then used in the conditioning scenes. Patients are instructed to relax and imagine as vividly as possible a typical situation in which they are about to use alcohol or drugs. In the imaginal scene, immediately after the patient has used alcohol or drugs, he or she is provided with a specific and disgusting description of the aversive consequences of the substance use. Such scenarios might include graphic descriptions of nausea, vomiting, hangovers, heart racing, the hurt or frightened look from their children, or other feared results of use. The imaginal scene may also include the suggestion that the patient will have relief from these symptoms by leaving the situation and avoiding using alcohol or drugs in the future. Such scenes are repeatedly paired until the unpleasant images become associated with alcohol and drug use, and the urge for using the substances has been extinguished.

Data on the long-term efficacy of covert sensitization has been mixed (Institute of Medicine, 1990; Lawson & Boudin, 1992; Nathan & Niaura, 1985; O'Leary & Wilson, 1987; Rimmele, Howard, & Hilfrink, 1995). Rimmele et al. (1995) noted that the most encouraging results are found in those studies that have specific sensitization procedures and have verified the presence of conditioned aversion. Although the results of covert sensitization's efficacy are mixed, there is optimism about its viability as an outpatient treatment option. Especially when compared to electrical and chemical aversion treatments, it has the advantages of being less intrusive and less physically stressful, and can be administered on an outpatient basis. It may not be useful for all patients, especially those who have difficulty with visualizations. (For more specific information about a covert sensitization treatment protocol, see Rimmele et al., 1995.)

Cue Exposure

The intent of cue exposure is to extinguish conditioned responses, such as craving, heart rate, sweating, shakiness, and ultimately substance use. As one would expect from the classical conditioning paradigm, extinction occurs through repeated exposures of the conditioned stimuli (e.g., stress, sight of cocaine, sight of drug paraphernalia, smell of beer) without the patient being able to execute the conditioned response (i.e., drinking or drug use). Thus, as craving for alcohol and drugs becomes extinguished, the urge to use these substances is eliminated.

However, it appears that exposure alone does not account for significant long-term effects (Childress, Ehrman, Rohsenow, Robbins, & O'Brien, 1992; Monti et al., 1993). Other elements that must be addressed include self-efficacy, personally relevant cues for substance use, and coping skills training. Despite these caveats, empirical support for cue exposure treatments in the areas of phobia and obsessive–compulsive disorders (Foa & Kozak, 1986) and bulimia (Wilson, Rossiter, Kleinfield, & Lindholm, 1986) offer conceptual and theoretical optimism for the use of exposure treatment with substance abuse disorders as well.

In providing cue exposure treatment, patients are given a rationale about the importance of reducing craving so that they are better able to cope with high-risk triggers. Patients are also given a simple description of the classical conditioning paradigm. In order to individualize treatment, a detailed description is needed of the patient's preferred drinks and drugs of abuse as well as details about situations in which the use occurs. Treatment typically consists of six to eight sessions, provided in an inpatient facility. Each session begins and ends with an assessment of the patient's subjective and physiological responses to the alcohol cues. Patients receive a series of brief exposures to an alcoholic beverage. Patients can also be exposed to alcohol cues after they have been induced into a negative mood state. (For those readers interested in a more detailed cue exposure protocol, see Monti, Rohsenow, Colby, & Abrams, 1995.)

The literature on efficacy of cue exposure is still relatively small. Uncontrolled studies have provided promising results (Institute of Medicine, 1990), although a recent review suggests that there is little consistent evidence for the efficacy of cue exposure as currently delivered (Conklin & Tiffany, 2002).

Behavioral Self-Control Training

Behavioral self-control training (BSCT) has been one of the most widely studied treatments in the alcohol field (Institute of Medicine, 1990; Miller & Wilbourne, 2002). BSCT has been described as a brief, educationally oriented approach in which patients can achieve a goal of nonproblematic drinking or abstinence. BSCT can either be implemented by a therapist (therapist-directed) or by the patient in the form of a self-help manual (self-directed). There are several advantages to using BSCT over traditional treatment with alcohol-abusing patients. One advantage is that some patients will refuse to accept an abstinence goal without at least attempting moderated nonproblematic drinking. A second rationale is that BSCT has the potential to reach a larger, broader population of individuals who are having problems with drinking. It has been suggested that there are many more problem drinkers than those who are diagnosably dependent on alcohol (Cahalan, 1987; Institute of Medicine, 1990). In fact, a majority of those with alcohol problems never have any treatment contact with self-help groups or professional services (Cunningham, 1999; Institute of Medicine, 1990). Thus, a treatment approach that offers a choice of goals may be more attractive for those who are not yet ready for abstinence and who might not otherwise consider treatment.

The active ingredients of BSCT are believed to be self-efficacy and self-control. The patient maintains the primary responsibility for making decisions throughout treatment. BSCT is brief—usually lasting from 6 to 12 sessions—with each session being 90 minutes in length. Follow-up "booster" sessions are scheduled to solidify gains and to assess whether patients need additional intervention. According to Hester (1995), BSCT is made up of steps that occur in the following order: (1) setting limits on the number of drinks per day and on peak blood alcohol concentrations (BACs), (2) self-monitoring of drinking behaviors, (3) changing the rate of drinking, (4) practicing assertiveness in refusing drinks, (5) setting up a reward system for achievement of goals, (6) learning which antecedents result in excessive drinking, and (7) learning other coping skills instead of drinking. Homework, role playing, and practice are emphasized in BSCT.

Although a great deal of research has been generated on BSCT over the past 20 years, results have been mixed. Studies have looked at different treatment populations (e.g., DWI offenders; chronic, alcohol-dependent veterans; early-stage problem drinkers), different treatment settings (inpatient vs. outpatient), different treatment goals (abstinence vs. moderation), and varied treatment delivery (self-directed vs. therapist-directed). Many controlled studies suggest that BSCT fares no worse than abstinence-oriented treatments in terms of drinking outcomes and that patients have shown significant improvement when compared to control groups. One study by Foy, Nunn, and Rychtarik (1984) reported that BSCT patients had worse short-term outcomes when compared to an abstinence-oriented treatment, but also pointed out that at long-term follow-up there were no significant differences between groups. Several factors likely contribute to the mixed results with BSCT. Treatment packages that are defined as BSCT can vary a good deal in terms of what treatment techniques are used. Also, BSCT has been used with a heterogeneous population and there may be certain types of patients who respond better or worse than others.

Overall, results of controlled empirical studies have suggested that BSCT is generally effective for treating those with alcohol problems. However, more definitive information is needed to identify the effective active ingredients of BSCT and for which patients it is most effective. (For those readers interested in a more detailed description of BSCT, see Hester, 1995.)

Social Skills Training

Social skills training addresses not only a patient's substance use but also other problem areas that might be associated with excessive alcohol/drug use. The rationale for providing social skills training is the belief that the initiation and maintenance of addictive disorders is related to problems with coping. That is, addictive behavior is seen as a habitual maladaptive way of coping with stress that can be alleviated through social skills training.

In social skills treatment, patients identify high-risk situations to use substances, such as negative emotional states, urges/cravings, social pressure, and experiencing interpersonal conflicts. Patients are taught behavioral strategies to cope with these situations, which include coping with urges/cravings, managing thoughts about substance use, developing drink/drug refusal skills, developing problem-solving skills, planning for emergencies, increasing pleasant activities, developing a sober support network, and training in assertiveness, relaxation, and effective communication. As with other behavioral treatments, it is important to have the patient practice these coping skills *in vivo* in order to enhance self-efficacy and broaden generalization of the skills.

Recent results from Project MATCH suggest treatment utilizing social skills training was a potent intervention for alcoholics in outpatient and aftercare treatments. Overall, the controlled literature has shown strong support for social skills training in a variety of settings (Carroll, 1996; Institute of Medicine, 1990; Irwin, Bowers, Dunn, & Wang, 1999; Miller, & Wilbourne, 2002; Monti et al., 1995; Morgenstern, Blanchard, Morgan, Labouvie, & Hayaki, 2001; Project MATCH Research Group, 1998). (For detailed protocols for social skills training, see Kadden et al., 1992; Monti, Abrams, Kadden, & Cooney, 1989; and Monti et al., 1995.)

Contingency Management

Environmental contingencies have an extremely powerful effect on behavior. Substance abuse treatment that uses the operant conditioning paradigm emphasizes reinforcing desirable behavior (abstinence) while punishing undesirable behavior (substance use). Many patients enter treatment as part of an implicit contingency contract, such as a spouse who comes to treatment rather than face a divorce, or a motorist who enters treatment in order to get his or her driver's license back. However, at the same time it is ironic that in spite of strong contingencies, people often continue to use substances. Nathan and Niaura (1985) explain this paradox by noting that people have unique differences and that what is rewarding or punishing for one individual is not necessarily rewarding or punishing for another. Additionally, the authors emphasize the need for contingencies to be mutually agreed on, carefully observed, and consistently implemented. The consistent involvement of collaterals and institutions connected with the patient is essential for an effective contingency contract, but can be difficult to obtain. The effectiveness of contingency management programs will be mixed, depending on the type of contingency being used (e.g., revocation of professional licenses, increase in methadone dosages) and the consistency with which they are applied. Nonetheless, these approaches have begun to garner significant research support for their efficacy, particularly in combination with cognitive-behavioral approaches. For this reason, contingency management approaches have been afforded a section of their own in this volume (Chapters 9 and 10), and the reader is referred to those chapters for a more extended discussion of these important behavioral approaches.

SPECIFIC ISSUES IN IMPLEMENTING SUBSTANCE ABUSE TREATMENT FROM A BEHAVIORAL PERSPECTIVE

Sequencing of Technique Use

Brownell, Marlatt, Lichtenstein, and Wilson (1986) conceptualize recovery from substance abuse disorders in three phases in which specific techniques are more appropriate during certain phases. For an individual seeking to make any behavioral change, the first phase of treatment is becoming motivated and committed to making a change. This area of treatment has been described in detail earlier in the section "Enhancing Motivation to Change."

The second phase of treatment, lasting 3–6 months, is initiating early changes. This early phase is particularly crucial as roughly 66% of relapses occur within the first 3 months (Hunt, Barnett, & Branch, 1971). During this phase of treatment, several tasks and techniques are most appropriate. First, there is a strong emphasis on actions that facilitate abstinence. These actions include setting up external supports for abstinence, such as residential treatment, medication (to curb cravings or create aversion to use), and contingencies with spouses, employers, or legal authorities. During this phase the treatment techniques should be those that assist in initial abstinence. The patient and clinician should identify high-risk situations for substance use and develop specific plans to deal with these situations. Such skills include drink/drug refusal skills, managing urges and cravings, understanding seemingly irrelevant decisions, and managing negative thoughts about substance use.

The third phase of treatment is the maintenance of behavioral changes. Most patients can make short-term changes relatively easily. However, it is much more difficult to maintain new behaviors over time. Mark Twain, an inveterate smoker, was quoted as saying, "Quiting smoking is easy . . . I've done it a thousand times." The point is that the maintenance of change is indeed a difficult task. Clinicians can facilitate this maintenance by encouraging the patient to self-monitor, remain aware of high-risk situations, and regularly weigh the advantages and disadvantages of both sobriety and returning to substance use. This is often difficult for the patient, who has gone a length of time without using substances. The patient's level of confidence is often high and the patient's need to be concerned about recovery issues, as was the case early in treatment, is not strong.

Another area of focus is to help the patient develop and maintain a social network that is supportive of sobriety. For many this will include members of a 12-step program such as AA or NA. Other patients who do not utilize 12-step programs may also develop support networks through their church or synagogue, family members, or other recovery-based self-help groups (such as Women for Sobriety, Secular Organizations for Sobriety, and S.M.A.R.T. Recovery). The crucial factors in these support groups are that they are supportive of sobriety and that group members are not substance users themselves (Beattie & Longabaugh, 1999; Gordon & Zrull, 1991; Longabaugh, Beattie, Noel, Stout, & Malloy, 1993).

How Problems Are Addressed and in What Order

Substance abuse patients come into treatment with a variety of concomitant problems, which are often a consequence of the substance use itself. Extreme stress related to unemployment, financial problems, relationship difficulties, pending legal action, or severe psychiatric symptomology is often found in those who present for substance abuse treatment. Individuals may feel depressed, guilty, and ashamed as they recount the toll their substance use has taken on themselves and others. In addition, some patients have preexisting psychiatric conditions that become prominent as the patient begins abstaining from alcohol and/or drugs.

If at all possible, the initial focus of treatment should be on assisting the patient in making changes in his or her substance use. Patients can rarely make headway with other problems while they continue to use alcohol and drugs. A slogan from the 12-step programs is relevant: the patient must remember to keep "first things first." However, it may be difficult for the clinician to focus on the problem of substance use. Some patients come into sessions each week with a personal crisis that is begging for immediate attention. Other times, patients insist on dealing with relationship problems or feelings of anxiety rather than their problems with substance use. Thus, it is understandably difficult for a caring clinician not to become engaged with a patient who begins to painfully talk about the abuse/trauma that he or she has suffered.

How can a clinician walk the fine line between remaining focused on substance abuse and recovery while also tending to significant issues that the patient brings into treatment? There are several strategies one can employ:

1. Initially, when briefing the patient about what to expect in treatment, make it clear that the first order of business in treatment is to address his or her substance use. Reminding the patient of the consequences of continued use will be useful in emphasizing the importance of dealing with the substance use first.

2. The clinician can structure the session into "minisessions" where the first third of the session is reserved for non-substance-abuse concerns, while the remaining two-thirds of the session is used to focus on initiating and maintaining changes in the patient's substance use. The advantage in this strategy is that the patient does have some time to vocalize problems that are important to him or her. Additionally, the clinician may have access to more material that can be used in the substance-focused part of the session. However, a disadvantage of breaking up the session in this way is that the transition between these parts can become incongruous. This also necessitates that the clinician have good assertiveness skills.

3. When the clinician finds him- or herself in sessions where the treatment is constantly focusing on non-substance-use material, this should be a signal to pause and reevaluate the treatment. It may be that in avoiding discussions of substance use, the patient might be expressing ambivalence about changing his or her behavior. It may also be that there are issues more painful

or pressing for the patient that were not initially assessed. In such cases it is useful to reevaluate the patient's treatment goals and modify them accordingly.

4. Finally, when a patient's psychiatric symptomology is consistently interfering with the tasks of substance abuse treatment, it is usually an indication that a referral for a psychiatric consultation is in order. Based on the evaluation, it may be that medication, concurrent psychiatric therapy, or a higher level of care is indicated.

How Denial, Resistance, and Lack of Progress Are Addressed

The concept of denial has long been the cornerstone of traditional alcohol- and drug-dependency treatment. Denial has been said to be the "cardinal and integral feature of chemical dependency and the fatal aspect of alcoholism and other drug dependencies" (Hazelden, 1975, p. 9). Likewise, a substance abuser's lack of "motivation" has been used to explain failure to enter, continue in, comply with, and succeed in treatment. Although confrontation of denial has been historically relied on as the essential first step in resolving substance abuse problems, this method has fallen out of favor.

From a behavioral perspective, "denial" or "resistance" are not seen as patient traits (Miller, 1985), but rather as a condition where the patient's versus the therapist's definition of the problem is simply not congruent. If the patient and clinician have differing definitions of the problem, progress in treatment will stall. Thus, rather than defining "resistance" as a patient characteristic, it is more accurate (and helpful) to define it as a problem in the therapeutic process (i.e., a "lack of progress"). Viewing resistance this way, rather than arguing to get the patient to accept the problem from the clinician's viewpoint, is also more likely to engage the patient in resolving differences.

In working with patients from the behavioral perspective there are two things to keep in mind regarding patient–clinician agreement on treatment goals. First, it is important to routinely assess the patient's commitment to his or her original treatment goals. We cannot assume that once a decision is made that it is static and etched in stone. Rather, it is hoped in developing a therapeutic relationship and outlining the expectations of treatment that the clinician has stressed how important it is for the patient to bring up changes he or she wants to make in his or her treatment goals. Patients are often reluctant to initiate a discussion about changing treatment goals, especially if they have been having urges or thoughts about returning to drinking. Thus the clinician needs to routinely ask how the patient is feeling about the original goal choice and whether he or she has entertained thoughts about returning to limited alcohol or drug use. Also, when progress is not forthcoming, the clinician should pause and reassess the treatment plan. Having an open objective discussion about the patient's treatment goals is paramount.

How Lapses/Relapses Are Viewed and Used in Treatment

Addiction is characterized by chronic episodes of relapse that Prochaska, DiClemente, and Norcross (1992) describe as being "the rule rather than the exception" (p. 1104). According to Hunt et al. (1971), approximately 66% of patients who complete treatment for smoking, alcohol, and heroin addiction relapse within the first 90 days. The frequency of return to drinking (although not necessarily full-blown relapse) has been estimated to be between 70 and 74% within the first year (Hunt et al., 1971; Miller & Hester, 1980; Miller, Walters, & Bennett, 2001). Because relapse is so prevalent, Prochaska et al. (1992) discuss how they have modified their stages-of-change model to include relapse as a stage of change.

From a behavioral perspective, clinicians should address the potential of relapse in the early stages of treatment. The clinician should initially discuss with the patient the distinction between a "lapse" and a "relapse." Marlatt and Gordon (1985) define a *relapse* as a return to a previous state, characterized by the perception of loss of control. However, a *lapse* is viewed as an event or situation in which one can take corrective action and not lose control. The cognitive and affective reactions to the first slip or lapse after a period of abstinence exert a significant influence over whether or not the lapse is followed by a complete return to the former level of use. The clinician should highlight the difference between a lapse and a relapse and emphasize that a relapse is not an inevitable result of a lapse. Rather, the clinician should advise the patient that lapses, or "slips," are part of the recovery process for many individuals. If one was to occur, the patient should have an "emergency plan" ready to implement that would keep the lapse from becoming a full-blown relapse. The clinician should convey to the patient the message that a lapse can be used as a leaning experience by reviewing what happened, identifying where the patient may have been caught off-guard, and reexamining the patient's decision to change.

The advantage of this open discussion of lapses and relapses is that it provides an honest appraisal of what the patient might expect. Patients can expect that if they slip all is not lost and they can use it as a way of learning more about themselves and the plans they have to stay sober.

How to Integrate Other Treatment Supports Such as Self-Help Groups and Medication

Utilization of support groups can be a valuable adjunct to a behaviorally oriented substance abuse treatment. Although there has been little empirical support for the efficacy of self-help groups on their own, clinically we know that participation in such groups can be extremely helpful for many patients. Research in the areas of social support and recovery also suggests that individuals have better treatment outcomes when they are involved with social networks supportive of abstinence (Beattie & Longabaugh, 1999; Gordon & Zrull, 1991; Longabaugh et al., 1993).

Self-help groups have been a prominent part of the treatment field for many years. Twelve-step groups such as AA and NA have been cornerstones of traditional treatment and are well known to substance abuse counselors. In addition, the development of alternative self-help groups has broadened in recent years with the emergence of Self-Management and Recovery Training (S.M.A.R.T.) and Rational Recovery groups to offer alternatives that are more theoretically compatible with the behavioral/social learning model. (For a more detailed description of alternative self-help groups, see McCrady & Delaney, 1995, for an excellent comprehensive review.)

The use of medication in substance abuse treatment has often been a part of the treatment for patients with a concurrent psychiatric disorder. There is a large overlap between psychiatric and substance use disorders. The National Comorbidity Study (Kessler, McGonagle, & Shanyang, 1994) found that between 17% and 24% of individuals who had a current substance abuse disorder also met criteria for another DSM-III psychiatric diagnosis (American Psychiatric Association, 1987). In dually diagnosed patients, severe anxiety, depression, sociopathy, or psychotic symptomology may be present and may thus become a significant aspect of treatment.

The use of psychotropic medications will be appropriate in many cases in order to effectively treat the psychiatric disorder. Because symptoms resulting from the chronic use of substances often mimic psychiatric symptoms (such as depression, anxiety, and paranoia) it is important to conduct a thorough assessment of the patient's psychiatric history and allow sufficient periods of abstinence to determine whether the psychiatric symptoms resolve with sobriety. There will be instances where patients have a preexisting psychiatric condition, exacerbated by their substance use, that will likely remain, even in recovery. Referral to a psychiatrist who has experience treating patients with addictions would be ideal. Those patients who participate in 12-step recovery meetings may feel uncomfortable in taking medication, as they might believe they are not totally drug-free. However, today most 12-step groups accept the need for some individuals to be taking medications for psychiatric conditions. In fact, Alcoholics Anonymous World Services has published a pamphlet specifically regarding the use of medications and recovery (Alcoholics Anonymous, 1984).

It should also be mentioned that medications are being used successfully to treat substance use disorders directly. Disulfiram (Antabuse) has long been used as a treatment for alcohol dependence, and other medications (e.g., acamprosate, naltrexone) are currently being used as well in addictions treatment. (See chapter 13, this volume, for a more detailed presentation of the role of medications in addictions treatment.)

SUMMARY

Of the many treatment approaches available, those that have the most empirical support are behaviorally based (Miller & Wilbourne, 2002). The behavioral model, with its emphasis on assessment and evaluation, lends itself well to studies of effectiveness. In addition, the health care system continues to demand accountability and quality treatment, and behavioral treatments are a good match given this climate. The behavioral approach offers patients options and flexibility in treatment. However, in treating substance use disorders from a behavioral perspective, one of its strengths is also one of its biggest drawbacks. By individualizing treatment, it is difficult to study "treatment" because the "package" varies from individual to individual. In the future, there needs to be continued efforts to focus research attention on the active elements in successful behavioral treatment (Morgenstern & Longabaugh, 2000). There also is a need for translation, dissemination, and training of these empirically supported behavioral approaches to frontline substance abuse counselors. The future of behavioral treatment is likely to include more focus on harm reduction (Marlatt et al., 1993) and providing brief interventions to populations of people who have less severe substance use problems. Finally, there is an interest in examining the efficacy of behavioral treatments when combined with pharmacological interventions.

CASE ILLUSTRATION

The following is a case example using cognitive-behavioral treatment techniques in the treatment of alcohol and cannabis dependence. Certain information of the case was altered in order to protect the privacy of the patient and to highlight important aspects of the treatment.

Background and History

Teri is a 43-year-old married white female who was self-referred to outpatient treatment as she felt her drinking had recently gotten "out of control." Teri had stopped drinking a week before the initial interview and hoped she could eventually learn how to drink moderately. Teri lives with her husband, Neil, in a house they have owned for 15 years. She and Neil have been married for 20 years and have no children. Teri is a college graduate and works as loan processor for a large mortgage company. Neil dropped out of college after 2 years and currently works as a meter reader for the local gas and electric company.

Assessment Procedure

In addition to the clinical interview, Teri completed the Inventory of Drinking Situations (IDS; Annis, 1982) and the University of Rhode Island Change Assessment Scale (URICA; DiClemente & Hughes, 1990). The IDS is a 100-item questionnaire that asks about the likelihood a patient will drink heavily in a variety of drinking situations. The URICA is a 32-item questionnaire that asks patients about their intentions to make changes regarding a problem behavior. A patient's score can be converted to a "readiness" indicator or to a change profile that shows an individual's score on each of the stages of change. The URICA stages include precontemplation, contemplation, action and maintenance.

Past Alcohol and Drug Use History

Teri stated that she first used alcohol at age 15 when she drank some of her father's vodka with friends while her parents were out of the house. During high school, Teri reported that she would drink once or twice a month, typically at social events on weekends. She did not report any excessive drinking episodes or problems due to her drinking during high school. During college, Teri drank regularly on the weekends. She reported limiting herself to two or three glasses of wine or three to four beers over the course of a drinking day. When she started to date Neil, she continued to limit her drinking to the weekends. However, the amount she drank increased to five or six beers over the course of a drinking day. Since getting married and working full time, Teri's drinking has gradually increased in quantity and frequency. For the past 2 years she has used alcohol nearly every day. During the week, she typically has three drinks of vodka (approximately 3 ounces per drink) after work. On the weekends, Teri will usually drink a bottle of wine plus four beers over the course of the weekend. In the past 6 months, Teri stated that she found herself drinking occasionally in the morning before work and having several drinks during lunch. Teri reported that her longest period of abstinence occurred 4 months ago. Her abstinence lasted 2 weeks and she felt pleased she could stop drinking on her own.

Teri reported a history of marijuana and cocaine use. She stated that she had experimented with cocaine "a few times" during her freshman year in college. Teri described feeling jumpy and uncomfortable when she used cocaine and felt more attracted to the effects of marijuana. Teri described her use of marijuana as "infrequent," typically once a month, and generally at large social events. When she met Neil during her sophomore year, her use of marijuana increased and became more regular. She described studying hard and abstaining from alcohol and marijuana during the week, but then "partying" all weekend long with Neil. Since her marriage, Teri stated that she and Neil smoked marijuana 3 to 4 times per month. Most often they got high when going to concerts or when they socialized with certain friends. Teri reported that she occasionally would smoke marijuana at home after a particularly stressful day at work.

Initial Phase of Treatment

During these sessions, the primary focus of treatment was to develop a therapeutic relationship, conduct a functional analysis of Teri's alcohol and drug use, and enhance her commitment to make changes in her use of substances.

DEVELOPING A THERAPEUTIC RELATIONSHIP

During the initial session, I explored Teri's expectations for treatment. She reported that this was her first treatment episode for drinking and drug use. She stated that she had several friends (one her mail carrier) whom she knew were recovering from addictions. She had attended an AA meeting with one of her friends but felt her drinking "wasn't that bad." As I discussed the expectations for our treatment, Teri seemed surprised. She feared I would tell her she had to stop drinking and dictate how to get and stay sober. I described how we would work together to understand her drinking and marijuana use from a variety of perspectives. We would talk also about possible treatment goals, but the ultimate decision about drinking and drug use would be up to her.

FUNCTIONAL ANALYSIS

Over the course of the first four sessions, using both the assessment questionnaires and information from our treatment sessions, Teri reported that the following situations were associated with heavier alcohol and marijuana use: (1) negative emotional states such as anxiety, depression, and anger; (2) pleasant times with others in social situations; and (3) free time spent with Neil. Table 8.1 shows three of Teri's self-monitoring exercises, which detail the functional analysis for high-risk situations during the initial phase of treatment.

COMMITMENT AND MOTIVATION TO CHANGE

In listening to Teri's perceptions of her drinking and noting her responses on the URICA, it appeared as if she was in the action stage of abstaining from marijuana and alcohol. She acknowledged that her alcohol and drug use were problems, was committed to abstaining during treatment, and was faithful in completing practice assignments between sessions. However, there were times

TABLE 8.1. Examples of Teri's Functional Analysis Worksheets

Thoughts/ feelings	Response	Positive consequence	Negative consequence
Trigger: End of work week			
Restless and bored. "A drink will help calm me down."	Started house projects. Read in a bubble bath.	Satisfied with accomplishments. Felt proud of self.	None
Trigger: Dinner with Neil and father-in-law			
Tense. "I want to loosen up and have fun." "A drink will help me socialize."	Drank 2 "Virgin Marys" and soda with dinner	Felt more awake. Felt "with it." Proud of myself. Neil was very happy.	Felt like I didn't belong. Felt like an outcast.
Trigger: Funeral			
Sad and helpless. "This is a heavy experience." "A drink will help me be less upset."	Drank two (3 oz.) glasses of vodka after the funeral.	Brief relief.	Felt more sad and helpless. Disappointed in self for "slipping."

when her ambivalence toward abstinence from alcohol became evident, especially when considering the long term. During this time, Teri and I worked together to complete a decisional balance worksheet using a modified version of the Carlson model (Carlson, 1991). Table 8.2 shows Teri's decisional balance worksheet.

As noted in Table 8.2, Teri listed a number of drawbacks of continuing to drink. She was most concerned about the emotional consequences, such as feeling "out of control" when she drank. Additionally Teri was concerned about the strain on her marriage with Neil, her difficulty concentrating at work, and her failure to accomplish tasks around the house. In discussing the advantages of drinking, Teri was quick to point out that she felt more comfortable in social situations when drinking. She also noted that drinking helped her escape uncomfortable feelings such as anger, tension, and grief, and helped her fall asleep after a stressful day. Finally, Teri noted that drinking made her feel "normal" when she was with her friends, and she didn't want to have to explain to them why she had quit.

Table 8.2 also describes Teri's list of advantages and disadvantages of sobriety. Teri had been sober for about 5 weeks and noted she felt better physically, had lost some weight, was accomplishing more at home and work, and felt her relationship with Neil had improved. Teri was able to note several drawbacks of her sobriety. She acknowledged that changing her thoughts and behavior was hard work, requiring a good deal of attention and energy. For

Teri, additional drawbacks of sobriety included feeling more intensely her frustration with Neil's drinking, her grief around the death of family members, and her embarrassment that she was "abnormal" by being abstinent.

Initial Behavior Change

The next phase of treatment included making initial behavioral changes to support Teri's goal of abstinence. We used information from the functional analysis, decisional balance worksheet, and IDS to focus on "high-risk" situa-

TABLE 8.2. Teri's Decisional Balance Worksheet

Disadvantages of using alcohol/drugs	Advantage of using alcohol/drugs	Achieving the same benefits without using alcohol/drugs
1. Emotional consequences: feeling guilty, depressed, and angry. 2. Failed obligations at home (laundry, care for the dog, bills). 3. Physical problems such as "fuzzy" thinking the next day. 4. Strained relationship with Neil. 5. Feeling "out of control"	1. Feels relaxed in social situations. 2. Escapes feelings such as anger, anxiety, boredom, and grief. 3. Helps to fall asleep. 4. Provides a break from responsibilities. 5. Feels "normal"	1. Think through situations where she has drank in the past. Linking alcohol use to more stress in the long term. 2. Develop alternative activities to cope with negative feelings, such as reading, walking the dog, and talking with friends. 3. Relaxation exercises and meditation. 4. Use alternative activities (noted above) to take a break. Work toward more balance and guilt-free leisure time.

Advantages of abstinence	Drawbacks of abstinence	Coping with the difficulties of abstinence and early recovery
1. Feeling proud and having a sense of accomplishment. 2. Feeling better physically. 3. Losing weight. 4. Getting more accomplished at work and home. 5. Getting more involved with family and friends.	1. Belief that "I'm not normal." 2. Requires a lot of time and energy to recover. 3. Seeing Neil might have a problem with alcohol. 4. Uncomfortable to experience painful feelings like anger, grief, and frustration while sober.	1. Talk with others in recovery and challenge this belief. 2. Balance lifestyle with self-care activities. 3. Talk to Neil about her concerns and disengage from shared activities where he drinks heavily. 4. Examine thoughts that contribute to negative feelings. Talk to others about her feelings and utilize alternative coping strategies.

tions. Of the two primary risk situations for Teri, one involved drinking in so-cial situations with friends and Neil, and the other was drinking in response to negative emotional states, such as depression, anxiety, and boredom. Due to space limits, I will describe the strategies developed for only one of Teri's high-risk situations: social pressure to drink.

Teri described a social life that was active and highly involved with alco-hol use. Teri and Neil had a regular restaurant they went to on Friday nights, where they would often have dinner at the bar. Additionally, at least two or three times a week Teri and Neil would socialize with friends or family where heavy drinking would be typical. There were three specific coping strategies we focused on in treatment to address these high-risk social situations: (1) drink refusal, (2) problem solving, and (3) challenging thoughts about the role of drinking. As one might expect, the discussion and development of these coping strategies were often closely related and overlapped during the treat-ment sessions.

DRINK REFUSAL

Teri stated that she had only told a few of her friends about her decision to ab-stain from alcohol. She feared going out socially as she was unsure how people would respond to her choice. We used the example of her Friday night dinner to prepare her to have dinner but to drink a nonalcoholic beverage. We dis-cussed a variety of options, beginning with making an intentional decision *not* to have dinner at the bar for the time being. Also, we rehearsed how Teri would respond to the server asking for her drink order. This would be some-what challenging as Teri was a familiar face at the restaurant and servers would often assume she wanted "the usual," a bottle of imported beer. Teri agreed to decide before she entered the restaurant what nonalcoholic beverage she planned to drink. When they were seated, Teri would ask the server to bring her this beverage. Teri noted it would be more challenging for her to refuse al-coholic drinks when she and Neil were with friends. Several friends were quite heavy drinkers and Teri feared they would push her to drink if she de-clined. We role-played such a scenario and focused on how she could immedi-ately and directly say "No," having an explanation prepared. Teri didn't feel comfortable telling these friends she had a drinking problem. She did, however, think it would be effective to explain that she wasn't drinking because she was trying to lose weight and was watching her diet. Teri also agreed that it would be helpful if she didn't make plans to socialize with these friends, at least for the next few months.

PROBLEM SOLVING

Teri found that working through problem-solving exercises was particularly helpful in coping with social situations without drinking. As we examined specific problem areas, Teri was quite engaged in generating possible solutions and deciding on realistic applications. Teri acknowledged that one problem area was that her social network was made up mostly of heavy drinkers. We examined a variety of potential solutions. One solution was for Teri to develop new friendships with individuals who didn't drink. In the past year, Teri had attended some AA meetings but did not feel that they were helpful. I encouraged Teri to try a few more AA meetings as well as to attend a few local S.M.A.R.T. recovery groups. Another solution we discussed was to renew old friendships with individuals who didn't drink. Eventually, Teri began to spend more time with a friend, Rebecca, who was also in recovery and regularly attending AA. In fact, Teri and Neil began to socialize more frequently with Rebecca and her husband.

CHALLENGING THOUGHTS ABOUT THE ROLE OF DRINKING

Use of a daily monitoring form to assess urges and thoughts about drinking served as a way Teri and I could discuss her beliefs about the role of drinking in her life. For example, she noted the following thoughts during the early part of our treatment: "I need a drink to relax" and "I deserve a drink to celebrate." I acknowledged Teri's need to relax and celebrate. However, I also asked her to identify other ways she might accomplish these goals. I challenged her belief that alcohol was the *only* way to achieve them. Through her initial period of abstinence, Teri had several experiences where she celebrated good times with friends and family without drinking. These experiences made it easier for her to challenge the old beliefs she had that linked alcohol with celebrating. Teri was quite successful at quickly finding and utilizing activities to help her relax. For example, she rediscovered her interest in reading novels and found it enjoyable to take the family dog out for long walks.

Maintenance and Termination Phase

The final stage of treatment with Teri focused on reestablishing sobriety after experiencing a slip. She had experienced the deaths of three close family members over the last 2 months of treatment. After the most recent funeral, she went home and drank 9 ounces of vodka. Teri was able to return to abstinence immediately after her lapse and we focused on how she might learn from this experience. What became apparent, particularly with her reactions to these deaths, was Teri's lack of support for her spiritual self. She began talking about how she might reconnect with her church or explore other places of worship. Teri felt she needed to address her spiritual needs in order to have a more balanced life and a stronger recovery.

During the termination phase of treatment, Teri and I discussed her progress and the specific skills she felt were most helpful. She reported regularly using the problem-solving method I had taught her with problems at home, with work, and with her parents. Teri also reported that she was consistently taking time for self-care activities and assertively communicating with Neil and colleagues at work. Finally, Teri stated she was spending a lot of time with her friend Rebecca and was socializing more with people who weren't drinkers.

Teri and I also discussed relapse warning signs and wrote out a detailed emergency plan she could follow in case she experienced another lapse. Teri identified specific relapse warning signs including (1) increases in arguments with Neil, (2) isolating herself from friends and family, and (3) reducing her self-care activities. Teri stated that if she experienced problems with sobriety, she would utilize her friend Rebecca as a support and/or reach out to me for a consultation. Toward the end of treatment Teri and I spoke more about her concern with Neil's drinking. We discussed how she could assertively communicate her concerns to him, as well as how couple treatment might be of some help.

References

Alcoholics Anonymous. (1984). *The A.A. member: Medications and other drugs.* New York: Alcoholics Anonymous World Services.

American Psychiatric Association. (1987). *Diagnostic and statistical manual of mental disorders* (3rd ed., rev). Washington, DC: Author.

Annis, H. M. (1982). *Inventory of drinking situations.* Toronto: Addiction Research Foundation of Ontario.

Beattie, M. C., & Longabaugh, R. (1999). General and alcohol-specific social support following treatment. *Addictive Behaviors, 24,* 593–606.

Booth, P. G., Dale, B., & Ansari, J. (1984). Problem drinker's goal choice and treatment outcome: A preliminary report. *Addictive Behaviors, 9,* 357–364.

Brownell, K. D., Marlatt, G. A., Lichtenstein, E., & Wilson, G. T. (1986). Understanding and preventing relapse. *American Psychologist, 41,* 765–782.

Cahalan, D. (1987). *Understanding America's drinking problem: How to combat the hazards of alcohol.* San Francisco: Jossey-Bass.

Carlson, V. B. (1991). *Testing a decisional balance worksheet for substance abusers: Factors related to intentions regarding treatment and abstinence.* Unpublished doctoral dissertation, Rutgers, The State University of New Jersey, 1991. *Dissertation Abstracts International, 52,* 5526B.

Carroll, K. M. (1996). Relapse prevention as a psychosocial treatment: A review of controlled clinical trials. *Experimental and Clinical Psychopharmacology, 4,* 46–54.

Childress, A. R., Ehrman, R., Rohsenow, D. J., Robbins, S. J., & O'Brien, C. P. (1992). Classically conditioned factors in drug dependence. In J. H. Lowinsohn, P. Ruiz, & R. B. Millman (Eds.), *Comprehensive textbook of substance abuse* (2nd ed., pp. 56–69). New York: Williams & Wilkins.

Conklin, C. A., & Tiffany, S. T. (2002). Applying extinction research and theory to cue-exposure addiction treatments. *Addiction, 97,* 155–167.

Connors, G. J., Carroll, K. M., DiClemente, C. C., Longabaugh, R., & Donovan, D. M. (1997). The therapeutic alliance and its relationship to alcoholism treatment participation and outcome. *Journal of Consulting and Clinical Psychology, 65,* 588–598.

Cunningham, J. A. (1999). Resolving alcohol-related problems with and without treatment: The effects of different problem criteria. *Journal of Studies on Alcohol, 60,* 463–466.

Davies, D. L. (1962). Normal drinking by recovered alcoholics. *Quarterly Journal of Studies on Alcohol, 23,* 94–104.

DiClemente, C. C., & Hughes, S. O. (1990). Stages of change profiles in outpatient alcoholism treatment. *Journal of Substance Abuse, 2,* 217–235.

Donovan, D. M. (1999). Assessment strategies and measures in addictive behaviors. In E. E. Epstein & B. S. McCrady (Eds.), *Addictions: A comprehensive guidebook* (pp. 187–215). New York: Oxford University Press.

Foa, E. B., & Kozak, M. S. (1986). Emotional processing of fear: Exposure to corrective information. *Psychological Bulletin, 99,* 20–35.

Foy, D. W., Nunn, B. L., & Rychtarik, R. G. (1984). Broad-spectrum behavioral treatment for chronic alcoholics: Effects of training in controlled drinking skills. *Journal of Consulting and Clinical Psychology, 52,* 218–230.

Gordon, A. J., & Zrull, M. (1991). Social networks and recovery: One year after inpatient treatment. *Journal of Substance Abuse Treatment, 8,* 143–152.

Hazelden. (1975). *Dealing with denial.* Center City, MN: Hazelden Caring Community Services.

Hester, R. K. (1995). Behavioral self-control training. In R. K. Hester & W. R. Miller (Eds.), Handbook of alcoholism treatment approaches: Effective alternatives (2nd ed., pp. 148–159). Needham Heights, MA: Allyn & Bacon.

Hunt, G. L., & Azrin, N. H. (1973). A community-reinforcement ap proach to alcoholism. *Behaviour Research and Therapy, 11,* 91–104.

Hunt, W. A., Barnett, L. W., & Branch, L. G. (1971). Relapse rates in addictions programs. *Journal of Clinical Psychology, 27,* 455–456.

Institute of Medicine (1990). *Broadening the base of treatment for alcohol problems.* Washington, DC: National Academy Press.

Irvin, J. E., Bowers, C. A., Dunn, M. E., & Wang, M. C. (1999). Efficacy of relapse prevention: A meta-analytic review. *Journal of Consulting and Clinical Psychology, 67,* 563–570.

Kadden, R. M., Carroll, K., Donovan, D., Cooney, N., Monti, P., Abrams, D., et al. (1992). *Cognitive-behavioral coping skills therapy manual: A clinical research guide for therapists treating individuals with alcohol abuse and dependence.* (NIAAA Project MATCH Monograph Series, Vol. 3, DHHS Publication No. ADM 92-1895). Rockville, MD: National Institute on Alcohol Abuse and Alcoholism.

Kadden, R. M., & Skerker, P. M. (1999). Treatment decision making and goal setting. In E. E. Epstein & B. S. McCrady (Eds.), *Addictions: A comprehensive guidebook* (pp. 216–231). New York: Oxford University Press.

Kessler, R. C., McGonagle, K. A., & Shanyang, Z. (1994). Lifetime and 12-month prevalence of DSM-III-R psychiatric disorders in the United States: Results from the National Comorbidity Survey. *Archives of General Psychiatry, 51,* 8–19.

Lawson, D. M., & Boudin, H. M. (1992). Alcohol and drug abuse. In M. Hersen & A. S. Bellack (Eds.), *Handbook of clinical behavior therapy with adults* (pp. 293–318). New York: Plenum Press.

Lieberman, M. A., Yalom, I. D., & Miles, M. B. (1973). *Encounter groups: First facts.* New York: Basic Books.

Longabaugh, R., Beattie, M., Noel, N., Stout, R., & Malloy, R. (1993). The effect of social investment on treatment outcome. *Journal of Studies on Alcohol, 54,* 465–478.

MacDonough, T. S. (1976). Evaluation of the effectiveness of intensive confrontation in changing the behavior of alcohol and drug abusers. *Behavior Therapy, 7,* 408–409.

Marlatt, G. A., & Gordon, J. R. (Eds.). (1985). *Relapse prevention: Maintenance strategies in the treatment of addictive behaviors.* New York: Guilford Press.

Marlatt, G. A., Larimar, M. E., Baer, J. S., & Quigley, L. A. (1993). Harm reduction for alcohol problems: Moving beyond the controlled drinking controversy. *Behavior Therapy, 24,* 461–504.

McCabe, R. J. R. (1986). Alcohol-dependent individuals sixteen years on. *Alcohol and Alcoholism, 21,* 165–171.

McCrady, B. S. (2001). Alcohol use disorders. In D. H. Barlow (Ed.), *Clinical handbook of psychological disorders: A step-by-step treatment manual* (3rd ed., pp. 376–433). New York: Guilford Press.

McCrady, B. S., & Delaney, S. I. (1995). Self-help groups. In R. K. Hester & W. R. Miller (Eds.), *Handbook of alcoholism treatment approaches: Effective alternatives* (2nd ed., pp. 160–175). Needham Heights, MA: Allyn & Bacon.

Meyers, R. J., & Miller, W. R. (2001). *A community reinforcement approach to addiction treatment.* New York: Cambridge University Press.

Miller, W. R. (1985). Motivation for treatment: A review with special emphasis on alcoholism. *Psychological Bulletin, 98,* 84–107.

Miller, W. R., Benefield, R. G., & Tonigan, J. S. (1993). Enhancing motivation for change in problem drinking: A controlled comparison of two therapist styles. *Journal of Consulting and Clinical Psychology, 61,* 455–461.

Miller, W. R., & Caddy, G. R. (1977). Abstinence and controlled drinking in the treatment of problem drinkers. *Journal of Studies on Alcohol, 38,* 896–1003.

Miller, W. R., & Hester, R. K. (1980). Treating the problem drinker: Modern approaches. In W. R. Miller (Ed.), *The addictive behaviors: Treatment of alcoholism, drug abuse, smoking and obesity* (pp. 11–141). Elmsford, NY: Pergamon Press.

Miller, W. R., Leckman, A. L., Delaney, H. D., & Tinkcom, M. (1992). Long-term follow-up of behavioral self-control training. *Journal of Studies on Alcohol, 53,* 249–261.

Miller, W. R., & Rollnick, S. (Eds.). (2002). *Motivational interviewing: Preparing people for change* (2nd ed.). New York: Guilford Press.

Miller, W. R., Walters, S. T., & Bennett, M. E. (2001). How effective is alcohol treatment in the United States? *Journal of Studies on Alcohol, 62,* 211–220.

Miller, W. R., Westerberg, V. S., & Waldron, H. B. (1995). Evaluating alcohol problems in adults and adolescents. In R. K. Hester & W. R. Miller (Eds.), *Hand-*

book of alcoholism treatment approaches: *Effective alternatives* (2nd ed., pp. 61–88). Needham Heights, MA: Allyn & Bacon.

Miller, W. R., & Wilbourne, P. L. (2002). Mesa Grande: A methodological analysis of clinical trials of treatments for alcohol use disorders. *Addiction, 97,* 265–277.

Monti, P. M., Abrams, D. B., Kadden, R. M., & Cooney, N. L. (1989). *Treating alcohol dependence: A coping skills training guide.* New York: Guilford Press.

Monti, P. M., Rohsenow, D. J., Colby, S. M., & Abrams, D. B. (1995). Coping and social skills training. In R. K. Hester & W. R. Miller (Eds.), *Handbook of alcoholism treatment approaches: Effective alternatives* (2nd ed., pp. 221–241). Needham Heights, MA: Allyn & Bacon.

Monti, P. M., Rohsenow, D. J., Rubonis, A. V., Niaura, R. S., Sirota, A. D., Colby, S. M., Goddard, P., & Abrams, D. B. (1993). Cue exposure with coping skills treatment for male alcoholics: A preliminary investigation. *Journal of Consulting and Clinical Psychology, 61,* 1011–1019.

Morgenstern, J., Blanchard, K., Morgan, T. J., Labouvie, E., & Hayaki, J. (2001). Testing the effectiveness of cognitive behavioral treatment for substance abuse in a community setting: Within treatment outcomes. *Journal of Consulting and Clinical Psychology, 69,* 1007–1017.

Morgenstern, J., & Longabaugh, R. (2000). Cognitive-behavioral treatment for alcohol dependence: A review of evidence for its hypothesized mechanisms of action. *Addiction, 95,* 1475–1490.

Nathan, P. E., & Niaura, R. S. (1985). Behavioral assessment and treatment of alcoholism. In J. H. Mendelson & N. K. Mello (Eds.), *The diagnosis and treatment of alcoholism* (pp. 391–45). New York: McGraw-Hill.

Nordstrom, G., & Berglund, M. (1987). A prospective study of successful long-term adjustment in alcoholic dependence: Social drinking versus abstinence. *Journal of Studies on Alcohol, 48,* 95–103.

Ogborne, A. C. (1987). A note on the characteristics of alcohol abusers with controlled drinking aspirations. *Drug and Alcohol Dependence, 19,* 159–164.

O'Leary, K. D., & Wilson, G. T. (1987). Alcoholism and cigarette smoking. In K. D. O'Leary & G. T. Wilson (Eds.), *Behavior therapy: Application and outcome* (pp. 293–319). Englewood Cliffs, NJ: Prentice-Hall.

Onken, L. S., Blaine, J. D., & Boren, J. J. (Eds.). (1993). *Behavioral treatments for drug abuse and dependence* (NIDA Research Monograph Series No. 137). Rockville, MD: National Institute of Drug Abuse.

Orford, J., & Keddie, A. (1986). Abstinence or controlled drinking in clinical practice: A test of the dependence and persuasion hypothesis. *British Journal of Addictions, 81,* 495–504.

Polich, J. M., Armor, D. J., & Braiker, H. B. (1981). *The course of alcoholism: Four years after treatment* (National Institute on Alcohol Abuse and Alcoholism). Santa Monica, CA: Rand Corporation.

Prochaska, J. O., DiClemente, C. C., & Norcross, J. C. (1992). In search of how people change: Applications to addictive behaviors. *American Psychologist, 47,* 1102–1114.

Project MATCH Research Group. (1998). Matching alcoholism treatments to client heterogeneity: Project MATCH three-year drinking outcomes. *Alcoholism: Clinical and Experimental Research, 22,* 1300–1311.

Rimmele, C. T., Howard, M. O., & Hilfrink, M. L. (1995). Aversion therapies. In R. K. Hester & W. R. Miller (Eds.), *Handbook of alcoholism treatment approaches: Effective alternatives* (2nd ed., pp. 134–147). Needham Heights, MA: Allyn & Bacon.

Rogers, C. R. (1957). The necessary and sufficient conditions for therapeutic personality change. *Journal of Consulting Psychology, 21,* 95–103.

Rosenberg, H. (1993). Prediction of controlled drinking by alcoholics and problem drinkers. *Psychological Bulletin, 113,* 129–139.

Rychtarik, R. G., Foy, D. W., Scott, T., Lokey, L., & Prue, D. M. (1987). Five–six-year follow-up of broad-spectrum behavioral treatment for alcoholism: Effects of training controlled drinking skills. *Journal of Consulting and Clinical Psychology, 55,* 106–108.

Sanchez-Craig, M., Annis, H. M., Bornet, A. R., & MacDonald, K. R. (1984). Random assignment to abstinent and controlled drinking: Evaluation of a cognitive-behavioral program for problem drinkers. *Journal of Consulting and Clinical Psychology, 52,* 390–403.

Sobell, M. B., & Sobell, L. C. (1976). Second-year treatment outcome of alcoholics treated by individualized behavior therapy: Results. *Behavior, Research and Therapy, 14,* 195–215.

Sobell, L. C., Toneatto, A., & Sobell, M. B. (1992). Behavior therapy. In R. B. Millman & J. G. Langrod (Eds.), *Substance abuse: A comprehensive textbook* (pp. 479–505). Baltimore: Williams & Wilkins.

Vaillant, G. E., & Milkofsky, E. S. (1982). Natural history of male alcoholism: IV. Paths to recovery. *Archives of General Psychiatry, 39,* 127–133.

Valle, S. K. (1981). Interpersonal functioning of alcoholism counselors and treatment outcome. *Journal of Studies on Alcohol, 42,* 783–790.

Wilson, G. T., Rossiter, E., Kleinfield, E., & Lindholm, L. (1986). Cognitive-behavioral treatment of bulimia nervosa: A controlled evaluation. *Behaviour Research and Therapy, 24,* 277–288.

9

Behavioral Economic Concepts in the Analysis of Substance Abuse

Rudy E. Vuchinich
Jalie A. Tucker

This chapter describes some aspects of basic research and theory on behavioral allocation (choice) and how those ideas have been extended to studying substance abuse and addiction. We begin with the historical development of the matching law, the conceptual innovations to which it led, and how those innovations connected with economic theory to produce behavioral economics. We then present the basic concepts and empirical relations in the behavioral economics of substance abuse, with an emphasis on intertemporal choice, temporal discounting, and the development of behavior patterns. Finally, we provide sketches of three formal theories of addiction that have been developed from the choice perspective. Our extensive discussion of some basic science issues may challenge the reader's patience in making the connection with substance abuse, which comes later in the chapter. We justify this organization on the grounds that full appreciation of the contributions of behavioral economics to studying substance abuse depends on a clear understanding of basic concepts. The reader, of course, is the final arbiter of the utility of this strategy.

THE MATCHING LAW

The original and still viable behavioral theory of choice is the matching law (Herrnstein, 1970), which is now over 30 years old. The seminal nature of the matching law is reflected in subsequent conceptual and empirical developments that currently are theoretically, methodologically, and quantitatively quite complex and sophisticated (e.g., Mazur, 2001). Discussion of the complexities of this contemporary work is beyond our present scope and purpose.

Moreover, the basic concepts concerning the matching law have been much more important than their nuances for extending these ideas to the substance abuse field.

The primary empirical arena of basic behavioral research on choice is the operant laboratory with animal subjects, although virtually all of the empirical generalizations found regarding animal choice also have been found to hold regarding human choice (e.g., Rachlin, 1987). In these laboratory preparations, animals are exposed to two schedules of reinforcement (the choice alternatives) simultaneously; relative frequency (rate) of responding to the two schedules is the primary dependent variable. Herrnstein's (1961) seminal study varied the relative frequency of reinforcement available from each of the two alternatives—that is, across conditions, more frequent reinforcement was provided by one alternative and then by the other.

The critical issue in Herrnstein's experiment was how the relative frequency of responding was distributed across the two response alternatives as a function of how the relative frequency of reinforcement was distributed across the two alternatives. The results were the surprisingly simple equality expressed in Equation 1.

$$\frac{B_1}{B_2} = \frac{FR_1}{FR_2} \tag{1}$$

In Equation 1, B_1 and B_2 represent the number of responses allocated to alternatives 1 and 2, respectively, and FR_1 and FR_2 represent the frequency or number of reinforcements received from alternatives 1 and 2, respectively. Thus, the animals' behavior was distributed over the response options in direct proportion to the frequency of reinforcement received from those options. For example, if one-third of the total reinforcements were received from alternative 1, then one-third of responding was allocated to alternative 1, and so on for different distributions of responding and reinforcement across the alternatives.

Subsequent research investigated how variations in dimensions of reinforcement other than frequency would affect relative behavioral allocation. Catania (1963) studied schedules in which the frequency of reinforcement was held constant and the amount of food per reinforcement was manipulated. He found that behavioral allocation matched relative reinforcement amounts, as reflected in Equation 2.

$$\frac{B_1}{B_2} = \frac{AR_1}{AR_2} \tag{2}$$

In Equation 2, B_1 and B_2 are the same as in Equation 1, and AR_1 and AR_2 represent the amounts of food received per reinforcement from options 1 and 2, respectively. Thus, relative behavioral allocation was directly proportional to relative reinforcement amount. So, for example, if the amount of food received per reinforcement from option 1 was twice that of option 2, then twice as many responses were allocated to option 1 than to option 2.

Chung and Herrnstein (1967) studied the effects of delay of reinforcement on behavioral allocation, and found a matching relation in which relative behavioral allocation matched the inverse of the relative delays of reinforcement, as depicted in Equation 3.

$$\frac{B_1}{B_2} = \frac{DR_2}{DR_1} \tag{3}$$

In Equation 3, B_1 and B_2 are as before, and DR_1 and DR_2 represent the delays of receipt of reinforcement from options 1 and 2, respectively. Thus, behavioral allocation was inversely proportional to the relative delays of reinforcement. So, if reinforcement for option 1 was delayed twice as long as that for option 2, then half as many responses would be allocated to option 1 than to option 2. Research on behavioral allocation in choice situations involving different amounts and delays of reinforcement (e.g., Rachlin & Green, 1972) has had significant implications for understanding impulsiveness and self-control. We return to this topic later in the chapter in the context of understanding addictive behavior.

These early empirical results regarding choice were sufficiently general for Herrnstein (1970) to propose the matching law as a general analytical framework for describing behavioral allocation to any particular response option in any situation. This general version of the matching law is expressed in Equation 4.

$$\frac{B_1}{B_O} = \frac{R_1}{R_O} \tag{4}$$

In Equation 4, B_1 and R_1 refer to behavior allocated to and (the combined dimensions of) reinforcement received from a particular response option, and B_O and R_O refer to behavior allocated to and reinforcement received from all other response options in that situation. Thus, Equation 4 states that the proportion of behavior allocated to any given response option (B_1) will be a joint function of reinforcement received from that option (R_1) and reinforcement received from all other sources (R_O).

CONCEPTUAL INNOVATIONS
DERIVED FROM THE MATCHING LAW

The matching law is a straightforward equation that originated in a simplified laboratory preparation. Although the law and the initial empirical arena are simple, the conceptual innovations initiated by the matching law have not been simple. In fact, these innovations involved revisions in some fundamental assumptions about what controls behavior. As described next, these conceptual innovations emanate from the relativism and molarity of the matching law.

Relativism of the Matching Law

The relativism of the matching law was a significant departure from the ideas that dominated learning theory in experimental psychology at the time (cf. Rachlin & Laibson, 1997). The principle of the reflex was the overarching concept, in which each particular response was thought to correspond to a particular environmental or internal stimulus. Thus, the stream of behavior was decomposed into a series of *reflexes*, that is, individual responses in reaction to individual stimuli, and theory was concerned with understanding the strength of individual stimulus–response connections (e.g., Hull, 1943) or of individual responses (e.g., Skinner, 1938). Given this focus on individual responses, with the reflex as the primary organizing concept, the determinants of any particular response were thought to reside in the eliciting or discriminative stimuli that immediately preceded it, the consequent stimuli that immediately followed it, or in some mechanism that mediated between stimuli, responses, and consequences. Little attention was paid to the more general context of other behavior and other consequences that surrounded a particular response. But Herrnstein's (1970) research and equations clearly indicated that behavior allocated to a particular response option could be altered by modifying the reinforcement for other options. This did not accord well with an account based on reflexes.

Assume, for example, that we want to increase the frequency of B_1 in Equation 4, which we could easily do by enriching R_1. An account based on individual responses would argue that the enriched R_1 strengthened the reflex of which B_1 is a part, and thereby increased its occurrence. This is fine as far as it goes, but it ignores the more general context in which B_1 and R_1 are occurring. Because the matching law focuses on that context, Equation 4 provides a somewhat different interpretation of such a change: enriching R_1 would increase the reinforcement ratio on the right side of the equation, which would realign the behavior ratio on the left side of the equation so that B_1 constituted a larger fraction of behavioral output. Thus, according to the matching law, enriching R_1 increases B_1 because R_1 is now relatively more valuable in this context, and not because the reflex of which B_1 is a part has gotten stronger.

Moreover, in Equation 4, B_1 and B_O exhaust the response possibilities, and total behavioral output cannot exceed their sum. Thus, a decrease in B_O necessarily involves an increase in B_1. So, the matching law states that we also could increase the frequency of B_1 by decreasing R_O, the reinforcement for behavior other than B_1. Decreasing R_O, like increasing R_1, also would increase the reinforcement ratio (i.e., make R_1 relatively more valuable) on the right side of Equation 4. This, in turn, would realign the behavior ratio on the left side of the equation so that a larger fraction of behavioral output would be comprised of B_1. Such indirect behavior modification due to the relativism inherent in the matching law was not easily handled by accounts that focused on individual responses (Rachlin & Laibson, 1997).

Molarity of the Matching Law

The matching law is a molar account of behavior in that it relates aggregates of behavior to aggregates of reinforcement as measured over some extended temporal interval (cf. Vuchinich, 1995). It cannot and does not attempt to account for the occurrence of particular B_1 or B_O responses, which would be the goal of a molecular account of behavior. Abandoning any theoretical effort aimed at accounting for the occurrence of particular responses was a significant departure from what was regarded as an acceptable explanation for behavior at the time (Lacey & Rachlin, 1978). Other influential behavioral theories in that era (e.g., Hull, 1943; Skinner, 1938) were molecular and were designed, at least in principle, to explain the occurrence of particular responses. In contrast, the matching law is concerned with understanding the distribution of behavior over time to response alternatives, in relation to the contextually determined value of the consequences of those alternatives.

THE ECONOMIC CONNECTION

The general implications of the relativism and molarity of the matching law were developed by Herrnstein (1970) and others (e.g., Lacey & Rachlin, 1978) during the several years after its formulation. These developments raised conceptual and empirical issues quite different from those raised by molecular accounts. In general, each response alternative and its associated consequences came to be viewed not as a reflex, but as a package with a certain benefit/cost ratio based on the consequences produced over time by a given level of behavioral output over time. Behavior is assumed to be allocated to a particular response alternative according to the value of its benefit/cost ratio relative to the ratios for the set of response alternatives. In general, changing the benefit or cost of an alternative would change its value relative to the set, which would change the behavior allocated to it—for example, increasing the benefit or lowering the cost of an alternative would raise its value relative to the set. The relative value of a given alternative also would change even if its own benefits and costs did not change, but if the more general context of benefit/cost ratios of other response alternatives changed.

Given this shift in orientation, the field became concerned with understanding the manner in which behavioral allocation over time entrains with the availability of valued consequences over time. As this choice literature developed, several scientists (e.g., Hursh, 1980; Rachlin, Green, Kagel, & Battalio, 1976) recognized that this type of general question was very similar to the questions addressed by consumer demand theory in economics. That is, animals in operant experiments and human consumers in the economy both allocate limited resources (e.g., time, behavior, money) to gain access to activities of variable value (e.g., eating, drinking, leisure) under conditions of variable environmental constraint. Recognizing this commonality led to a merger of the behavioral analysis of choice and of microeconomic theory, now known as "behavioral economics" (e.g., Hursh, 1980; Kagel, Battalio, & Green, 1995).

BEHAVIORAL ECONOMICS OF SUBSTANCE USE AND ABUSE: BASIC CONCEPTS AND EMPIRICAL RELATIONS

The relevance of behavioral economics for studying substance abuse was recognized early in its development (e.g., Vuchinich, 1982), and research applications to human substance abuse are growing (e.g., Bickel, Madden, & Petry, 1998; Vuchinich, 1997). Behavioral economics is a system of specific concepts that applies the general principles of relativism and molarity to understanding substance abuse. As such, behavioral economics has focused on studying patterns of substance abuse as they emerge, develop, and change over extended time frames in the context of variability in access to substance use and to other activities.

In general, the value of substance use, and thus the extent to which it is preferred, is a function of the benefit/cost ratio of substance use in relation to the benefit/cost ratios of other available activities. This section summarizes behavioral economic research on substance abuse and is organized into three broad topics: (1) substance use as a function of its own benefit/cost ratio (e.g., constraints on access to the abused substance, such as price), (2) substance use as a function of the benefit/cost ratio of other activities (e.g., constraints on access to and price of valuable activities other than substance use), and (3) intertemporal choice situations, in which individuals choose between outcomes that vary in amount as well as in the delay to which they are received. Our emphasis is on intertemporal choice, because the first two topics have been amply summarized elsewhere (Bickel et al., 1998; Vuchinich, 1997).

Substance Use as a Function of Its Own Benefit/Cost Ratio

Demand, the amount of a commodity that is purchased, is the primary dependent variable in microeconomics (Kagel et al., 1995). Because excessive consumption is the crux of the problem in substance abuse, this focus on demand renders behavioral economics immediately relevant (Hursh, 1993). Early research demonstrated that consumption of abused substances varies inversely with their cost (cf. Vuchinich & Tucker, 1988). Behavioral economic concepts and research have organized and expanded upon these relations through the analysis of demand curves. A *demand curve* plots consumption of a commodity as a function of its price. In general, there is an inverse relation between consumption and price.

This relation is shown by the solid line in Figure 9.1, which is a demand curve for a hypothetical commodity A. A key concept for describing this consumption–price relation is *own-price elasticity of demand*, which is the ratio of proportional changes in consumption to proportional changes in price (cf. Hursh, 1993). Thus, own–price elasticity of demand quantifies how consumption changes as price changes. The dotted line in Figure 9.1 shows "unit elasticity" ($\varepsilon = -1.0$), wherein demand decreases by the same proportion that price increases. Demand elasticities fall along a continuum from inelastic demand

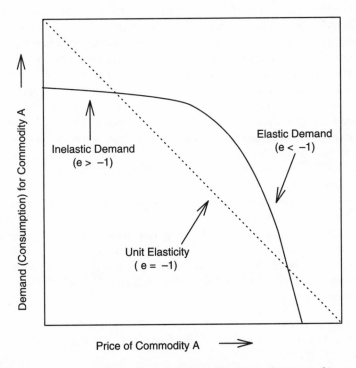

FIGURE 9.1. Demand for hypothetical Commodity A as a function of its own price (solid line). Own–price elasticity of demand (e) is defined as the ratio of proportional changes in consumption of A to proportional changes in the price of A. The dotted line shows unit elasticity, in which consumption decreases by the same proportion as price increases. The demand curve for A shows the typical mixed elasticity, with relatively inelastic demand at low prices and relatively elastic demand at high prices.

($\varepsilon > -1.0$), which shows little or no changes in consumption as price changes (the left part of the demand curve in Figure 9.1), to elastic demand ($\varepsilon < -1.0$), which shows substantial changes in consumption as price changes (the right part of the demand curve in Figure 9.1). Demand typically shows mixed elasticity across a range of price changes, being more inelastic at low prices and more elastic at high prices, as depicted by the solid line in Figure 9.1. For example, rising gas prices will not produce substantial changes in gas purchases and driving until they get quite high.

Behavioral economic research in this area initially focused on two questions: (1) Does demand for abused substances show an inverse relation with price? (2) Do the quantitative properties of demand curves (i.e., own-price elasticity) aid in the description of the determinants of substance consumption? Both of these questions have been answered "Yes." Bickel, DeGrandpre, and colleagues (e.g., DeGrandpre, Bickel, Hughes, Layng, & Badger, 1993) reanalyzed data from numerous drug self-administration experiments with relevant data that had not previously been inspected using demand curve analyses (including studies of cocaine, codeine, d-amphetemine, ethanol, ketamine, methohexital, morphine, pentobarbital, phencyclidine, and procaine self-administration). Rearranging the data into demand curves revealed the typical mixed elasticity for all drugs studied: demand was inelastic at lower prices and elastic at higher prices (see Figure 9.1). Similar relations were found when data from 17 studies of human cigarette smoking were reanalyzed (DeGrandpre, Bickel, Hughes, & Higgins, 1992). This same inverse relation between substance consumption and price also has been observed in the natural environment for alcoholic beverages (e.g., Leung & Phelps, 1993), cigarettes (e.g., Chaloupka, 1991), and illicit drugs (e.g., Saffer & Chaloupka, 1999).

Overall, research on substance use as a function of its own benefit/cost ratio has consistently found a quantifiable inverse relation between consumption and cost (cf. DeGrandpre & Bickel, 1996). The relation generalizes across species, substances, normal and clinical populations, and laboratory and natural environments. The findings indicate that the consumption of abused substances can be usefully described with the same analytic tools that apply to all commodities.

Substance Use as a Function of the Benefit–Cost Ratio of Other Activities

The relativism inherent in behavioral economics implies that the value of substance use will depend on the more general context of what other activities are also available for engagement and on variability in their benefit/cost ratios. This more general context is a key issue in substance abuse research, because strong preferences for abused substances arise in natural environments that presumably contain opportunities to engage in a variety of other activities. Understanding the conditions under which substance consumption emerges as a highly preferred activity from among an array of qualitatively different activities is a basic problem for substance abuse research (Vuchinich & Tucker, 1988). In general, the choice perspective suggests that demand for abused substances will vary inversely with the benefit/cost ratios of other activities. Numerous laboratory studies with animals and humans have demonstrated this important qualitative relationship (reviewed by Carroll, 1996; Vuchinich & Tucker, 1988).

Quantifying how drug demand interacts with the availability of and demand for other reinforcers can be approached using the economic concept of *cross-price elasticity of demand*, which refers to how demand for one commodity changes when the price for another commodity changes (Hursch, 1993; Kagel et al., 1995). This is represented in Figure 9.2, which shows two possible ways that demand for (hypothetical) commodity B may change as a

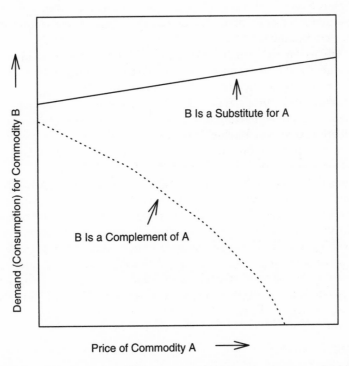

FIGURE 9.2. Demand for hypothetical Commodity B as a function of the price of Commodity A. Cross-price elasticity of demand is defined as the ratio of proportional changes in consumption of B to proportional changes in the price of A. Positive cross-price elasticity (solid line) indicates that B is a substitute for A (consumption of B increases as consumption of A decreases). Negative cross-price elasticity (dotted line) indicates that B is a complement of A (consumption of B decreases as consumption of A decreases).

function of the price of commodity A. If demand varies inversely, the commodities are *substitutes* (the solid line in Figure 9.2), and if demand varies directly, they are *complements* (the dashed line). Positive and negative cross-price elasticities indicate economic substitutes and complements, respectively.

Bickel, DeGrandpre, and Higgins (1995) evaluated the utility of this concept in a reanalysis of 16 drug self-administration studies that permitted the determination of substitutability relations between drug consumption (including caffeine, nicotine, cocaine, etonitazene, ethanol, heroin, methadone, morphine, pentobarbital, and phencyclidine [PCP]) and alternative drug and nondrug reinforcers (e.g., food, sucrose, water). Demand for the drugs entered into relations with other reinforcers at all points along the substitutability continuum. In separate studies, for example, substitute relations were found between sucrose and ethanol, etonitazene and water, and PCP and ethanol, whereas complement relations were found between heroin and cigarettes, alcohol and cigarettes, heroin and food, and ethanol and water. Thus, behavioral economic concepts concerning substitutability relations are useful for describing how demand for drugs interacts with demand for other commodities.

Variability in the benefit/cost ratios of activities other than substance use presumably also are important in understanding variability in substance abuse in the natural environment. Vuchinich and Tucker (1996b) applied this reasoning to a prospective analysis of relapse episodes among alcohol-dependent males after treatment. Relapses occurred more often and tended to be more severe when valued nondrinking rewards in the posttreatment environment became more constrained. In related research, Tucker, Vuchinich, and colleagues (Tucker, Vuchinich, & Gladsjo, 1994; Tucker, Vuchinich, & Pukish, 1995; Tucker, Vuchinich, & Rippens, 2002a) investigated the environmental contexts associated with successful long-term resolution of drinking problems in treated and untreated problem drinkers. Resolution can be conceptualized as involving the reverse process compared to relapse, wherein the reward structure in the natural environment shifts toward greater availability of nondrinking rewards. Such relationships were observed between stable resolution and increased access to valued nondrinking rewards in the natural environments of former problem drinkers. This pattern was not found for active problem drinkers, whose life circumstances tended to worsen over time.

Intertemporal Choice, Temporal Discounting, Impulsiveness, and Substance Abuse

BACK TO THE MATCHING LAW

So far this chapter has been concerned with behavioral allocation in situations in which the outcomes of the choice alternatives were immediately available.

In the natural environment, however, outcomes of choices typically do not occur immediately: behavior is typically allocated to current activities that produce outcomes that occur sometime in the future. Behavioral allocation in these conditions is termed *intertemporal choice* because the outcomes of the choice alternatives are spread out in time. Intertemporal choice is especially important for understanding substance abuse, since individuals presumably are repeatedly choosing between a readily available but relatively small reward (substance use) and engaging in activities that will produce delayed but more valuable rewards in various life-health areas (e.g., positive intimate, family, or social relations; vocational or academic success).

Equation 2 and Equation 3 showed matching with respect to amount and delay of reinforcement. Variability in these two dimensions of reinforcement can be combined multiplicatively (e.g., Rachlin & Green, 1972), as in Equation 5.

$$\frac{B_1}{B_2} = \frac{A_1}{A_2} \times \frac{D_2}{D_1} \tag{5}$$

Equation 5 describes preference in intertemporal choice situations involving different amounts of reinforcement that are available after different delays. If the smaller reinforcer is available relatively sooner and the larger reinforcer is available relatively later, then intertemporal choice in this situation can be described as either impulsive or self-controlled. Choice of the smaller, sooner reinforcer (SSR) is labeled "impulsive," and choice of the larger later reinforcer (LLR) is labeled "self-controlled." Equation 5 states that preference will be directly proportional to the amount of reinforcement and inversely proportional to the delay of reinforcement. The critical importance of this form of the matching law for understanding intertemporal choice is the manner in which the value of rewards is predicted to vary as a function of delay to their receipt. As articulated next, the matching law predicts that preference between the two reinforcers will depend on the temporal distance to their receipt in relation to when behavioral allocation occurs. At some choice points the individual will be impulsive, and at other choice points the individual will be self-controlled.

TEMPORAL DISCOUNTING

As a concrete example from the animal laboratory (e.g., Rachlin & Green, 1972), say alternative 1 (the LLR) is 6 seconds of food ($A_1 = 6$) and alternative 2 (the SSR) is 2 seconds of food ($A_2 = 2$), and that the LLR is available 8 seconds after the SSR. These relations are shown in Figure 9.3, with time along the abscissa, reward value along the ordinate, and the rewards represented as vertical boxes at the times they are available. In Figure 9.3, the 2-second food reward (A_2) is available at time 14, and the 6-second food reward (A_1) is available at time 22. As derived from Equation 6, the value of a delayed rein-

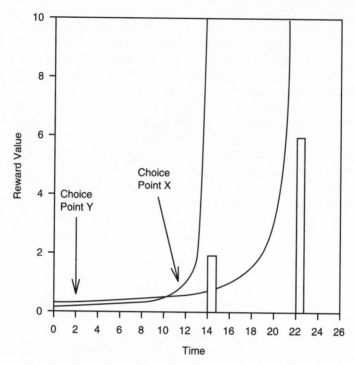

FIGURE 9.3. Intertemporal choice between 2 seconds of food available at time 14 and 6 seconds of food available at time 22. Value curves to the left of the rewards were drawn from Equation 7. See text for explanation.

forcer at a particular point in time is given by the A/D fraction, as shown in Equation 6.

$$v_1 = \frac{A_i}{D_i} \qquad (6)$$

In Equation 6, v_i is the present value of a reward of amount A_i that is available after a delay of D_i. In Figure 9.3, the curves to the left of the rewards trace the respective A/D fractions for the rewards as delay changes; thus, these curves represent the value of the rewards during the times before they are available. This change in reward value as a function of delay is termed *temporal discounting* because the present value of a delayed reward is discounted below what its value will be at the time it is received in the future. Equation 6 is one form of a temporal discounting function because it describes how reward value changes with delay.

In Equation 5, the B_1/B_2 ratio measures whether the subject prefers alternative 1 or alternative 2: a behavior ratio greater than unity (i.e., 1.0) indicates a preference for alternative A_1, while a behavior ratio less than unity indicates a preference for alternative A_2. At Choice Point X at time 12 in Figure 9.3, the LLR is delayed by 10 seconds ($A_1 = 6$, $D_1 = 10$), and the SSR is delayed by 2 seconds ($A_2 = 2$, $D_2 = 2$). Inserting these amount and delay values into Equation 5 yields a B_1/B_2 ratio of .60, indicating a preference for alternative 2, the SSR, or the impulsive choice. At Choice Point X, the absolute values (from Equation 6) of alternative 1 and alternative 2 would be .600 and 1.000, respectively. But preference is predicted to change if both rewards are further delayed by 10 seconds, so that the choice occurs at a greater temporal distance from both rewards. This is shown as Choice Point Y at time 2 in Figure 9.3. Now alternative 1 is 6 seconds of food delayed by 20 seconds ($A_1 = 6$, $D_1 = 20$), and alternative 2 is 2 seconds of food delayed by 12 seconds ($A_2 = 2$, $D_2 = 12$). Inserting these modified amount and delay values into Equation 5 yields a B_1/B_2 ratio of 1.80, indicating a preference for alternative 1, the LLR, or the self-controlled choice. At Choice Point Y, the absolute values of alternatives 1 and 2 (from Equation 6) would be .300 and .167, respectively. Thus, the values of both rewards are less at Choice Point Y than at Choice Point X because of temporal discounting. Importantly, the shape of the discount function inherent in the matching law predicts that preference between the rewards will reverse simply with the passage of time.

Although the matching law implies that reward value will vary over time according to the simple A/D fraction in Equation 6, subsequent research (e.g., Mazur, 1987) has provided strong support for the slightly different temporal discounting function shown in Equation 7.

$$v_i = \frac{A_i}{1 + kD_i} \tag{7}$$

In Equation 7, v_i, A_i, and D_i are the same as in Equation 6. The k parameter in Equation 7 is a constant that is proportional to the degree of temporal discounting, with higher and lower k values describing greater and lesser degrees of discounting, respectively. Inclusion of 1 and k in the denominator of Equation 7 resolved two problems with the simple A/D fraction (Equation 6). First, with 1 in the denominator of Equation 7, the value of a reinforcer never exceeds its amount (as in Figure 9.3 at very short delays), even when it is immediately available (i.e., if $D_i = 0$, then $v_i = A_i$). Second, variability in the k parameter allows for greater or lesser degrees of temporal discounting, which can incorporate differences between individuals in how much they value delayed rewards. This discount function is in the form of a hyperbola; hence it is termed "hyperbolic temporal discounting".

TEMPORAL DISCOUNTING AND SUBSTANCE ABUSE

Ainslie (1975, 1992), Rachlin (1995), and others (e.g., Loewenstein & Prelec, 1992) have written extensively on the general implications of hyperbolic dis-

counting for understanding impulsiveness and self-control. These intertemporal choice dynamics also are important for understanding substance
abuse. In Figure 9.4, the SSR is analogous to an alcohol or drug consumption
episode, and the LLR is analogous to a more valuable but delayed nondrinking
or nondrug activity. The choice dynamics that result from hyperbolic discounting are consistent with two general and important aspects of substance
abuse patterns. First, even when reward availability does not change, individuals often display ambivalence in that their preference for substance use will
vary over time depending on the temporal distance to the availability of the
substance and the alternative activity. The LLRs will be preferred before the
point where the reward value curves cross, and substance use will be preferred
after that point. But once the person exits the situation involving imminent

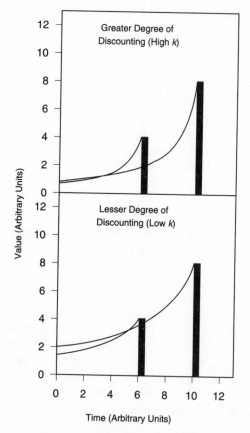

FIGURE 9.4. Both panels show an intertemporal choice between a smaller and a
larger reward available at time 6 and time 10, respectively. The upper and lower panels
show greater and lesser degrees of hyperbolic temporal discounting, respectively.

substance availability, preference will revert back to the LLRs, and the individual may regret the substance use episode. Such ambivalence is a key feature of substance use problems (e.g., Miller, 1998). Second, the LLRs that enter into these intertemporal choice dynamics with substance use will likely differ across individuals and across time for the same individual (Vuchinich & Tucker, 1996a, 1996b). Such variability is consistent with the diverse life-health problems associated with substance abuse in populations of alcohol and drug abusers (e.g., Maisto & McCollum, 1980).

This behavioral economic theoretical framework also makes a straightforward prediction regarding differences in the degree of temporal discounting between substance-abusing and normal populations. This prediction is displayed graphically in Figure 9.4, which again shows an intertemporal choice between an SSR that is available at time 6 and an LLR that is available at time 10. The reward value curves in both panels of Figure 9.4 were drawn using the hyperbolic function in Equation 7, with the top and bottom panels showing the curves for relatively high and relatively low values of k, respectively. The higher k used in the top panel produces steeper value curves than the lower k used in the bottom panel. Preference between the SSR and the LLR reverses with the passage of time in both panels, with higher and lower discounting producing sooner and later preference shifts, respectively. As suggested by Figure 9.4, an individual with a high degree of temporal discounting (top panel) would spend more time preferring the SSR (i.e., substance use) than an individual with a low degree of discounting (bottom panel). This leads to the prediction that k values would be larger among substance abusers compared to nonabusers.

This prediction has been supported in several recent studies. When compared to normal individuals, greater temporal discounting has been found among alcohol abusers (Vuchinich & Simpson, 1998), heroin addicts (e.g., Kirby, Petry, & Bickel, 1999), smokers (e.g., Mitchell, 1999), and compulsive gamblers (Petry & Casarella, 1999). Moreover, Tucker, Vuchinich, and Rippens (2002b) reported a 2-year longitudinal study of predictors of successful natural resolutions of alcohol problems by problem drinkers in the natural environment. They found that a measure of temporal discounting derived from monetary spending patterns during the year prior to initial resolution was a significant predictor of stable resolution throughout the 2-year follow-up period. Those participants who reported a higher proportion of preresolution discretionary expenditures on savings than on alcoholic beverages were more likely to remain continuously resolved compared to those who relapsed. This differential allocation pattern to savings and drinking reflects behavior controlled by delayed versus immediate consequences, respectively, and is presumed to reflect a discounting process. Thus, the relationship between substance abuse and temporal discounting appears to have considerable generality across substance-abusing populations and across laboratory and natural environments.

Objects of Choice: Particular Acts or Temporally Extended Patterns of Acts

The preceding discussion of intertemporal choice and temporal discounting characterized the objects of choice (i.e., SSRs and LLRs) as discrete events that occur at a particular time, much like food reinforcement for an animal in the laboratory. In this conception, if an individual prefers the LLR, he or she forgoes the SSR and then the LLR arrives later at a given point in time (as in Figures 9.3 and 9.4). Many SSRs in the natural environment, like a drugs or alcohol-consumption episode, may reasonably be viewed as discrete, tangible, and temporally circumscribed events. However, most naturally occurring LLRs, like vocational success, are not so reasonably viewed in this way (Rachlin, 1995; Vuchinich & Tucker, 1996b). Real LLRs in peoples' lives (e.g., "vocational success," "marital happiness," "health") are not discrete, tangible, and temporally circumscribed events. Rather, they are better viewed as abstractions that comprise many smaller rewards that occur over an extended temporal interval in a complex but coherent pattern. An individual's behavior is allocated over time to activities that produce a series of relatively small but

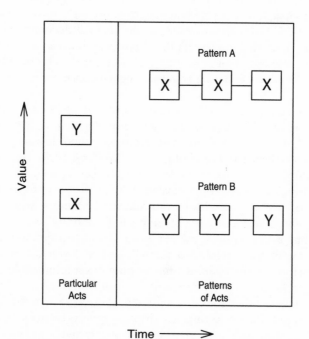

FIGURE 9.5. Figure represents the relative value of particular acts (X and Y) when considered in isolation (left side), and the relative value of temporally extended patterns of behavior (A and B) that contain Acts X and Y as components (right side).

immediate gratifications (e.g., SSRs associated with alcohol consumption), or that may produce a more temporally extended but more valuable gratification (e.g., the LLR associated with "vocational success"). But even if an individual let every discrete drinking opportunity (the SSR) pass by, "vocational success" (the LLR) would not suddenly arrive fully formed at a specific future time. Rather, vocational success takes time to develop and maintain. As more acts are emitted that are consistent with the molar pattern of vocational success (e.g., continuously improving work products), and as less behavior is devoted to activities that may undermine vocational success (e.g., excessive drinking), then more of the constituent parts of the overall LLR will be accrued over an extended interval.

Rachlin (1995) proposed a shift in the view of intertemporal choice situations that attempts to accommodate those considerations. Hyperbolic discounting produces temporal inconsistencies between short-term and long-term preferences, but perhaps the key distinction is between the value of *discrete acts* and the value of *patterns of acts*, rather than between the value of a discrete SSR and the value of a discrete LLR. Rachlin argued that the temporal inconsistencies often found between individuals' preferences at different points in time are better characterized as differences between the value of discrete acts that determine short-term preferences and the value of temporally extended patterns of acts that determine long-term preferences. In this view, obtaining the higher valued, long-term preferences entails temporally extended patterns of behavior. But the development and maintenance of such patterns may be undermined because their component acts often are relatively less valuable than alternative particular acts that are inconsistent with the pattern. Thus, a key issue becomes whether the objects of choice are perceived as discrete acts or as patterns of acts.

These relations are illustrated in Figure 9.5. The left side of Figure 9.5 shows the value of Act X and Act Y when they are considered as discrete, particular acts. The right side of Figure 9.5 shows the value of temporally extended behavior Pattern A and Pattern B, which are comprised of a series of Act X's and Act Y's, respectively. When considered as particular acts in a choice between discrete outcomes, Act Y has greater value than Act X. When considered as single components of wider behavior patterns, Pattern A (which includes Act X) has greater value than Pattern B (which includes Act Y). When the choice is perceived as being between particular acts in the present, Act Y is more valuable (in the short term) than Act X, so Act Y tends to be preferred. When the choice is perceived as being between temporally extended patterns of acts that extend into the future, Pattern A (comprised of a series of X's) is more valuable (in the long term) than Pattern B (comprised of a series of Y's), so Pattern A tends to be preferred. Thus, patterns of behavior that are more valuable over long temporal intervals may be comprised of single component acts that individually are less valuable than alternative particular acts. Conversely, patterns of behavior that are less valuable over long temporal intervals may be comprised of single component acts that alone are more valuable than alternative particular acts.

For example, suppose that the long-term, higher valued Pattern A in Figure 9.5 represents a satisfying family life, and that some of the particular acts (X) that constitute that pattern are quiet but mildly enjoyable evenings at home with family members. Further suppose that the long-term, lower valued Pattern B represents alcohol abuse, and that some of the particular acts (Y) that constitute that pattern are raucous and highly enjoyable evenings out of the home that involve heavy drinking with friends. In a discrete choice between Act X and Act Y, the value of an evening out with friends (Act Y) may be much higher than the value of an evening at home with the family (Act X). However, over an extended interval, the pattern that produces a satisfying family life (Pattern A) would almost certainly be preferred to the pattern of alcohol abuse (Pattern B) and all its resulting problems. Thus, if the objects of choice are perceived as temporally extended patterns of behavior (A and B), then Pattern A would likely be preferred because it has greater value over an extended temporal horizon. On the other hand, if the objects of choice are perceived as individual acts (X and Y), then Act Y would likely be preferred because it has more value in the temporally circumscribed present. The degree of temporal extension with which the objects of choice are perceived therefore may be critically important in the allocation of behavior that leads to patterns of substance abuse or to the realization of more valuable LLRs.

Viewing the primary unit of analysis as a patterns of acts, rather than as a particular act, is a recent development and one that has not been well researched. There is, however, some evidence relevant to the value of behavior patterns. In laboratory studies using both humans and animals, Rachlin (1995) found that, if contingencies are established that generate cohesive patterns in participants' behavior, then behavioral allocation is more consistent with long-term preferences. Other studies (e.g., Loewenstein & Prelec, 1992, 1993) showed that, if future events are part of a temporally extended sequence or pattern, then their value is greater than if they are independent events in separate, discrete choices. Pursuing the conceptual and empirical implications of the discrete act versus pattern of acts distinction will be important in the continued development of behavioral economics generally and in its applications to substance abuse.

THEORIES OF ADDICTION

The key challenge to any theory of addiction is explaining why some individuals continue a behavior pattern of excessive consumption when that pattern produces a variety of sometimes extremely negative consequences. Theories of addiction based on other literatures (e.g., neuroscience research; see Robinson & Berridge, 1993) sometimes argue that consumption has somehow gotten outside the individual's volitional control. Indeed, the ubiquitous term "addiction" often implies this characteristic and is a reason why behavioral accounts prefer other terms, such as "addictive behavior" or "substance use disorder." Regardless of terminology, appealing to nonvolitional forces is not an option for a theory of addiction based on choice. Thus, the challenge of developing a theory of addiction is particularly acute in the choice literature because of the orienting assumption that individuals "freely choose" their behavioral allocation patterns based on some function of the consequences of those patterns.

The temporal inconsistencies in preference caused by hyperbolic temporal discounting are an important element in explaining addiction from this perspective. Hyperbolic discounting alone, however, is widely regarded as an insufficient explanation by itself (e.g., Monterosso & Ainslie, 1999). Thus, other choice dynamics have been proposed to explain the apparently self-defeating behavior pattern of addiction. In this section, we sketch three formal theories of addiction: (1) melioration addiction theory (Herrnstein & Prelec, 1992), (2) relative addiction theory (Rachlin, 1997), and (3) rational addiction theory (Becker & Murphy, 1988). Melioration and relative addiction theory originated in the psychological literature, while rational addiction theory originated in the economic literature.

Before sketching the theories, we must mention two important commonalities and one important distinction among them. The first commonality is that long-term behavioral allocation patterns of consumption of the abused substance and other activities are the focus of each theory. The second commonality is the notion that consumption of addictive commodities during one time period reduces the utility derived in later time periods from consumption of the addictive commodity and from other commodities. Consumption of the addictive commodity in one time period reduces utility of the same level of consumption in future periods through tolerance. The utility derived from nonaddictive commodity consumption in one time period is reduced by earlier addictive commodity consumption because the latter disrupts the ability to engage the former. Thus, each theory proposes a sort of intertemporal dependency between consumption and utility in different time periods that is critical in accounting for addiction.

Each theory also is based on some form of utility maximization. Indeed, the important distinction among them is the type of utility that is maximized. Rational and relative addiction theory argue that overall utility is maximized, while melioration theory argues that local utility is maximized. *Local utility* is the benefit derived from engaging in an activity during the time of that engagement. *Overall utility* is the sum of the local utilities over a more extended time period. In the context of the matching law discussed earlier (i.e., Equation 1), the local utility of alternative 1 is the rate of R_1 while engaging in B_1, and the local utility of alternative 2 is the rate of R_2 while engaging in B_2. Overall utility is the sum of R_1 and R_2 over the length of the session. Maximization of local utility is termed *melioration* (Herrnstein, 1982), and maximization of overall utility is simply termed *maximization* (Rachlin et al., 1976).

Melioration Theory of Addiction

The melioration theory (Herrnstein & Prelec, 1992) holds that the maximization of local utility derived from substance use and from other activities can lead to addiction. In this theory, all non-substance-use activities are considered together as one choice option, so the individual is allocating behavior to substance-use or to non-substance-use activities. These choice options are mutually exclusive and exhaustive. The local utility of substance-use activity is the benefit derived during consumption, and the local utility of non-substance-use activities is the utility derived while engaged in them. Overall utility is the sum of the local utilities of substance-use and non-substance-use activities. According to melioration theory, the individual's behavioral allocation is insensitive to overall utility and completely sensitive to the comparison of local utilities.

As noted earlier, a key element of the melioration theory of addiction is that substance use lowers the utility derived from such substance use and from non-substance-use activities. This process is depicted graphically in Figure 9.6 (Figures 9.6–9.8 are based on similar figures in Rachlin, 1997). In Figure 9.6, utility is along the ordinate, and the relative allocation of behavior to substance-use and non-substance-use activities is along the abscissa. Movement to the right along the abscissa signifies relatively more behavior being allocated to substance use and less to other activities (the process of addiction); the converse is true for movement to the left. The local utility of substance use, the local utility of other activities, and overall utility are signified by lines 2–3, 1–4, and 1–3, respectively. Melioration maintains that behavior is allocated according to which choice option provides the highest local utility. As seen in Figure 9.6, even though both local utilities and overall utility are being reduced by substance use, the individual continues to use the substance. Increasing levels of addictive commodity consumption—that is, movement to the right along the abscissa of Figure 9.6—reduces both local and overall utility, but the melioration process continues to drive addictive consumption because the local utility of that consumption remains higher than the local utility of not consuming. Although the process of melioration has considerable empirical support in basic laboratory experiments (Rachlin & Laibson, 1997), there is no direct evidence in addiction studies that favor it over other theories of addiction.

Relative Theory of Addiction

Rachlin's (1997) relative theory of addiction is based on maximization of overall utility derived from substance use and social interaction. A basic assumption

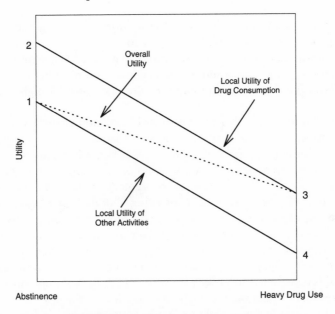

FIGURE 9.6. Processes in the melioration theory of addiction. Utility of substance use and other activities are shown as a function of the relative behavioral allocation to substance use and other activities.

of relative addiction theory is that substances of abuse (e.g., alcohol, nicotine, cocaine) are mutually substitutable with social interaction (see Figure 9.2). Because demand for economic substitutes varies inversely, increased demand for the addictive substance is associated with decreased demand for social interaction, and decreased demand for the addictive substance is associated with increased demand for social interaction. Relative addiction theory proposes a process whereby patterns of consumption over time modify the benefit/cost ratios of addictive consumption and social interaction in a way that accounts for the excessive drug use that characterizes addiction.

Two key processes of relative addiction theory are known as *price habituation* and *price sensitization*, which refer to changes over time in the benefit/cost ratios of activities as more or less of them is consumed. With price-habituated commodities, there is a negative relation between consumption and the benefit/cost ratio. The more a price-habituated commodity is consumed, the less benefit is derived from a given unit of behavioral allocation (e.g., tolerance to alcohol). With price-sensitized commodities, there is a positive relation between consumption and the benefit/cost ratio. The more a price-sensitized commodity is consumed, the more benefit is derived from a given unit of behavioral allocation (e.g., enjoyment derived from interacting with a friend). According to relative addiction theory, addictive substances are price-habituated, and social interaction is price-sensitized. Because addictive substances and social interaction are mutual substitutes, maximization of utility from the two commodities will lead to consumption of the one with the highest benefit/ cost ratio.

The central choice dynamic of relative addiction theory is the rate of price habituation of the addictive substance in relation to the rate of price sensitization of social interaction. This process is depicted in Figure 9.7. Utility is along the ordinate, and the relative allocation of behavior to substance use and social interaction is along the abscissa. Movement to the right along the abscissa signifies relatively more behavior being allocated to substance use and less to social interaction (the process of addiction); the converse is true for movement to the left. The utility derived from a given unit of behavioral allocation to substance use and to social interaction are signified by lines 1–3 and 2–4, respectively. The price habituation and price sensitization of substance use and social interaction, respectively, are shown with lines sloping down to the right. Movement to the right and left raises and lowers the price of both commodities, respectively. According to relative addiction theory, individuals maxi-

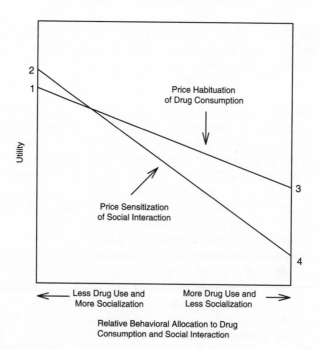

FIGURE 9.7. Processes in the relative theory of addiction. Utility of substance use and social interaction are shown as a function of relative behavioral allocation to substance use and social interaction.

mize the utility derived from these two commodities by consuming the one with the highest benefit/cost ratio.

As an example, assume that over a period of time an individual's behavior is at a stable allocation pattern of drinking and social interaction at the point of intersection of lines 1–3 and 2–4 in Figure 9.7. This behavioral allocation pattern involves relatively more social interaction and less substance use. However, an event (e.g., marital separation) then occurs that makes social interaction more expensive or more difficult to obtain (cf. Vuchinich & Tucker, 1996a, 1996b), which reduces the behavioral allocation to social interaction. Because drinking and social interaction are mutually substitutable, after the event the individual begins to drink more to make up for less social interaction (movement to the right along the abscissa in Figure 9.7). Because of the price habituation of drinking and the price sensitization of social interaction, drinking more and socializing less will decrease the benefit/cost ratios of both drinking and socializing. A critical aspect of relative addiction theory is that if the rate of price sensitization of social interaction is higher than the rate of price habituation of the addictive substance (relative price sensitization), then the benefit/cost ratio of the addictive commodity will be greater than the benefit/cost ratio of social interaction. This is shown in Figure 9.7 with the steeper slope of line 2–4 (social interaction) than of line 1–3 (substance use). Movement along the abscissa to the right of the point of intersection results in relatively more utility being derived from substance use than from social interaction. Because the two commodities are mutually substitutable, the addictive commodity is always preferred, leading to the "runaway consumption" considered characteristic of addiction in economic accounts.

It is important to note that the relative rates of price sensitization and price habituation are critical in this theory. If the rate of price habituation of the addictive substance were higher than the rate of price sensitization of social interaction (relative price habituation), at some point the benefit/cost ratio of addictive substance consumption would fall below the benefit/cost ratio of social interaction. This would be represented in Figure 9.7 if line 1–3 were steeper than line 2–4. At that point the individual would begin to socialize more and drink less, and therefore move to the left along the abscissa. Rachlin (1997) reviewed some evidence that cigarette smoking and social interaction have some features that are compatible with the assumptions of relative addiction theory. Moreover, the social function of Alcoholics Anonymous (AA) may be conceptualized in this framework. Beyond this, however, little evidence from addiction studies exists in favor of relative addiction theory over other accounts.

Theory of Rational Addiction

The theory of rational addiction (Becker & Murphy, 1988) has become a dominant force in the relevant economic literature. It is based on the common economic assumption that the allocation of limited resources to available commodities is governed by a choice process that maximizes some lifetime utility function, given the discounting of future utilities and a constrained budget. The "rational" in rational addiction theory primarily means that individuals are proposed to take into account the future effects of current consumption when making decisions about current consumption. The incorporation of future effects on current consumption was a significant step beyond earlier ("myopic") economic models of addiction (e.g., Pollack, 1970) in which only past consumption was thought to effect present consumption.

Like melioration theory, rational addiction theory groups all non-substance-use activities into one category, and views the individual as allocating behavior to substance use or some other activity (without specifying the other activity). Like both melioration and relative addiction theory, rational addiction theory assumes that past (and present) substance use lowers the present (and future) utility derived from a given level of substance use, and that addictive commodity consumption lowers the utility derived from other activities. An important distinction is made between total and marginal utility derived from a given level of commodity consumption. *Total utility* is the benefit derived from a given level of consumption during a given time period. *Marginal utility* is the contribution to total utility made by consumption of the next unit of a commodity. For example, if one ate three peaches in a day, the marginal utility of the third peach would be that amount of utility added to total utility by its consumption. In general, marginal utility diminishes as more of a commodity is consumed—for example, the third peach adds less marginal utility to total utility than the second peach.

The theory of rational addiction models the effect of past and present consumption on present and future consumption and utility through the accumulation of a "stock of consumption capital." This addictive stock is analogous to the relative behavioral allocations to substance use and other activities in melioration and relative addiction theory (i.e., the abscissas in Figures 9.6 and 9.7). Addictive stock increases with consumption and depreciates at a rate that varies across individuals and commodities. Stock accumulation entails a consumption rate higher than the depreciation rate, and lowers total utility derived from substance use and other activities, while raising the marginal utility of consumption of the addictive good. The latter feature, termed "adjacent complementarity," is a key feature of rational addiction in that it proposes that substance use in adjacent time periods are complements (see Figure 9.2). That is, consumption levels in one time period will produce similar consumption levels in adjacent time periods. The price of the addictive good, degree of adjacent complementarity, rate of stock depreciation, and degree of temporal discounting are key aspects of the theory that determine whether addiction will occur (Becker & Murphy, 1988).

These relations are shown in Figure 9.8. Utility is along the ordinate, and the stock of addictive capital is along the abscissa. A rate of substance use greater or less than the rate of stock depreciation would move the individual to the right or left along the abscissa, respectively. The utility derived from a given level of substance use and the utility of engagement in other activities are signified by lines 2–3 and 1–4, respectively. The marginal utility of an instance of substance use is represented by the distance between line 1–4 and line 2–3 (adjacent complementarity). As substance use occurs and stock accumulates, the persons moves to the right along the abscissa. Such movement reduces the total utility derived from substance use and other activities, but raises the marginal utility of each instance of substance use. This increase in marginal utility leads to more substance use and further movement along the abscissa, the process of addiction.

Empirical evaluations of rational addiction theory have consisted primarily of demand equations that regress past, current, and future prices, and past and future consumption, onto current consumption. The theory has met with considerable success in studies involving the consumption of alcohol (e.g., Grossman, Chaloupka, & Sirtalan, 1998), cigarettes (e.g., Chaloupka, 1991), and cocaine (e.g., Grossman & Chaloupka, 1998). While this empirical focus on

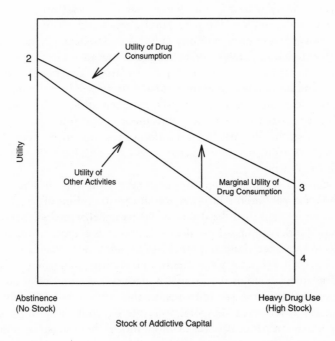

FIGURE 9.8. Processes in the theory of rational addiction. Utility of substance use and other activities are shown as a function of the stock of addictive capital.

price–consumption relations has generally yielded positive results, other critical elements of rational addiction theory remain unevaluated. Variability in
consumption due to the degree of adjacent complementarity and the rate of
stock depreciation has not been studied, and the discounting–consumption relation has received meager empirical attention in the economic literature (e.g.,
Chaloupka, 1991).

SUMMARY AND CONCLUSIONS

Contemporary scientific thinking on substance abuse and addiction has been
dominated by molecular approaches (cf. Vuchinich, 1995), which are inherently reductive, and have produced the current focus on cognitive and
neurophysiological mechanisms as the controlling variables of excessive consumption (Vuchinich, 1995). This scientific activity has made major advances,
and its past, present, and future contributions have been and will continue to
be important in the field. But such molecular, reductive explanations of addiction are only part of the story, because they lead to an understanding of forces
that act from inside the individual at the time of drug or alcohol consumption.
Another part of the story will involve an understanding of forces that act from
outside the individual over a time frame much broader than particular consumption episodes, such as intimate, family, and social relationships, and the
structure and function of community, cultural, and societal practices and institutions (Vuchinich & Tucker, 1996a). Developing an understanding of how
excessive consumption fits into the behavior patterns generated by these outside forces will be an advance in the field and likely will lead to more effective
clinical, public health, and public policy interventions. This "contextual-
ization" of substance abuse contrasts with theories that place the causes of addiction in either the pharmacological action of the substances themselves or in
biological, personality, or genetic characteristics of individuals that heighten
their risk of addiction.

Readers most interested in applications to prevent or treat substance
abuse probably will find the broad, reorienting assumptions of behavioral economics more relevant than the details of the basic behavioral science that supports them. Understanding those details, however, is important for sound applications to substance abuse and other health behavior problems (cf. Bickel &
Vuchinich, 2000). For example, it seems unlikely that the nuances of melioration and relative addiction theory will be reconciled empirically, but the debate draws deserved attention to two issues that have considerable applied significance: (1) Over what temporal intervals do individuals organize their
behavior allocation patterns (local or more molar), how stable or unstable are
their time horizons, and what variables influence the horizon duration? (2)

How can behavioral economics advance understanding of the role of social interaction in relation to substance use and abuse? Are these activities substitutes, as suggested by relative addiction theory and by the appeal of mutual help groups like AA during the recovery process?

In a related vein, psychological research in both the laboratory and the field has yielded evidence that is at odds with key assumptions of rational addiction theory. First, the "runaway consumption" considered characteristic of addiction in economic models has not been supported empirically. A large body of research has reliably demonstrated the sensitivity of substance use to environmental contingencies along the entire continuum of problem severity (reviewed by Griffiths, Bigelow, & Henningfield, 1980). Second, research on temporal discounting indicates that a hyperbolic function describes the relation between choice and delay better than the exponential function that underlies rational addiction theory (reviewed by Bickel & Marsch, 2001). This fact is important because hyperbolic discounting predicts that preference between an SSR and an LLR will reverse simply with the passage of time, whereas exponential discounting predicts a constant relation in their values over time. As any clinician knows, a hallmark of substance abuse is the variability over time between abuse, use, and abstinence. These temporal dynamics are not modeled well in economic theories that rest on an exponential discounting function and that predict runaway consumption. Whether these data will have a corrective effect on economic theory remains to be seen, but awareness of the discrepancies is relevant to applications with substance abusers.

In addition to supporting a contextualist perspective on substance abuse, behavioral economics has shifted our views of reinforcement, has made rich connections with economic theory, and has yielded concepts and terms that have applicability across clinical, public health, economic, and policy arenas. Although the methods and tools of these perspectives differ greatly, sharing a common scientific language should facilitate multidisciplinary interchange that is critical to address a complex behavioral health problem like substance abuse that ramifies through individuals, families, communities, and economies. The promise of behavioral economics as an organizing framework that can span multiple levels of application is beginning to emerge in the substance abuse intervention field and in behavioral medicine generally (Bickel & Vuchinich, 2000). Chapter 10 (this volume) describes some of these applied developments.

ACKNOWLEDGMENT

Manuscript preparation was supported in part by Grant Nos. R01 AA08972 and K02 AA00209 from the National Institute on Alcohol Abuse and Alcoholism.

REFERENCES

Ainslie, G. (1975). Specious reward: A behavioral theory of impulsiveness and self-control. *Psychological Bulletin, 82,* 463–496.
Ainslie, G. (1992). *Picoeconomics: The strategic interaction of successive motivational states within the person.* Cambridge, UK: Cambridge University Press.
Becker, G. S., & Murphy, K. M. (1988). A theory of rational addiction. *Journal of Political Economy, 96,* 675–700.
Bickel, W. K., DeGrandpre, R. J., & Higgins, S. T. (1995). The behavioral economics of concurrent drug reinforcers: A review and reanalysis of drug self-administration research. *Psychopharmacology, 118,* 250–259.
Bickel, W. K., Madden, G. J., & Petry, N. M. (1998). The price of change: The behavioral economics of drug dependence. *Behavior Therapy, 29,* 545–565.
Bickel, W. K., & Marsch, L. A. (2001). Toward a behavioral economic understanding of drug dependence: Delay discounting processes. *Addiction, 96,* 73–86.
Bickel, W. K., & Vuchinich, R. E. (Eds.). (2000). *Reframing health behavior change with behavioral economics.* Mahwah, NJ: Erlbaum.
Carroll, M. E. (1996). Reducing drug abuse by enriching the environment with alternative nondrug reinforcers. In L. Green & J. Kagel (Eds.), *Advances in behavioral economics: Vol. 3. Substance use and abuse* (pp. 37–68). Norwood, NJ: Ablex.
Catania, A. C. (1963). Concurrent performances: A baseline for the study of reinforcement magnitude. *Journal of the Experimental Analysis of Behavior, 6,* 299–300.
Chaloupka, F. J. (1991). Rational addictive behavior and cigarette smoking. *Journal of Political Economy, 99,* 722–742.
Chung, S.-H., & Herrnstein, R. J. (1967). Choice and delay of reinforcement. *Journal of the Experimental Analysis of Behavior, 10,* 67–74.
DeGrandpre, R. J., & Bickel, W. K. (1996). Drug dependence as consumer demand. In L. Green & J. H. Kagel (Eds.), *Advances in behavioral economics: Vol. 3. Substance use and abuse* (pp. 1–36). Norwood, NJ: Ablex.
DeGrandpre, R. J., Bickel, W. K., Hughes, J. R., & Higgins, S. T. (1992). Behavioral economics of drug self-administration: III. A reanalysis of the nicotine regulation hypothesis. *Psychopharmacology, 108,* 1–10.
DeGrandpre, R. J., Bickel, W. K., Hughes, J. R., Layng, M. P., & Badger, G. (1993). Unit price as a useful metric in analyzing effects of reinforcer magnitude. *Journal of the Experimental Analysis of Behavior, 60,* 641–666.
Griffiths, R. R., Bigelow, G. E., & Henningfield, J. E. (1980). Similarities in animal and human drug taking behavior. In N. K. Mello (Ed.), *Advances in substance abuse: Behavioral and biological research* (Vol. 1, pp. 1–90). Greenwich, CT: JAI Press.
Grossman, M., & Chaloupka, F. J. (1998). The demand for cocaine by young adults: A rational addiction approach. *Journal of Health Economics, 17,* 427–474.
Grossman, M., Chaloupka, F. J., & Sirtalan, I. (1998). An empirical analysis of alcohol addiction: Results from the Monitoring the Future panels. *Economic Inquiry, 36,* 39–48.
Herrnstein, R. J. (1961). Relative and absolute strength of response as a function of

frequency of reinforcement. *Journal of the Experimental Analysis of Behavior, 4,* 267–272.

Herrnstein, R. J. (1970). On the law of effect. *Journal of the Experimental Analysis of Behavior, 13,* 243–266.

Herrnstein, R. J. (1982). Melioration as behavioral dynamism. In M. L. Commons, R. J. Herrnstein, & H. Rachlin (Eds.), *Quantitative analyses of behavior: Vol. II. Matching and maximizing accounts* (pp. 433–458). Cambridge, MA: Ballinger.

Herrnstein, R. J., & Prelec, D. (1992). A theory of addiction. In G. Loewenstein & J. Elster (Eds.), *Choice over time* (pp. 331–360). New York: Russell Sage Foundation.

Hull, C. L. (1943). *Principles of behavior.* New York: Appleton-Century.

Hursh, S. R. (1980). Economic concepts for the analysis of behavior. *Journal of the Experimental Analysis of Behavior, 34,* 219–238.

Hursh, S. R. (1993). Behavioral economics of drug self-administration: An introduction. *Drug and Alcohol Dependence, 33,* 165–172.

Kagel, J. H., Battalio, R. C., & Green, L. (1995). *Economic choice theory: An experimental analysis of animal behavior.* New York: Cambridge University Press.

Kirby, K. N., Petry, N. M., & Bickel, W. K. (1999). Heroin addicts have higher discount rates for delayed rewards than non-drug-using controls. *Journal of Experimental Psychology: General, 128,* 78–87.

Lacey, H. M., & Rachlin, H. (1978). Behavior, cognition, and theories of choice. *Behaviorism, 6,* 177–202.

Leung, S. F., & Phelps, C. E. (1993). "My kingdom for a drink . . . ?": A review of the estimates of the price sensitivity of demand for alcoholic beverages. In M. E. Hilton & G. Bloss (Eds.), *Economics and the prevention of alcohol-related problems* (NIAAA Research Monograph No. 25, NIH Publication No. 93-3513, pp. 1–31). Rockville, MD: National Institutes of Health.

Loewenstein, G. F., & Prelec, D. (1992). Anomalies in intertemporal choice: Evidence and an interpretation. *Quarterly Journal of Economics, 107,* 573–597.

Loewenstein, G. F., & Prelec, D. (1993). Preferences for sequences of outcomes. *Psychological Review, 100*(1), 91–108.

Maisto, S. A., & McCollam, J. B. (1980). The use of multiple measures of life health to assess alcohol treatment outcome: A review and critique. In L. C. Sobell, M. B. Sobell, & E. Ward (Eds.), *Evaluating alcohol and drug abuse treatment effectiveness* (pp. 15–76). New York: Pergamon Press.

Mazur, J. (1987). An adjusting procedure for studying delayed reinforcement. In M. Commons, J. Mazur, J. A. Nevin, and H. Rachlin (Eds.), *Quantitative analysis of behavior: Vol. 5. The effect of delay and of intervening events on reinforcement value* (pp. 55–76). Hillsdale, NJ: Erlbaum.

Mazur, J. E. (2001). Hyperbolic value addition and general models of animal choice. *Psychological Review, 108,* 96–112.

Miller, W. R. (1998). Enhancing motivation for change. In W. R. Miller & N. Heather (Eds.), *Treating addictive behaviors* (2nd ed., pp. 121–132). New York: Plenum Press.

Mitchell, S. H. (1999). Measures of impulsivity in cigarette smokers and non-smokers. *Psychopharmacology, 146,* 455–464.

Monterosso, J., & Ainslie, G. (1999). Beyond discounting: Possible experimental models of impulse control. *Psychopharmacology, 146,* 339–347.

Petry, N. M., & Casarella, T. (1999). Excessive discounting of delayed rewards in substance abusers with gambling problems. *Drug and Alcohol Dependence, 56,* 25–32.

Pollack, R. A. (1970). Habit formation and dynamic demand functions. *Journal of Political Economy, 78,* 745–763.

Rachlin, H. (1987). Animal choice and human choice. In L. Green & J. Kagel (Eds.), *Advances in behavioral economics* (Vol. 1, pp. 48–64). Norwood, NJ: Ablex.

Rachlin, H. (1995). Self-control: Beyond commitment. *Behavioral and Brain Sciences, 18,* 109–159.

Rachlin, H. (1997). Four teleological theories of addiction. *Psychonomic Bulletin and Review, 4,* 462–473.

Rachlin, H., & Green, L. (1972). Commitment, choice, and self-control. *Journal of the Experimental Analysis of Behavior, 17,* 15–22.

Rachlin, H., Green, L., Kagel, J., & Battalio, R. (1976). Economic demand theory and psychological studies of choice. In G. Bower (Ed.), *The psychology of learning and motivation* (pp. 129–154). New York: Academic Press.

Rachlin, H., & Laibson, D. I. (1997). *The matching law: Papers in psychology and economics by Richard Herrnstein.* Cambridge, MA: Harvard University Press.

Robinson, T. E., & Berridge, K. C. (1993). The neural basis of drug craving: An incentive-sensitization theory of addiction. *Brain Research Reviews, 18,* 247–291.

Saffer, H., & Chaloupka, F. J. (1999). Demographic differentials in the demand for alcohol and illicit drugs. In F. J. Chaloupka, W. K. Bickel, M. Grossman, & H. Saffer (Eds.), *The economic analysis of substance use and abuse: An integration of econometric and behavioral economic perspectives* (pp. 187–212). Chicago: University of Chicago Press.

Skinner, B. F. (1938). *The behavior of organisms: An experimental analysis.* Englewood Cliffs, NJ: Prentice-Hall.

Tucker, J. A., Vuchinich, R. E., & Gladsjo, J. A. (1994). Environmental events surrounding natural recovery from alcohol-related problems. *Journal of Studies on Alcohol, 55,* 401–411.

Tucker, J. A., Vuchinich, R. E., & Pukish, M. A. (1995). Molar environmental contexts surrounding recovery from alcohol problems by treated and untreated problem drinkers. *Experimental and Clinical Psychopharmacology, 3,* 195–204.

Tucker, J. A., Vuchinich, R. E., & Rippens, P. D. (2002a). Environmental contexts surrounding resolution of drinking problems among problem drinkers with different help-seeking experiences. *Journal of Studies on Alcohol, 63,* 334–341.

Tucker, J. A., Vuchinich, R. E., & Rippens, P. D. (2002b). Predicting natural resolution of alcohol-related problems: A prospective behavioral economic analysis. *Experimental and Clinical Psychopharmacology, 10,* 248–257.

Vuchinich, R. E. (1982). Have behavioral theories of alcohol abuse focused too much on alcohol consumption? *Bulletin of the Society of Psychologists in Substance Abuse, 1,* 151–154.

Vuchinich, R. E. (1995). Alcohol abuse as molar choice: An update of a 1982 proposal. *Psychology of Addictive Behaviors, 9,* 223–235.

Vuchinich, R. E. (1997). Behavioral economics of drug consumption. In B. A. Johnson & J. D. Roache (Eds.), *Drug addiction and its treatment: Nexus of neuroscience and behavior* (pp. 73–90). Philadelphia: Lippincott-Raven.

Vuchinich, R. E., & Simpson, C. A. (1998). Hyperbolic temporal discounting in social drinkers and problem drinkers. *Experimental and Clinical Psychopharmacology, 6*, 292–305.

Vuchinich, R. E., & Tucker, J. A. (1988). Contributions from behavioral theories of choice to an analysis of alcohol abuse. *Journal of Abnormal Psychology, 97*, 181–195.

Vuchinich, R. E., & Tucker, J. A. (1996a). The molar context of alcohol abuse. In L. Green & J. Kagel (Eds.), *Advances in behavioral economics: Vol. 3. Substance use and abuse* (pp. 133–162). Norwood, NJ: Ablex Press.

Vuchinich, R. E., & Tucker, J. A. (1996b). Alcoholic relapse, life events, and behavioral theories of choice: A prospective analysis. *Experimental and Clinical Psychopharmacology, 4*, 19–28.

10

Contingency Management in the Substance Abuse Treatment Clinic

Alan J. Budney
Stacey C. Sigmon
Stephen T. Higgins

Individuals who seek treatment for substance abuse problems are notoriously difficult to retain in treatment and motivate to change. Even when clients make initial progress, frequently their motivation wanes and relapse occurs. Contingency management interventions represent one approach that has great potential to effectively motivate and facilitate change in this challenging clinical population. A recent resurgence of clinical trials examining the efficacy of contingency management across multiple types of drug dependence and clinical populations provides compelling empirical support for the efficacy of this treatment approach (Higgins & Silverman, 1999).

Contingency management interventions are based on extensive basic science and clinical research evidence demonstrating that drug use and abuse is heavily influenced by learning and conditioning and is quite sensitive to systematically applied environmental consequences (Griffiths, Bigelow, & Henningfield, 1980; Higgins, 1997; Stitzer & Higgins, 1995). The goal of contingency management interventions is to systematically weaken drug use and strengthen drug abstinence. These interventions arrange the environment such that reinforcing or punishing events occur contingent on drug use or other behavior deemed therapeutic such as counseling attendance or compliance with adjunct medication protocols. Typically, contingency management has been used as a component of a more comprehensive treatment intervention.

This chapter begins with a brief overview of the conceptual and empirical underpinnings of the contingency management approach. A review of the basic principles that guide the development and application of effective use of contingencies in the substance abuse treatment clinic provides a context for the range of interventions that comprise contingency management. We then review selected clinical research studies that showcase the efficacy of various models of contingency management interventions across different subtance-dependent populations. Last, a detailed case study illustrating a specific application of a contingency-based intervention for cocaine dependence is used to highlight the technical and clinical issues involved in implementing this treatment approach.

BASIC THEORY AND PRINCIPLES

Conceptual Framework

Within an operant framework, drug use is considered a case of operant behavior that is maintained, in part, by the pharmacological actions of the drug in conjunction with social and other nonpharmacological reinforcement derived from the drug-abusing lifestyle (Higgins & Katz, 1998). Reliable scientific observations indicate that abused drugs function as reinforcers with humans and laboratory animals (Griffiths et al., 1980). Most drugs that are abused by humans are voluntarily self-administered by a variety of species. These commonalities across species and drugs provide strong support for the position that reinforcement is a fundamental determinant of drug use and abuse.

Within this model, then, drug use is considered a normal learned behavior that falls along a continuum ranging from patterns of little use and few problems to excessive use and dependence. All healthy humans are assumed to possess the necessary neurobiological systems to experience drug-produced reinforcement and to have the potential to develop patterns of use or abuse. Clearly, genetic or acquired characteristics (e.g., family history of substance dependence, other psychiatric disorders) can affect the probability of developing drug abuse, but this model assumes that such special characteristics are not necessary for drug abuse to develop.

An important feature of this conceptual model of drug abuse is that it facilitates a direct connection between clinical practice and the scientific disciplines of behavior analysis and behavioral pharmacology. Those disciplines include an extensive research literature demonstrating principles and procedures that can be applied to modify behavior of all kinds, including drug abuse. A major strength of conceptualizing drug use and abuse as a "biologically normal" learned human behavior is that as such it is amenable to change via the same processes and principles as other types of human behavior irrespective of its etiology. Indeed, controlled studies with humans and laboratory animals have shown that drug use is an orderly form of behavior that is affected by environmental context and the reinforcement contingencies under which it occurs. Alterations in drug availability, drug dose, response requirement needed to obtain drug, and the availability of other nondrug reinforcers each have orderly and generalizable effects on drug use (Griffiths et al., 1980; Higgins, 1997).

The contingency management approach to treating drug dependence capitalizes on knowledge that drug seeking and drug use are behaviors that can be directly modified by manipulating the relevant environmental contingencies. Within this framework, treatment is designed to assist in reorganizing the physical and social environments of the user. The goal is to systematically weaken the influence of reinforcement derived from drug use and the related lifestyle, and to increase the frequency and magnitude of reinforcement derived from healthier alternative activities, especially those that are incompatible with continued drug use.

Basic Principles of Contingency Management

Contingency management interventions involve the use of positive reinforcement, negative reinforcement, positive punishment, or negative punishment contingencies to motivate increases and decreases in the frequency of target behavior. *Positive reinforcement* involves delivery of a desired consequence contingent on the individual meeting a therapeutic goal. Examples of desired consequences that have been used in effective contingency management programs for substance dependence are vouchers/tokens exchangeable for retail items, methadone take-home privileges, access to affordable housing, and increased opportunity to win a prize. The behavioral goal that must be achieved in order to receive these consequences has usually been abstinence from use of a specific substance that is documented by a biological marker of drug use such as urine toxicology testing. Other less frequently employed goals have been counseling attendance, achievement of a specific treatment goal or homework task, or medication compliance.

Negative reinforcement involves removing an aversive or confining circumstance contingent on meeting a therapeutic goal. Examples of such circumstances in the substance abuse treatment setting that can function as negative reinforcers are a reduction in the intensity of criminal justice supervision or schedule of counseling. Again, the contingent behavior required to remove these circumstances would typically be drug abstinence, attendance at counseling sessions, or achievement of other therapeutic goals.

Positive punishment involves delivery of a punishing consequence contingent on evidence of undesirable behavior. Punishing consequences employed in some substance abuse treatment programs include increases in treatment participation requirements, termination of treatment, suspension of employment, or a specified period of incarceration. Undesirable behaviors that could be followed by punishment include positive urine or breath alcohol tests, or failure to attend counseling sessions.

Negative punishment involves removal of a positive circumstance or condition contingent on evidence of the occurrence of an undesirable behavior. Examples of positive conditions that could be removed include the reduction in the monetary value of vouchers that could be earned for drug abstinence or removal of a preferred schedule of medication dosing or counseling sessions.

Both reinforcement and punishment contingencies can be effective tools in substance abuse treatment programs, but the former are generally preferred over the latter by both patients and clinicians. An important limitation of punishment contingencies is that they can increase treatment dropout, which is an outcome to be avoided in substance abuse treatment. This is less of an issue in some circumstances (e.g., court-mandated treatment) and can likely be offset by inclusion of reinforcement contingencies. Below we illustrate how creative and careful programming of a combination of contingencies can generate effective outcomes within programs readily accepted by patients and therapists alike.

Principles of Application

Whether the contingencies employed in the clinic setting involve reinforcement, punishment, or both, the efficacy of the intervention will be influenced by the schedule according to which the consequence is delivered, the magnitude of the consequence, and the method and schedule of monitoring the target behavior. Familiarity with these concepts is recommended prior to the design and implementation of contingency management programs in a clinical setting. A wide variety of examples of various contingency management interventions can be found in a recently published text on this topic (Higgins & Silverman, 1999). General overviews on the application of general behavior analytic principles can be found in a number of sources (Miller, 1984; Sulzer-Azaroff & Meyer, 1991). Here we offer an abbreviated summary of these principles and examples of their application in a substance abuse setting.

The *schedule of reinforcement or punishment* refers to the temporal relation between the target behavior and the delivery of the consequence. The efficacy of the contingency will generally increase as the temporal delay between the occurrence of the target behavior and delivery of the scheduled consequence decreases. Reinforcement or punishment should be applied as close in time to the detection of the target behavior as possible. For example, all else being equal, a clinic that provides positive reinforcement for cocaine abstinence 5 minutes after a client submits a cocaine-negative urine specimen would generate greater rates of cocaine abstinence than a clinic that waits 4 days after the submission of the specimen before reinforcement is delivered. Indeed, patients who experienced longer delays between submitting drug-free urine specimens and receipt of tokens exchangeable for retail items achieved less drug abstinence than those receiving the same tokens but with shorter delays (Rowan-

Szal, Joe, Chatham, & Simpson, 1994). Additional studies have demonstrated that substance abusers' ratings of the value of various reinforcers are negatively affected by temporal delays to an even greater extent than those of individuals who do not have substance abuse problems (Kirby, Petry, & Bickel, 1999; Petry, Bickel, & Arnett, 1998).

Similarly, more frequent schedules of reinforcement (e.g., three times per week) are preferable to less frequent (once per week) schedules in establishing an initial target behavior like drug abstinence or regular attendance at counseling sessions. A more frequent schedule allows additional opportunities to reinforce and thereby strengthen the target behavior. Once a target behavior (e.g., abstinence) is established, a less frequent schedule of reinforcement that is delivered on a fixed or variable schedule may be used for maintenance purposes.

A good example of the application of these principles is a contingency management intervention for cocaine dependence that provides positive reinforcement in the form of vouchers contingent on cocaine-negative urinalysis results (Budney & Higgins, 1998; Higgins, Budney, & Bickel, 1994). A fixed schedule of three times per week urinalysis monitoring is used during the first 12 weeks of treatment. A voucher is delivered immediately (2–5 minutes) after drug-negative results are documented. The vouchers are then exchanged for retail items within 24–48 hours. During the second 12 weeks of treatment, the urinalysis testing schedule is reduced to twice weekly and the magnitude of the vouchers is reduced to a $1 lottery ticket.

Second, the *magnitude of the reinforcing or punishing consequence* provided is important. Basic laboratory research demonstrates that the magnitude of a reinforcer directly affects the amount of work an individual will do to achieve a specific target goal (Catania, 1998). For example, if a patient's goal is drug abstinence as indicated by a drug-negative urine test, the scheduled delivery of a voucher worth $10.00 for each negative specimen is more likely to motivate drug cessation than a voucher worth $2.50. Silverman, Chutuape, Bigelow, and Stitzer (1999) demonstrated the importance of magnitude with methadone-maintenance patients showing that high-value vouchers produced more cocaine abstinence than low-value vouchers, which were superior to zero-value vouchers. Similarly, two studies examining tobacco smoking also demonstrated greater rates of abstinence related to the increased magnitude of monetary reinforcers made contingent on nicotine abstinence (Stitzer & Bigelow, 1983, 1984b). Counseling and job-training attendance rates are also sensitive to the magnitude of reinforcement provided for engaging in these clinical activities (Kidorf, Stitzer, Brooner, & Goldberg, 1994; Silverman, Chutuape, Bigelow, & Stitzer, 1996).

Choice of what magnitude of reinforcement to use requires careful consideration of the severity of the behavior targeted for change and the difficulty patients experienced trying to change such behavior. An effective reinforcer must compete with the reinforcement derived from the behavior targeted for change (Higgins, 1997). Given the resilience of substance-use habits typically developed over many years, and especially when treating individuals who use relatively large quantities of a drug, strong reinforcers are likely to be necessary. The importance of magnitude notwithstanding, creative use of relatively low magnitude reinforcers has been successful in modifying a wide variety of target behaviors among drug abusers, especially when used in combination with other treatment interventions (Higgins & Silverman, 1999).

Contingency management programs must also employ an effective *monitoring system* such that reinforcement or punishment can be applied systematically. Precise information on the occurrence of the therapeutic target response is necessary to implement a successful intervention. With drug abusers, this is usually whether they have used drugs recently and involves some form of biochemical verification of drug abstinence. Urinalysis testing is the most common verification procedure in contingency management treatments for drug abuse. Such objective monitoring is necessary for fair and effective implementation of contingency management programs. When choosing other behavioral targets, such as medication compliance, attending counseling sessions, increasing social activities, and completion of skills-training homework, the treatment provider program must always keep in mind the need to have a method to objectively verify whether the target behavior occurred. Reliance on patient self-reports of whether or not drug use has occurred or whether a therapeutic task has been completed would not be adequate for these purposes.

Alcohol Abuse and Dependence

One of the first examples of contingency management to appear in the substance abuse treatment literature addressed the problem of chronic public drunkenness among "skid row" alcoholics (Miller, 1975). Public inebriates who received shelter, employment, food, clothing, and other services from local social agencies *contingent* on sobriety documented via negative breath-alcohol tests (100 ml/BAC) and staff observation showed reduced alcohol use, increased employment, and fewer legal problems than those who received these services regardless of alcohol use (usual care group). When alcohol use was detected in a contingent-group participant, social services were immediately suspended for 5 days. This study provided an illustration of how a treatment organization that serves underprivileged or homeless alcohol abusers might enhance the efficacy of the services they provide.

Another study demonstrated how positive reinforcement of disulfiram ingestion among severe alcohol-dependent outpatients can enhance compliance with the medication schedule and reduce alcohol use (Azrin, Sisson, Meyers, & Godley, 1982). Here a concerned other agreed to observe ingestion of disulfiram each day and provided a desirable consequence (e.g., appreciation or praise, a cooked meal, a hug) if disulfiram was taken as scheduled.

Concurrent alcoholism among methadone-maintained, opiate-dependent patients is commonly regarded as one of the major factors associated with treatment failure. One method found effective in reducing alcohol use in this population is to require identified patients to take disulfiram (medication to treat alcohol dependence) under nursing supervision prior to receiving their daily dose of methadone (medication to treat opiate dependence) (Liebson, Tommaselo, & Bigelow, 1978). In this case, methadone was used to reinforce disulfiram ingestion. Patients who did not take the mandatory doses of disulfiram as scheduled had their daily dose of methadone reduced until it reached zero and then were discontinued from the program. This study showed that treatment efficacy can be enhanced by making desired treatment services (methadone dose) contingent on compliance with therapeutic goals (disulfiram ingestion).

To our knowledge, little clinical research using contingency management to treat alcohol dependence appeared in the literature during the 1980s or 1990s. However, the growth of positive findings with contingency management in the treatment of illicit drug abuse in the 1990s (reviewed below) stimulated a recent study demonstrating the efficacy of intermittent positive-reinforcement procedures to enhance treatment outcome with alcohol-dependent patients (Petry, Martin, Cooney, & Kranzler, 2000). Patients in an intensive outpatient substance abuse clinic received standard treatment plus contingency management or standard treatment only. The contingent group earned the chance to win a prize (with a value from $1 to $100) for each negative breath sample they submitted and for each of three preset therapeutic activities that they completed during the week. Treatment retention and relapse rates were superior in the contingent group. Perhaps this innovative and successful application of positive reinforcement principles will rekindle an interest in contingency management strategies for the treatment of alcohol abuse and dependence.

THE METHADONE CLINIC

Contingency management interventions for opiate dependence have received relatively sustained scientific attention and refinement over the past 25 years. Methadone, an oral, long-acting opioid substitution medication, is the recommended treatment for opiate dependence as it effectively reduces heroin and other illicit opioid use, related withdrawal symptomatology, criminal activity, and risk of infectious disease. Methadone therapy typically is administered through clinics that provide daily doses of methadone and various types of adjunct counseling. Although effective, it does not directly address the full range of problems that most clients bring to treatment. A number of potential reinforcers and punishments directed at decreasing drug use or increasing other prosocial behavioral targets can be identified within the structure of a daily methadone-dispensing clinic (Kidorf & Stitzer, 1999).

Methadone Take-Home Procedures

The methadone take-home privilege involves providing an extra daily dose of methadone for ingestion at home so that patients do not need to attend the clinic as frequently. Attending the clinic daily can be burdensome, sometimes interfering with vocational or family responsibilities. Hence, take-home privileges are desirable to patients because simply skipping a daily dose is likely to result in adverse withdrawal symptoms and increased risk for using heroin or other opiates. Take-home doses are not provided to all patients because they have the potential for abuse either through the patient ingesting the take-home dose prior to the scheduled dosing time or by selling it on the street. Thus, the take-home privilege offers a convenient and valued incentive for use in contingency management programs and is one of the most potent positive reinforcers available within the context of routine clinic operation (Stitzer & Bigelow, 1978).

The most common use of take-homes has been to reinforce abstinence from other drug use among methadone-dependent patients, as multiple substance abuse is common in this population. Numerous studies have demonstrated that making take-home doses contingent on abstinence from secondary drug(s) is an effective method for reducing drug use in this difficult treatment population (e.g., Magura, Casriel, Goldsmith, Strug, & Lipton, 1988; Milby, Garrett, English, Fritschi, & Clarke, 1978; Stitzer, Bigelow, Liebson, & Hawthorne, 1982; Stitzer, Iguchi, & Felch, 1992).

Take-home privileges have also been used to enhance attendance at counseling sessions with fairly dramatic results. Contingent take-home interventions can increase counseling attendance from two fold to six fold compared with conditions that have no contingencies on attendance (Iguchi et al., 1996; Stitzer et al., 1977). Additional studies have demonstrated the potential for contingent take-home doses to impact other treatment-related behaviors such as compliance with clinic regulations, pursuit of vocational training, and payment of clinic fees (Magura, Casriel, Goldsmith, & Lipton, 1987; Stitzer & Bigelow, 1984a). The methadone take-home procedure exemplifies how treatment providers can creatively use contingency management strategies within existing clinic settings to positively influence treatment participation and outcomes.

Methadone Dose Alterations

The dose of methadone provided to clients can also function as a positive reinforcer within a contingency management program (Kidorf & Stitzer, 1999).

Multiple studies have employed a combination of contingencies that provide methadone dose increases or decreases dependent on achievement of specific target behaviors (Glosser, 1983; Higgins, Stitzer, Bigelow, & Liebson, 1986; Stitzer, Bickel, Bigelow, & Liebson, 1986). In one creative dosing program patients could earn 4 points per day for completing treatment goals, attending sessions, and drug abstinence (Glosser, 1983). If all 4 points were earned, a dose increase of 4 mg could be requested (positive reinforcement). If less than 4 points were earned, the dose was decreased in direct relation to the number of points not earned (negative punishment). The contingent-dosing group remained in treatment twice as long and submitted 25% more drug-negative urine samples compared with the standard treatment group..

Another dose alterations study illustrated the preference for using positive reinforcement rather than negative punishment when possible (Stitzer et al., 1986). One patients group could earn 5mg dose *increases* for each drug-negative sample up to a ceiling level of 160% of their initial dose (positive reinforcement). Drug-positive specimens resulted in a return to the baseline dose. A second group received 5mg dose *decreases* for each drug-positive specimen with a maximum of a 40% reduction from baseline dose (negative punishment). Both groups responded well to the interventions; however, the contingent dose *increase* group had a lower dropout rate.

Dose alteration contingencies have also been used to impact other clinic behaviors. For example, informing patients that their dose would be lowered if they did not bring a supportive, non–drug-using significant other in to participate in counseling sessions greatly increased significant other attendance (Kidorf, Brooner, & King, 1997). In this case, doses that were reduced because of failure to comply returned to baseline when the contingency was met. Dose alterations have also been used to prompt gainful employment (Kidorf, Hollander, King, & Brooner, 1998). Unemployed patients had 2 months to show objective evidence of 20 employment hours per week. If they remained unemployed, they had to enter intensive counseling, and eventually received a dose taper until employment was secured. This program resulted in a 75% employment rate in a previously unemployed sample.

VOUCHER–BASED REINFORCEMENT PROGRAMS FOR COCAINE DEPENDENCE

In the early 1990s, Higgins and colleagues developed an effective 24-week behavioral treatment for cocaine dependence that integrated the community reinforcement approach (CRA; Azrin, 1976) with an abstinence-based voucher program targeting cocaine abstinence (Higgins, Budney, Bickel, et al., 1994; Higgins et al., 1993; Higgins et al., 1991; see Budney & Higgins, 1998, for a clinician manual for implementing this treatment). The voucher program provides a classic example of the use of a contingency management intervention that utilizes positive reinforcement and a negative punishing contingency to engender drug abstinence and increase sources of alternative nondrug reinforcement. A case illustration using this intervention is presented later in this chapter.

Briefly, the voucher-based intervention is an incentive program designed to increase treatment retention and cocaine abstinence. Clients provide urine specimens on a thrice-weekly schedule and vouchers are earned for each cocaine-negative urine specimen submitted. Vouchers have a monetary value that increases with each consecutive cocaine-negative specimen, beginning with $2.50 for the first cocaine-free sample. If a client should have an unexcused absence from a scheduled urine test or a cocaine-positive test result, the value of the vouchers is reset to the initial low level. This schedule of reinforcement is designed to promote initial abstinence by providing frequent reinforcement for cocaine abstinence. The schedule also promotes continuous periods of abstinence by increasing the amount of reinforcement earned in direct relation to the number of consecutive cocaine-negative specimens submitted, and by resetting the value of the vouchers back to low amounts of reinforcement if cocaine use occurs. Vouchers are exchangeable for retail goods or services in the community; cash is never provided to clients. Clinic staff purchase items requested by clients; purchases are only approved if therapists deem them to be in concert with treatment goals. During the first 12 weeks of the program, clients can earn a maximum of approximately $1,000 in vouchers if they provide all scheduled urine specimens and all test negative for cocaine. No vouchers are earned if a specimen is cocaine-positive or if the patient fails to submit a scheduled specimen. To give patients who slip an incentive to keep working toward cocaine abstinence, submission of five consecutive cocaine-negative specimens following a positive specimen returns the voucher amount to the value prior to the reset, from which it can escalate again.

The efficacy of CRA plus vouchers has been demonstrated in three randomized trials for cocaine dependence (Higgins, Budney, Bickel, et al., 1994; Higgins et al., 1993; Higgins, Wong, Badger, Ogden, & Dantona, 2000). In the first study, CRA plus vouchers resulted in greater treatment completion and longer periods of sustained abstinence than standard drug abuse counseling. Importantly, cocaine abstinence did not show a precipitous decrease following the end of the voucher program (Higgins et al., 1993). The second trial comparing CRA alone to CRA plus vouchers demonstrated that the contingent voucher component contributed to the positive effects of CRA plus vouchers (Higgins, Budney, Bickel, et al., 1994). The third trial demonstrated that the positive effects of the voucher program were due to its direct effects on cocaine abstinence rather than merely an effect of increasing treatment retention (Higgins, Wong, et al., 2000). A retrospective study of outcomes across these trials suggests that the mechanism by which the contingent voucher affects

positive outcome is in its ability to engender substantial periods of initial abstinence in a greater percentage of patients than comparison treatment groups
(Higgins, Badger, & Budney, 2000). This positive effect is then maintained
posttreatment, and rates of relapse do not appear to differ between the contingent voucher treatment and the comparison interventions.

The generality of this voucher program for engendering cocaine abstinence has been demonstrated with inner-city intravenous cocaine abusers enrolled in a methadone maintenance program (Silverman et al., 1996; Silverman
et al., 1998). Moreover, these studies showed that this intervention also increased rates of abstinence from illicit opiates even though the vouchers were
delivered contingent on cocaine abstinence only.

Modifications to the schedule, magnitude, and form of reinforcement of
the original voucher program have been implemented with positive results in
cocaine-abusing populations. For example, a voucher program using lower
magnitude vouchers was effective with inner-city crack users, but one with
lower frequency *and* magnitude was not (Kirby, Marlowe, Festinger, Lamb, &
Platt, 1998). Also, the same intermittent reinforcement schedule technique described earlier in this chapter that enhanced treatment outcome for alcohol
dependence has also demonstrated efficacy for increasing cocaine abstinence
for cocaine-dependent outpatients (Petry & Martin, 2002).

Voucher Programs with Other Drugs of Abuse and Polydrug Abuse

The efficacy of the voucher program for cocaine dependence prompted inves-
tigations of similar programs for other types of drug abuse problems. For example, voucher programs can improve marijuana abstinence rates when combined with motivational enhancement therapy or cognitive-behavioral coping
skills therapy for marijuana-dependent adults (Budney, Higgins, Radonovich,
& Novy, 2000). The voucher program used in that study was similar to the
original Higgins and colleagues program, except the total magnitude of
vouchers was approximately 50% of that used in the cocaine studies, and urinalysis monitoring was reduced from thrice to twice weekly.

Voucher-based reinforcement also has been demonstrated to enhance
treatment outcomes with opioid-dependent individuals (Bickel, Amass, Higgins, Badger, & Esch, 1997; Preston, Umbricht, & Epstein, 2000). One approach modified the voucher program such that one-half of the available
vouchers could be earned by providing opiate-negative specimens and the
other half by participating in therapeutic activities specified as part of CRA
therapy (Bickel et al., 1997). A strong correlation between completion of the
therapeutic activities and opioid abstinence ($r = .76$) was observed, underscor-
ing the role of competing sources of nondrug reinforcement in promoting

cessation of drug use. Another group also demonstrated that voucher programs targeting completion of treatment plan activities can improve outcomes (Iguchi, Belding, Morral, Lamb, & Husband, 1997).

Polydrug abuse is common among persons seeking treatment for cocaine or opiate dependence, and is typically thought to be a risk factor for relapse to cocaine or opiates. An initial voucher study examined a sequential approach to treatment of multiple drug use by first reinforcing abstinence from the primary drug of abuse (cocaine) with vouchers and then moving on to abstinence from a secondary drug (marijuana) (Budney, Higgins, Delaney, Kent, & Bickel, 1991). First, a voucher intervention was used to engender cocaine abstinence with patients using cocaine and marijuana regularly. Cocaine abstinence was achieved, but the patients continued to use marijuana regularly. Patients were then offered a voucher program that required abstinence from both cocaine and marijuana. Abstinence from both drugs was achieved, with the initiation of marijuana abstinence coinciding with the initiation of the modified voucher program.

More recently, Piotrowski et al. (1999) demonstrated modest treatment gains with an innovative voucher program addressing polydrug use in methadone patients. During the first month of treatment, voucher earnings were contingent on abstinence from both opiate and cocaine use. Use of other substances did not affect this contingency, but clinic staff reminded clients that they would need to cease use of other substances to earn vouchers during months 2–4 of treatment. A hierarchy of bonuses was created for achievement of "plateaus" defined as specific periods of abstinence. A reset procedure was used such that a drug-positive urine specimen resulted in a decrease in voucher value only to the previous "plateau" level achieved, providing less of a penalty for "slips" that occur during treatment.

Voucher-based interventions of similar magnitude to that used by Higgins et al. (1994), but that require simultaneous abstinence from multiple drugs of abuse in order to earn the vouchers, generally have not been successful (Downey, Helmus, & Schuster, 2000; Iguchi et al., 1997; Katz, Chatuape, Jones, & Stitzer, 2002). In these studies, methadone-maintained patients earned vouchers if they submitted urine specimens indicating abstinence from all drugs of abuse. Unfortunately, the majority of patients were unable to achieve even one drug-free urine specimen. The target goal, complete drug abstinence, was either too difficult for the patients to achieve or the reinforcer was not of sufficient magnitude to motivate them to abstain from all drug use. Indeed, most recently Dallery, Silverman, Chutuape, Bigelow, and Stitzer (2001) demonstrated that simultaneous abstinence from cocaine and opioids in treatment-resistant methadone patients can be achieved if the magnitude of the incentive is increased.

These studies of polydrug abuse highlight the importance of designing contingency management programs that provide ample opportunities to reinforce the target behavior. Abstinence from all drugs of abuse is a very difficult goal for most polydrug abusers. Programs for this difficult treatment population may need to consider using sequential strategies that require progressively more difficult abstinence goals, providing higher magnitude reinforcers for more difficult goals, or enlisting adjunct treatment strategies such as medication, short-term hospitalization, or more intensive counseling (Chutuape, Silverman, & Stitzer, 1999). Effective strategies for managing polydrug abuse are more likely to result from thoughtful, focused efforts than from sweeping goals of achieving simultaneous abstinence form all psychoactive drug use.

CONTINGENCY MANAGEMENT IN SPECIAL POPULATIONS

Drug abuse when combined with other medical, psychiatric, or social problems presents a particularly difficult challenge for treatment providers. Efforts to extend contingency management to the treatment of groups such as the homeless, pregnant women, and the severe mentally ill are currently under way at numerous sites throughout the United States.

Contingent Housing and Work Therapy for the Homeless

Recently, a creative contingency-management approach to treating homeless substance abusers demonstrated that a contingent housing and work therapy program combined with an intensive psychosocial treatment can decrease drug abuse and increase other important areas of functioning among homeless crack and other substance abusers (Milby et al., 2000; Milby et al., 1996). Cocaine-abusing homeless persons could earn access to a rent-free furnished apartment if they provided two consecutive weeks of cocaine-negative urine tests. Once living in the apartment, a cocaine-positive urine test resulted in immediate eviction and transportation to a shelter. Two consecutive drug-negative tests following eviction earned renewed access to the apartment. During the second phase of this program, participants could also participate in a paid work therapy program that involved construction (refurbishing apartments for the program) or food service work. Access to work was again contingent on 2 weeks of documented drug abstinence; once employed, drug-positive urine tests resulted in suspension from work.

Incentive Programs for Pregnant Substance Abusers

Pregnant drug abusers pose multiple risks to their fetuses not only from the direct pharmacological effects of the drugs on the fetus, but from the generally impoverished and neglectful lifestyle of the mother, including her poor compliance with prenatal care. The observation that pregnant drug abusers continue to use drugs despite knowledge of potential adverse consequences to the fetus suggests that the severity of their drug abuse and related problems pose a particularly difficult challenge to treatment providers. A number of projects have demonstrated that creative contingent incentive programs can decrease drug use and increase prenatal care in this important target population.

In an initial study, contingent reinforcement for evidence of reduced cocaine use and attendance at prenatal clinic visits enhanced treatment outcome (Elk et al., 1995). Ten dollars was provided for each successive decrease in cocaine use, $12 for each cocaine-free urine specimen, and $15 if all three weekly urine specimens indicated abstinence and they attended their scheduled prenatal clinic visit. Of note, this program utilized a *quantitative* method of urinalysis to test for reduced amounts of cocaine use in addition to cocaine abstinence. This allowed for "shaping" cocaine-use behavior in contrast to requiring complete abstinence to access the reinforcer. More recently, a program offering vouchers contingent on abstinence from cocaine, opioids, and treatment attendance demonstrated enhanced outcomes with pregnant methadone-maintained patients (Jones, Haug, Silverman, Stitzer, & Svikis, 2001).

Voucher programs are also being used to promote abstinence from cigarette smoking during pregnancy and postpartum. In one study, smoking cessation increased when pregnant women and their significant other received vouchers monthly during the pregnancy and for 2 months postpartum contingent on verified smoking abstinence (Donatelle, Prows, Champeau, & Hudson, 2002). Voucher magnitude was $50 per test for the pregnant smokers, and $50 for the first test and $25 for each subsequent test for the significant others. In another ongoing study, throughout pregnancy and 3 months postpartum pregnant smokers receive vouchers on a schedule similar to one used in the initial cocaine studies (Higgins, Alessi, & Dantona, 2002). A woman who entered this study at 12 weeks into her pregnancy, for example, and who sustained abstinence continuously through the pregnancy and postpartum period could earn $1,147 in vouchers, or approximately $127/month. To date, abstinence levels achieved with this program are much higher than those observed among those who received encouragement to quit from their health care provider and vouchers that were not contingent on abstinence from smoking.

Importantly, communities appear willing to financially support incentive programs for pregnant women. The costs of the vouchers in the Dontatello study described above were covered through donations from local health care organizations, businesses, and foundations. In another study, vouchers were redeemable at an onsite "voucher store" stocked with items obtained via a direct-mail fundraising campaign, and run by local volunteers (Amass, 1997). Donations for store items were solicited from corporations and local retailers, and included baby accessories, clothes, toys, maternity products, and entertainment and recreation equipment. Such community support is encouraging when thinking about dissemination issues such as how voucher/incentive programs might be funded in community-based clinics.

Another innovative application of contingency management with great potential for practical application is the reinforcement-based Therapeutic Workplace, an intervention that uses the opportunity to participate in paid work to reinforce abstinence (Silverman, Svikis, Robles, Stitzer, & Bigelow, 2001). The efficacy of this approach was demonstrated in a study of methadone-maintained pregnant women enrolled in treatment that included group and individual therapy, ob/gyn medical services, family planning, transportation to appointments, childcare, initial residential care, and day treatment during the 28 days following residential care. Therapeutic Workplace participants were invited to attend a workplace 3 hours per day in addition to receiving these other services. To gain access to this program, each day they were required to provide a urine specimen that tested negative for cocaine and opiates. If the specimen tested positive, they were not allowed to work that day. Those who gained entrance received basic skills education and job skills training. At the end of the shift they received a base pay voucher. Pay was dictated by an escalating reinforcement schedule. Additional vouchers could be earned for professional demeanor, meeting daily learning goals, and data-entry productivity. The majority of voucher earnings were available as base pay that was contingent on abstinence and attendance. This intervention provides a model for treatment of low-income pregnant abusers with strong potential for generality to other subpopulations of drug abusers. Indeed, this group is currently using a similar intervention with homeless alcoholics and HIV-positive drug abusers.

Contingency Management for People with Schizophrenia

Drug abuse among those with serious mental illness is three to six times higher than among the general population, and has been associated with increased severity of psychiatric symptoms, poor psychosocial functioning, high rates of rehospitalization, and noncompliance with pharmacological and psychosocial treatment for their mental illness (Hughes, Hatsukami, Mitchell, & Dahlgren, 1986; Regier et al., 1990). Shaner and colleagues (Shaner et al., 1995) documented a temporal relationship between arrival of disability payments and peaks in cocaine use, psychiatric symptoms, and hospital admissions among cocaine-dependent men with schizophrenia. Thus, the money intended to compensate for these patients' disability appeared to be contributing to the severity of their problems, spawning an idea that making such payments contingent on drug abstinence might reduce such misuse of funds. Indeed, feasibility studies have demonstrated that abstinence from cocaine, cigarette, and marijuana use among patients with schizophrenia can be increased with contingent positive reinforcement (Roll, Higgins, Steingard, & McGinley, 1998; Shaner et al., 1997; Sigmon, Steingard, Badger, Anthony, & Higgins, 2000; Tidey, O'Neill, & Higgins, 1999).

A potential mechanism for applying contingency management on a larger scale to address the problem of seriously mentally ill patients using disability income to support drug use is being implemented and tested (Ries & Comtois, 1997; Ries & Dyck, 1997). A model for this approach currently exists in some mental health centers in that they already use representative payees and a form of contingent disbursement of benefits for severely ill and dually diagnosed patients.

CLINICAL ILLUSTRATION

The purpose of the following case illustration is to provide additional detail on the technical aspects involved with implementing a contingency management program in a clinical setting. We've chosen to use an example from our CRA plus vouchers, manual-driven therapy for cocaine dependence (Budney & Higgins, 1998). This treatment integrates an abstinence-based voucher program with an intensive behavior therapy, CRA counseling. Clinical details of the case and the behavior therapy will be limited as the primary reason for this illustration is to highlight some of the application issues unique to the administration of a voucher program.

Sandy is a 30-year-old, single, white female who lives with her 8-year-old son. She is divorced but shares custody of her son with her ex-husband. At intake, she was unemployed but reported a history of employment as a cashier. Sandy reported several consequences of her cocaine use, including losing her job due to her alcohol and cocaine use, spending her savings on cocaine, and coping poorly with behavioral problems displayed by her son. She expressed concern that if her cocaine use continued, it would escalate and she would lose her son. At intake, Sandy met criteria for cocaine, alcohol, and nicotine dependence. She reported one previous episode of treatment for alcohol dependence and no prior cocaine treatment. She also reported a suicide attempt at age 18 and noted that she had received psychotherapy for depression at that time. At intake she reported only mild depressive symptomatology. Her first cocaine use occurred at age 17 and involved intranasal use of 2 grams of cocaine. Her preferred route of administration upon treatment entry was smoking cocaine. At intake she was using 2 grams of cocaine 3 days per week and typically did so with her friends either at their apartment or a bar.

Initial Rationale

After concluding a comprehensive intake assessment, a therapist provided Sandy with a description of the CRA-based counseling and then introduced her to the voucher program as follows:

"In addition to receiving counseling, you will be requested to provide urine samples three times per week during the first half of treatment and twice weekly during the second half of treatment. During the next 3 months, you also will have the opportunity to earn what we call "vouchers." Vouchers have a monetary value and you earn them every time you provide a urine sample that tests negative for recent cocaine use. In fact, you can earn almost $1,000 worth of vouchers during the next 3 months. These vouchers can be used in whatever way you and I agree would support the lifestyle changes that we discuss in our counseling sessions. For example, many people use their vouchers to buy ski-lift passes, fishing licenses, gift certificates to local restaurants, bicycle equipment, educational materials, and other positive things. In other words, anything that you think will help you remain cocaine-abstinent can be considered. You won't receive cash directly, but all you do is decide with me what items you'd like to spend your vouchers on, and the staff will make the purchase and have whatever you select waiting here for you.

"Our reason for using this incentive program is based on a few ideas. Prior to becoming involved with cocaine, many people engage in a variety of activities that aren't drug-related, such as going to the movies with their partner or working out at the gym. As they become more and more involved with drug-related activities and friends, they spend less time engaging in those positive activities. That is, they may start to hang out at bars or the apartment of someone who uses cocaine, and eventually they start partying with cocaine in addition to drinking or smoking marijuana. Sooner or later they find themselves hanging out getting high all the time rather than doing other things like going out to dinner or to a movie, or doing other prosocial non-drug-related activities.

"This voucher program aims to do two things. First, it immediately rewards you for not using cocaine and provides an extra incentive for remaining abstinent. Second, spending your vouchers on healthy activities can help reintroduce you to the things you used to enjoy that might help you stay away from cocaine. So, for example, you said that on Friday nights you often go out to a bar to meet some friends, have a few drinks, and then end up using cocaine there.

Your vouchers could be used to help you find other ways to unwind on a Friday night that don't involve going to the bar. You could purchase a gift certificate to take a friend out to dinner or take your son bowling or to a movie."

Abstinence Contract

After discussing the voucher program, the therapist then reviews a detailed abstinence contract with the client. This contract outlines the urine-monitoring schedule and voucher program such that the client knows precisely the requirements for earning vouchers.

"Next, I'd like to go over our abstinence contract, which reviews some important parts of treatment as well as the details of the voucher program. This contract represents an agreement between you and the clinic to help you maintain abstinence from cocaine. Like I mentioned earlier, you will be providing urine samples three times per week on a Monday, Wednesday, and Friday schedule during the first 12 weeks of treatment. Then urine samples will be collected twice per week on a Monday and Thursday schedule during the second half of treatment. Throughout treatment, a clinic staff member of your same sex will observe the urination. The reason behind this clinic policy is that urinalysis testing is an integral component of our treatment program. Our on-site testing procedures permit us to carefully monitor your progress toward drug abstinence, and help therapists design effective treatment plans each week. We realize that this is sometimes awkward at first, but we try to be sensitive to your comfort level while at the same time maintaining the integrity and credibility of the monitoring program. Do you have any questions about our procedure for collecting urine samples?

"Also, once per week we screen for a variety of drugs other than cocaine, but whether or not you earn vouchers is based only on urine sample tests for cocaine. If you ever need to go out of town for an emergency, just let us know in advance and we can excuse that sample and add it to the end of treatment. Also, if you ever have transportation problems or for some other reason can't make it to the clinic, just give us a call and we will provide assistance in getting you to the clinic or collecting a sample there. If for appropriate medical reasons you receive a prescription for a drug that is sometimes abused, let us know and bring us a copy of the prescription so that we can take note."

Voucher Schedule

"Now let me tell you more about the incentive program. For every cocaine-negative sample that you provide during the first half of treatment, you will earn points. For example, your first negative sample is worth 10 points, at $0.25 each, so that's $2.50 in vouchers. Every consecutive cocaine-negative sample collected after that will increase in value by 5 points (or $1.25) each time. So, your first negative sample is worth $2.50, your second is worth $3.75, the third is with $5.00, and so on. In other words, the longer you're abstinent, the more each urine sample is worth. You will also earn a $10 bonus for every third consecutive-negative sample you provide, which is even more of an incentive to string together long periods of abstinence. If you provide all cocaine-negative samples, you an earn $997.50 in vouchers during the first 12 weeks of treatment.

"On the other hand if you provide a urine sample that tests positive for recent cocaine use the following things will happen. For each cocaine-positive sample collected you will receive no voucher points. In addition, the voucher points earned for the next cocaine-negative sample will be reset to the initial value: 10 points, or $2.50. However, if you provide five consecutive cocaine-negative samples the voucher value will return to where it was prior to the cocaine 'slip.' In other words, this fifth cocaine-negative sample will be worth the same amount that was earned for the sample preceding the cocaine-positive one, and the system I described earlier will continue from there.

"If you fail to provide a urine sample on the scheduled urinalysis day without prior approval of your therapist, that sample will be treated as a cocaine-positive, like we just discussed. We are always more than happy to help you get to the clinic if you have transportation problems or to collect a sample at a place convenient to you. So there is almost never a reason for you to have a 'no-show.'

"Do you have any questions about treatment, the urinalysis testing, the voucher schedule, or how the vouchers work? If all this sounds good to you, we can both sign at the bottom."

Sandy had one question that is typical of many clients:

"Does that mean I can spend my money on anything I want?" The therapist responded: "Well, almost anything. One of the first things you and I will do is try to understand what usually happens when you use cocaine. By doing this, we will identify what activities, people, or places seem to be associated with your cocaine use. Then we will try and come up with some activities that you get involved with that could compete with or replace your cocaine-using activities. It's these alternative activities, in particular, for which voucher spending is most appropriate. So, like I mentioned earlier, maybe you will choose to use vouchers to join a gym or go to dinner and the movies. Mainly, vouchers are used to reward you for the progress you make in treatment with cocaine abstinence. Maybe you would decide to reward yourself with a massage, a haircut, or tickets to a play. You can also use vouchers for more practical items, like buying some new clothes for job interviews you set up through our Job Club or buying materials for an educational or recreational class that interests you.

"Examples of items that are not appropriate are cigarettes, alcohol, or gift certificates to places that are primarily bars, or items that don't really help you make healthy lifestyle changes, like televisions, VCRs, and the like. You and I will be work together to come up with all the possible, healthy ways you'd like to spend your vouchers."

Collection and Testing of Urine Samples

When the client arrives at the clinic on a scheduled urinalysis day, a urine sample is collected prior to meeting with his or her therapist. This is done to ensure that the voucher procedures are implemented and to provide the therapist with objective evidence relevant to his or her client's progress with cocaine abstinence. If the therapist doesn't have this information and the client reports cocaine abstinence despite having used cocaine, the therapist will mistakenly offer social praise for cocaine abstinence and the session will not focus on the problems that led to the cocaine use.

After the sample has been collected, the client remains in the testing area with the staff member while the urinalysis is performed. This offers several minutes to engage in pleasant conversation while the urine sample is being tested. Then, following each cocaine-negative sample, the staff offers social praise to the client ("Way to go, Sandy. You're negative again! That is four straight weeks, keep up the great work!"). This praise is an additional way to deliver positive reinforcement for providing cocaine-negative samples. The therapist then hands the client a voucher indicating the total amount earned for that day's sample as well as the total earned throughout treatment.

If the urine sample tests positive for cocaine use, the client receives immediate feedback of test results from the staff member in an empathic, nonjudgmental manner. She or he is then asked when the cocaine use occurred and the amount used ("Sandy, your sample tests positive for cocaine. Can you tell me when you last used and how much?"). This information is recorded and then communicated to the client's therapist. The staff member also reminds the client that by providing five consecutive cocaine-negative samples, the value of the vouchers will return to what they were prior to the slip. The staff member then terminates the conversation and facilitates contact between the client and their therapist ("Okay, Sandy. We're done back here. How about we get you to your therapist so you can discuss your cocaine use?"). The staff member also gives the therapist a brief call to provide the urinalysis results.

Integrating the Voucher Program with Behavior Therapy

As discussed earlier, the therapist can maximize the utility of the voucher program by guiding clients to spend their voucher earnings on items or activities that are in concert with their treatment goals related to increasing drug-free prosocial activities. Often, appropriate voucher spending is based on the therapist's knowledge of the client's cocaine use. For example, perhaps the client's cocaine use typically occurs on Friday night following a 50-hour work week. When the therapist and client conduct a functional analysis of his or her cocaine use, they might determine that the function of such use is to unwind from the long work week. The therapist can then encourage the client to use vouchers to purchase a massage or a gym membership, with the goal of helping him or her learn to relax or reduce stress without using cocaine. In this example, perhaps the client can plan on working out at a local gym on Friday evenings instead of going out to bars, thereby reducing his or her risk for using cocaine and meeting safe people at the gym at the same time.

In Sandy's case, she and her therapist had identified Tuesday nights as particularly high risk for cocaine use. On most Tuesdays she would go to a bar to play darts and have a few drinks with old friends. In response to this analysis, the therapist and Sandy scanned the current events section of the local newspaper to find potential alternative activities for Tuesday nights. Sandy saw an add for an aerobics class at a nearby gym that she would like to sample, and the therapist arranged for her to use her vouchers to register for the Tuesday evening class. They then planned each week for the aerobics class, which included solving transportation and childcare problems that might interfere with attending the class. The weekly aerobics class effectively competed with Sandy's previous Tuesday routine in the bar. Moreover, she met several women with whom she became friends, thereby expanding her social network to include friends outside of the bar scene.

Regarding voucher spending, therapists must also give consideration to whatever the client identifies as rewarding. For example, a client may desire to use vouchers to pay off fines in order to get a revoked driver's license reinstated. Achieving this goal would also facilitate transportation necessary to obtain full-time employment or increase contact with safe family or friends. In this case, the therapist may suggest that the client spend a portion of her vouchers on paying off fines. On the other hand, if the client has earned $350 in vouchers and wants to spend the entire sum on these fines, the therapist may suggest an alternative plan. Depleting the client's entire voucher earnings on paying off these fines may not be as helpful as saving half of the vouchers for the gym membership or to pay for dinners out with her significant other that she continually says are of interest to her. To facilitate such a compromise in voucher spending, the therapist would provide skills training focused on budgeting and money management, thereby helping the client to save money to put toward the fines, while retaining some vouchers to access other types of prosocial reinforcers.

In Sandy's case, she requested to use her vouchers on tanning sessions at a nearby salon. Although this use of vouchers didn't directly relate to a treatment goal, she identified it as something that she found rewarding. Her therapist recognized it as an activity that might enable her to relax in a way that did not involve alcohol or cocaine. Her therapist also viewed the tanning salon as a potential place to socialize and meet new friends. Sandy and her therapist developed a plan for her to approach a woman who worked there and start a casual conversation with the eventual goal of asking her out to coffee or to come along to her aerobics class. Making contact with this other person would indicate progress toward the "increasing social support" goal on Sandy's treatment plan.

Overall, therapists must keep in mind that the goal of this contingency management procedure is to utilize vouchers as a reward for cocaine abstinence as well as a means of increasing clients' involvement in drug-free prosocial activities. If the voucher spending is not rewarding to the client, it will have little effect. In other words, one must remember that an activity or item that is reinforcing for one client may not be so for another. The therapist and the client must decide *together* on voucher spending. Such collaboration will increase the probability of accomplishing the long-term goal of the voucher program, which is continuous participation in activities that are incompatible or that compete with the reinforcing effects of cocaine use.

Relapses

Therapists can use the voucher program to address cocaine use (slips) during treatment in two ways. First, if the client's motivation has waned, a review of potential future voucher earnings can contribute to a therapeutic discussion of this important issue. That is, the therapist reminds the client that five cocaine-negative samples in a row will return his or her voucher earnings to the value prior to the cocaine use. The therapist can make a hypothetical graph showing progress toward the fifth negative sample and the amount of vouchers that can still be earned if the client gets back on track with cocaine abstinence. In addition, the therapist may revisit the list of items that the client had previously identified as desirable purchases to make with voucher earnings. Here, the therapist might encourage the client to choose one he or she would like to work toward. Again, the therapist could graph hisor her progress toward that particular voucher-spending goal.

For example, when Sandy experienced an instance of cocaine use after a prolonged period of abstinence, she and her therapist reviewed other potential uses of vouchers that she had not yet requested and which might give her an incentive to get back on track. Sandy mentioned that she would eventually like to start purchasing savings bonds for her son's college education. The therapist agreed with this use of vouchers, and they decided that if she submitted four consecutive negative samples ($17.50 plus the $10 bonus), she would be able to use $25 in vouchers to purchase her son a $50 savings bond. The therapist also created a graph to monitor progress toward this goal, whereby each sample leading up to the fourth negative sample was graphed and a photo of Sandy's son was taped next to the target (fourth) sample. Sandy successfully reached her savings bond goal, during which time she and her therapist were able to make progress on other treatment goals as well.

The second strategic use of vouchers in response to cocaine use is to supplement the plans that follow from a functional analysis of the slip. For example, Sandy had a series of slips throughout treatment that were reflected by cocaine-positive urinalysis tests on Wednesdays. Hence the therapist initiated the following conversation with Sandy.

THERAPIST: Sandy, you've been doing relatively well with cocaine abstinence, although I see a few "slips" during the past month. Can you identify specifically what was going in your life or certain situations that arose that put you at risk for using cocaine?

SANDY: Not really. I just ran into some old friends, I guess.

THERAPIST: Well, let's take a look at your urinalysis graph. When I compare it with this month's calendar, it looks like these cocaine-positive samples were all on Wednesdays. Is there anything particular that's going on Monday or Tuesdays that might be associated with these positives on Wednesdays?

SANDY: Well, now that you mention it, I did join group of friends for a regular card game a few weeks ago. On Monday nights, we meet at the pub, have a few beers, and play cards all evening. I guess I got caught up in hanging out with those guys a few times and ended up partying with them like we used to do. It's not that I plan it, but just that once we all start hanging out and drinking and playing cards, it's hard to leave. I guess that could be a problem. I had noticed that since I'd been doing well with staying away from cocaine I hadn't spent much time in the pub like I used to.

Based on this information, the therapist and Sandy discussed a goal to minimize time spent in bars, paying particular attention to helping Sandy make plans for Monday nights. Together they decided that Sandy could ask her significant other to dinner, make the reservation at the restaurant, and make a voucher-spending request for a gift certificate for the dinner. This plan would reflect a commitment to engaging in a safer activity on Monday nights and would put her at lower risk for using cocaine.

If the therapist and client identify a needed change in the treatment plan that may prevent a future relapse to cocaine use (i.e., increasing activities on weekends or increased contact with safe friends), vouchers can be used effectively to support these changes. Vouchers can be useful in practically any effort to increase contact with sources of non-drug reinforcement that may compete with cocaine, particularly if a recent relapse indicates deprivation in a certain area.

Outcome

During the 24-week treatment, Sandy achieved 15 weeks of continuous cocaine abstinence and earned approximately $900 in vouchers. Her voucher uses included bowling and skiing passes, restaurant and movie gift certificates, tanning sessions, a membership to aerobics classes, and a $50 U.S. savings bond. In addition to promoting cocaine abstinence, the thoughtful, strategic uses for voucher spending helped Sandy minimize the amount of time she spent in bars, increased her involvement in healthy alternative activities, and increased her social network of non-drug-using friends. Sandy entered an aftercare program that initially involved once per month meetings with her counselor and urinalysis testing. During the first 5 months posttreatment, Sandy continued to maintain cocaine abstinence. During the sixth month, she returned to treatment requesting additional counseling for concerns about a recent night of binge drinking during which a cocaine slip had also occurred. Once per week counseling was initiated for 4 weeks to strengthen Sandy's plans for dealing with high-risk friends who asked her to go out drinking. Other than this slip, Sandy had maintained the progress made in treatment and had enrolled in continuing education classes at the local community college. At 12-month follow-up, Sandy reported one other similar alcohol/cocaine slip, but felt that she coped with it well by using the skills she had learned during treatment and did not require additional counseling. She reported no significant problems in other life areas.

Concluding Comments

This case illustration demonstrates how a voucher program can be integrated almost seamlessly with a behavioral therapy program for substance dependence. The use of the contingent vouchers to motivate drug abstinence and support lifestyle change appears logical and obviously facilitates the therapist's task of engaging clients in therapy and the client's task of finding alternative, nondrug sources of reinforcement. Nonetheless, contingency management, like many other drug abuse treatments that have been developed and shown to be effective in research settings, are not the models of intervention commonly used in community clinics (Miller et al., 1995). Most of the work described in this chapter has been implemented only in research settings.

A number of philosophical and practical factors contribute to this situation. As one can imagine, the logistics of initiating such a program in a typical community clinic may appear daunting. The costs of incentives, regular urine testing, and the personnel to run the program may seem beyond reasonable expectations, particularly given today's tight market on health care spending. Moreover, asking experienced therapists with histories of providing treatments that are based on a very different understanding of substance dependence also may appear problematic. Yet the need for more effective interventions in the drug abuse community is so great and the contingency management approach has so much to offer that it seems imperative that the field turn its attention to the issue of dissemination of such programs.

The practical and clinical obstacles such as funding programs, educating and training treatment providers, and convincing program developers and policymakers of the value of this approach to substance abuse treatment have been discussed in depth elsewhere (Crowley, 1999; Kirby, Amass, & McLellan, 1999). This chapter provided examples of how communities appear willing to become involved in funding voucher-based programs (Amass, 1997; Donatelle et al., 2002), and how such programs have the potential to become self-sustaining while simultaneously enhancing the vocational skills of the substance abuser (Silverman et al., 2001). Other examples highlighted how creative, low-cost contingency management strategies can be developed by using existing clinic privileges to enhance therapeutic outcomes (Kidorf & Stitzer, 1999).

The extant research suggests that investing in the development and dissemination of contingency management programs for substance abusers has the potential for a substantial, cost-effective payoff. The high cost of problems associated with drug dependence and its seemingly refractory course implore us to seek alternative strategies for intervening with this difficult treatment population. Contingency management strategies certainly do not provide "the answer" that will eradicate this societal problem. They do, however, offer an alternative approach with great promise to reach and effectively treat more people suffering from serious substance-use disorders.

ACKNOWLEDGMENT

Preparation of this chapter was supported in part by National Institute on Drug Abuse Grant Nos. DA12157, DA09378 and DA07242.

REFERENCES

Amass, L. (1997). Financing voucher programs for pregnant substance abusers through community donations. In L. S. Harris (Ed.), *Problems of drug dependence 1996: Proceedings of the 58th Annual Scientific Meeting of the College on Problems of Drug Dependence* (NIDA Research Monograph No. 174, pp. 59). Washington, DC: U.S. Government Printing Office.

Azrin, N. H. (1976). Improvements in the community reinforcement approach to alcoholism. *Behaviour Research and Therapy, 14*, 339–348.

Azrin, N. H., Sisson, W., Meyers, R., & Godley, M. (1982). Alcoholism treatment by disulfiram and community reinforcement therapy. *Journal of Behavior Therapy and Experimental Psychiatry, 13*, 105–112.

Bickel, W. K., Amass, L., Higgins, S. T., Badger, G. J., & Esch, R. A. (1997). Effects of adding a behavioral treatment to opioid detoxification with buprenorphine. *Journal of Consulting and Clinical Psychology, 65*, 803–810.

Budney, A. J., & Higgins, S. T. (1998). *A community reinforcement plus vouchers approach: Treating cocaine addiction.* Rockville, MD: U.S. Department of Health and Human Services.

Budney, A. J., Higgins, S. T., Delaney, D. D., Kent, L., & Bickel, W. K. (1991). Contingent reinforcement of abstinence with individuals abusing cocaine and marijuana. *Journal of Applied Behavior Analysis, 24*, 657–665.

Budney, A. J., Higgins, S. T., Radonovich, K. J., & Novy, P. L. (2000). Adding voucher-based incentives to coping-skills and motivational enhancement improves outcomes during treatment for marijuana dependence. *Journal of Consulting and Clinical Psychology, 68*, 1051–1061.

Catania, A. C. (1998). *Learning* (4th ed.). Upper Saddle River, NJ: Prentice-Hall.

Chutuape, M. A., Silverman, K., & Stitzer, M. L. (1999). Contingent reinforcement sustains post-detoxification abstinence from multiple drugs: A preliminary study with methadone patients. *Drug and Alcohol Dependence, 54*, 69–81.

Crowley, T. J. (1999). Research on contingency management treatment of drug drependence: Clinical implications and future directions. In S. T. Higgins & K. Silverman (Eds.), *Motivating behavior change among illicit-drug abusers* (pp. 345–370). Washington, DC: American Psychological Association.

Dallery, J., Silverman, K., Chutuape, M. A., Bigelow, G. E., & Stitzer, M. L. (2001). Voucher-based reinforcement of opiate plus cocaine abstinence in treatment-resistant methadone patients: Effects of reinforcer magnitude. *Experimental and Clinical Psychopharmacology, 9*(3), 317–325.

Donatelle, R. J., Prows, S. L., Champeau, D., & Hudson, D. (2002). Randomized controlled trial using social support and financial incentives for high risk pregnant smokers: Significant other supporter (SOS) program. *Tobacco Control,* *2*(III), iii67–iii69.

Downey, K. K., Helmus, T. C., & Schuster, C. R. (2000). Treatment of heroin-dependent poly-drug abusers with contingency management and buprenorphine maintenance. *Experimental and Clinical Psychopharmacology, 8,* 176–184.

Elk, R., Schmitz, J., Spiga, R., Rhoades, H., Andres, R., & Gabowski, J. (1995). Behavioral treatment of cocaine-dependent pregnant women and TB-exposed patients. *Addictive Behaviors, 20,* 533–542.

Glosser, D. S. (1983). The use of token economy to reduce illicit drug use among methadone maintenance clients. *Addictive Behaviors, 8,* 247–252.

Griffiths, R. R., Bigelow, G. E., & Henningfield, J. E. (1980). Similarities in animal and human drug-taking behavior. In N. K. Mello (Ed.), *Advances in substance abuse: Behavioral and biological research* (pp. 1–90). Greenwich, CT: JAI Press.

Higgins, S. T. (1997). The influence of alternative reinforcers on cocaine use and abuse: A brief review. *Pharmacology, Biochemistry, and Behavior, 57,* 419–427.

Higgins, S. T., Alessi, S. M., & Dantona, R. L. (2002). Voucher-based incentives. A substance abuse treatment innovation. *Addictive Behaviors, 27*(6), 887–910.

Higgins, S. T., Badger, G. J., & Budney, A. J. (2000). Initial abstinence and success in achieving longer-term cocaine abstinence. *Experimental and Clinical Psychopharmacology, 8*(3), 377–386.

Higgins, S. T., Budney, A. J., & Bickel, W. K. (1994). Applying behavioral concepts and principles to the treatment of cocaine dependence. *Drug and Alcohol Dependence, 34,* 87–97.

Higgins, S. T., Budney, A. J., Bickel, W. K., Foerg, F., Donham, R., & Badger, G. (1994). Incentives improve outcome in outpatient behavioral treatment of cocaine dependence. *Archives of General Psychiatry, 51,* 568–576.

Higgins, S. T., Budney, A. J., Bickel, W. K., Hughes, J. R., Foerg, F., & Badger, G. (1993). Achieving cocaine abstinence with a behavioral approach. *American Journal of Psychiatry, 150*(5), 763–769.

Higgins, S. T., Delaney, D. D., Budney, A. J., Bickel, W. K., Hughes, J. R., Foerg, F., et al. (1991). A behavioral approach to achieving initial cocaine abstinence. *American Journal of Psychiatry, 148,* 1218–1224.

Higgins, S. T., & Katz, J. L. (1998). *Cocaine abuse: Behavior, pharmacology, and clinical applications.* San Diego, CA: Academic Press.

Higgins, S. T., & Silverman, K. (1999). *Motivating behavior change among illicit-drug abusers: Research on contingency-management interventions.* Washington, DC: American Psychological Association.

Higgins, S. T., Stitzer, M. L., Bigelow, G. E., & Liebson, I. A. (1986). Contingent methadone delivery: Effects on illicit-opiate use. *Drug and Alcohol Dependence, 1,* 311–322.

Higgins, S. T., Wong, C. J., Badger, G. J., Ogden, D. H., & Dantona, R. (2000). Contingent reinforcement increases cocaine abstinence during outpatient treatment and 1 year of follow up. *Journal of Consulting and Clinical Psychology, 68,* 64–72.

Hughes, J. R., Hatsukami, D. K., Mitchell, J. E., & Dahlgren, L. A. (1986). Prevalence of smoking among psychiatric outpatients. *American Journal of Psychiatry, 143,* 993–997.

Iguchi, M. Y., Belding, M. A., Morral, A. R., Lamb, R. J., & Husband, S. D. (1997). Reinforcement operants other than abstinence in drug abuse treatment: An effective alternative for reducing drug use. *Journal of Consulting and Clinical Psychology, 65*(3), 421–428.

Iguchi, M. Y., Lamb, R. J., Belding, M. A., Platt, J. J., Husband, S. D., & Morral, A. R. (1996). Contingent reinforcement of group participation versus abstinence in a methadone maintenance program. *Experimental and Clinical Psychopharmacology, 4*, 315–321.

Jones, H. E., Haug, N., Silverman, K., Stitzer, M. L., & Svikis, D. (2001). The effectiveness of incentives in enhancing treatment attendance and drug abstinence in methadone-maintained pregnant women. *Drug and Alcohol Dependence, 61*, 297–306.

Katz, E. C., Chatuape, M. A., Jones, H. E., & Stitzer, M. L. (2002). Voucher reinforcement for heroin and cocaine abstinence in an outpatient drug-free program. *Experimental and Clinical Psychopharmacology, 10*, 136–143.

Kidorf, M., Brooner, R. K., & King, V. L. (1997). Motivating methadone patients to include drug-free significant others in treatment: A behavioral intervention. *Journal of Substance Abuse Treatment, 14*, 23–28.

Kidorf, M., Hollander, J. R., King, V. L., & Brooner, R. K. (1998). Increasing employment of opioid dependant outpatients: An intensive behavioral intervention. *Drug and Alcohol Dependence, 50*, 73–80.

Kidorf, M., & Stitzer, M. L. (1999). Contingent access to clinic privileges reduces drug abuse in methadone maintenance patients. In S. T. Higgins & K. Silverman (Eds.), *Motivating behavior change among illicit-drug abusers* (pp. 221–241). Washington, DC: American Psychological Association.

Kidorf, M., Stitzer, M. L., Brooner, R. K., & Goldberg, J. (1994). Contingent use of take-home doses reinforce adjunct therapy attendance of methadone maintenance patients. *Behavior Therapy, 27*, 41–51.

Kirby, K. C., Amass, L., & McLellan, A. T. (1999). Disseminating contingency management research to drug abuse treatment practitioners. In S. T. Higgins & K. Silverman (Eds.), *Motivating behavior change among illicit-drug abusers* (pp. 327–344). Washington, DC: American Psychological Association.

Kirby, K. C., Marlowe, D. B., Festinger, D. S., Lamb, R. J., & Platt, J. J. (1998). Schedule of voucher delivery influences initiation of cocaine abstinence. *Journal of Consulting and Clinical Psychology, 66*, 761–767.

Kirby, K. N., Petry, N. M., & Bickel, W. K. (1999). Heroin addicts discount delayed rewards at higher rates than non-drug using controls. *Journal of Experimental Psychology General, 128*, 78–87.

Liebson, I. A., Tommaselo, A., & Bigelow, G. E. (1978). A behavioral treatment of alcoholic methadone patients. *Annals of Internal Medicine, 89*, 342–344.

Magura, S., Casriel, C., Goldsmith, D. S., & Lipton, D. S. (1987). Contracting with clients in methadone treatment. *Social Casework: The Journal of Contemporary Social Work, 68*, 485–494.

Magura, S., Casriel, C., Goldsmith, D. S., Strug, D. L., & Lipton, D. S. (1988). Contingency contracting with polydrug-abusing methadone patients. *Addictive Behaviors, 13*, 113–118.

Milby, J. B., Garrett, C., English, C., Fritschi, O., & Clarke, C. (1978). Take-home methadone: Contingency effects on drug-seeking and productivity of narcotic addicts. *Addictive Behaviors, 3*, 215–220.

Milby, J. B., Schumacher, J. E., McNamara, C., Wallace, D., Usdan, S., McGill, T., et al. (2000). Initiating astinence in cocaine abusing dually diagnosed homeless persons. *Drug and Alcohol Dependence, 60*, 55–68.

Milby, J. B., Schumacher, J. E., Raczynski, J., Caldwell, E., Engle, M., & Michael, M. (1996). Sufficient conditions for effective treatment of substance abusing homeless persons. *Drug and Alcohol Dependence, 43*, 39–47.

Miller, L. K. (1984). *Behavior analysis for everyday life*. Pacific Grove, CA: Brooks/Cole.

Miller, P. M. (1975). A behavioral intervention program for chronic public drunkenness offenders. *Archives of General Psychiatry, 32*, 915–918.

Miller, W. A., Brown, J. M., Simpson, T. L., Handmaker, N. S., Bien, T. H., Luckie, L. F., et al. (1995). What works?: A methodological analysis of the alcohol treatment literature. In R. K. Hester & W. R. Miller (Eds.), *Handbook of alcoholism treatment approaches: Effective alternatives* (pp. 12–44). Boston: Allyn & Bacon.

Petry, N. M., Bickel, W. K., & Arnett, M. (1998). Shortened time horizons and insensitivity to future consequences in heroin addicts. *Addiction, 93*, 729–738.

Petry, N. M., & Martin, B. (2002). Low-cost contingency management for treating cocaine- and opioid-abusing methadone patients. *Journal of Consulting and Clinical Psychology, 70*(2), 398–405.

Petry, N. M., Martin, B., Cooney, J. L., & Kranzler, H. R. (2000). Give them prizes, and they will come: Contingency management for treatment of alcohol dependence. *Journal of Consulting and Clinical Psychology, 68*, 250–257.

Piotrowski, N. A., Tusel, D. J., Sees, K. L., Reilly, P. M., Banys, P., Meek, P., et al. (1999). Contingency contracting with monetary reinforcers for abstinence from multiple drugs in a methadone program. *Experimental and Clinical Psychopharmacology, 7*, 399–411.

Preston, K., Umbricht, A., & Epstein, D. (2000). Methadone dose increase and abstinence reinforcement for treatment of continued heroin use during methadone maintenance. *Archives of General Psychiatry, 57*, 395–404.

Regier, D. A., Farmer, M. E., Rae, D. S., Locke, B., Keith, S. J., Judd, L. L., et al. (1990). Comorbidity of mental disorders with alcohol and other drug abuse: Results from the Epidemiological Catchment Area Study. *Journal of the American Medical Association, 264*, 2511–2519.

Ries, R. K., & Comtois, K. A. (1997). Managing disability benefits as part of treatment for persons with severe mental illness and comorbid drug/alcohol disorders: A comparative study of payees and non-payee participants. *American Journal on Addictions, 6*, 330–338.

Ries, R. K., & Dyck, D. G. (1997). Representative payee practices of community mental health centers in Washington State. *Psychiatric Services, 48*, 811–814.

Roll, J. M., Higgins, S. T., Steingard, S., & McGinley, M. (1998). Use of monetary reinforcement to reduce the cigarette smoking of persons with schizophrenia: A feasibility study. *Experimental and Clinical Psychopharamacology, 6*, 157–161.

Rowan-Szal, G., Joe, G. W., Chatham, L. R., & Simpson, D. D. (1994). A simple reinforcement system for methadone clients in a community-based treatment program. *Journal of Substance Abuse Treatment, 11,* 217–223.

Shaner, A., Eckman, T. A., Roberts, L. J., Wilkins, J. N., Tucker, D. E., Tsuang, J. W., et al. (1995). Disability income, cocaine use, and repeated hospitalization among schizophrenic cocaine abusers: A government-sponsored revolving door? *New England Journal of Medicine, 333,* 777–783.

Shaner, A., Roberts, L. J., Eckman, T. A., Tucker, D. E., Tsuang, J. W., Wilkins, J. N., et al. (1997). Monetary reinforcement of abstinence from cocaine among mentally ill patients with cocaine dependence. *Psychiatric Services, 48,* 807–810.

Sigmon, S. C., Steingard, S., Badger, G. J., Anthony, S. L., & Higgins, S. T. (2000). Contingent reinforcement of marijuana abstinence among individuals with serious mental illness: A feasibility study. *Experimental and Clinical Psychopharmacology, 8,* 509–517.

Silverman, K., Chutuape, M. A., Bigelow, G. E., & Stitzer, M. L. (1996). Voucher-based reinforcement of attendance by unemployed methadone patients in a job skills training program. *Drug and Alcohol Dependence, 41,* 197–207.

Silverman, K., Chutuape, M. A.., Bigelow, G. E., & Stitzer, M. L. (1999). Voucher-based reinforcement of cocaine abstinence in treatment-resistant methadone patients: Effects of reinforcement magnitude. *Psychopharmacology, 146*(2), 128–138.

Silverman, K., Svikis, D., Robles, E., Stitzer, M. L., & Bigelow, G. E. (2001). A reinforcement-based therapeutic workplace for the treatment of drug abuse: Six-month abstinence outcomes. *Experimental and Clinical Psychopharmacology, 9*(1), 14–23.

Silverman, K., Wong, C. J., Umbricht-Schneiter, A., Montoya, I. D., Schuster, C. R., & Preston, K. L. (1998). Broad beneficial effects of reinforcement for cocaine abstinence in methadone patients. *Journal of Consulting and Clinical Psychology, 60,* 927–934.

Stitzer, M. L., Bickel, W. K., Bigelow, G. E., & Liebson, I. A. (1986). Effect of methadone dose contingencies on urinalysis test results of polydrug-abusing methadone maintenance patients. *Drug and Alcohol Dependence, 18,* 341–348.

Stitzer, M. L., & Bigelow, G. (1978). Contingency management in a methadone maintenance program: Availability of reinforcers. *International Journal of the Addictions, 13,* 737–746.

Stitzer, M. L., & Bigelow, G. E. (1983). Contingent reinforcement for carbon monoxide reduction: Effects of pay amount. *Behavior Therapy, 14,* 647–656.

Stitzer, M. L., & Bigelow, G. E. (1984a). Contingent methadone take-home privileges: Effects on compliance with fee payment schedules. *Drug and Alcohol Dependence, 13,* 395–399.

Stitzer, M. L., & Bigelow, G. E. (1984b). Contingent reinforcement for carbon monoxide reduction: Within-subjects effects of pay amounts. *Journal of Applied Behavior Analysis, 17,* 477–483.

Stitzer, M. L., Bigelow, G. E., Lawrence, C., Cohen, J., D'Lugoff, B., & Hawthorne, J. (1977). Medication take-home as a reinforcer in a methadone maintenance program. *Addictive Behaviors, 2,* 9–14.

Stitzer, M. L., Bigelow, G., Liebson, I., & Hawthorne, J. W. (1982). Contingent reinforcement for benzodiazepine-free urines: Evaluation of a drug abuse treatment intervention. *Journal of Applied Behavior Analysis, 15,* 493–503.

Stitzer, M. L., & Higgins, S. T. (1995). Behavioral treatment of drug and alcohol
abuse. In F. E. Bloom & D. J. Kupfer (Eds.), *Psychopharmacology: The fourth gen-
eration of progress* (pp. 1807–1819). New York: Raven Press.

Stitzer, M. L., Iguchi, M. Y., & Felch, L. (1992). Contingent take-home incentive:
Effects of drug use of methadone patients. *Journal of Consulting and Clinical
Psychology, 60,* 927–934.

Sulzer-Azaroff, B., & Meyer, G. R. (1991). *Behavior analysis for lasting change.* Fort
Worth, TX: Holt Rinehart & Winston.

Tidey, J. W., O'Neill, S. C., & Higgins, S. T. (1999). Effects of abstinence on cigarette smoking among outpatients with schizophrenics. *Experimental and Clinical Psychopharmacology, 7,* 347–353.

11

Theoretical Perspectives on Motivation and Addictive Behavior

Scott T. Walters
Frederick Rotgers
Bill Saunders
Celia Wilkinson
Tania Towers

Without an appreciation of the role of motivation, substance abuse treatment can read like a mystery novel with a missing page: How did the butler get that knife in his hand and what does he plan to do with it? Indeed, addiction counselors are often frustrated with exactly this sense of missing something. Laments one: "My client came in last week desperate to make a change. He finally got off parole and was really going to make it work this time. We spent the whole session talking about his plan for avoiding relapse, and now I found out he nearly OD'd this weekend!" The irony is clear: Why would a person persist in behavior that is clearly harming him- or herself and others?

To many in the addictions field, motivation is *the* magic bullet. Puzzling and elusive, the desire to change has long been a matter of interest in the addictions field (see, e.g., Lemere, O'Hollaren, & Maxwell, 1958; Mindlin, 1959; Sterne & Pittman, 1965). In the new century, motivation continues to sit squarely as the number-one client predictor of treatment outcome (DiClemente, Bellino, & Neavins, 1999), and its role is becoming increasingly emphasized in the literature and in practice (Dunn, Deroo, & Rivara, 2001). On the one hand, it is simple to say that individuals need to be motivated in order to change. On the other hand, the historically high treatment dropout rates in the addictions field have caused many to discard earlier straightforward notions of what motivation is. A survey of psychological textbooks will reveal a panoply of definitions, most of which refer to inner drive states, the operation of incentives, decision-making processes, or some form of intervening process that impels the individual to action. Although motivation is sometimes treated as a single construct, even a quick reflection suggests that people are moved to action by very different factors. People can be motivated reluctantly because of strong external pressure to act, or sacrificially because of deeply held values. Not surprisingly, Reber (1985) noted that the term "motivation" was "extremely important but definitionally elusive" (p. 454).

THE PSYCHOLOGY OF MOTIVATION

Drives as Motivation

Historically, motivation has been linked to the notion of drive states. From a drive reduction perspective, motivation is the product of physiological needs such as hunger, thirst, or sex. We are motivated to seek and get the things we need. From this standpoint, drug-seeking behavior is an attempt to reduce unpleasant withdrawal symptoms, and is sustained through negative reinforcement (e.g., the removal of a noxious stimulus). Also consistent with drive theory is evidence that there may be a "genetic predisposition" to become alcohol-dependent (Bierut et al., 1998), as well as long-lasting neurological changes as a result of continued drug use (Robinson & Berridge, 2000). The common thread in these findings is that there are certain identifiable physiological characteristics, such as levels of neurochemicals, that mediate the extent to which a person will pay attention to a drug or "want" it (Robinson & Berridge, 2000).

Historically, drive models were first challenged by, and then incorporated into, behaviorist or learning models of motivation. It is now widely agreed upon that genetic and biological factors do account for some proportion of the variance in alcohol dependence (Schuckit, 1985; Schuckit, Tsuang, Anthenelli, Tipp, & Nurnberger, 1996). Such models have made the use of medication more acceptable as an adjunct to substance abuse treatment (see Carroll, Chapter 13, this volume). However, at this point, findings from the biological and genetic literature are not well integrated with our philosophical ideas of free will in recovery. That is, whether genetic factors account for 1% or 99% of the variance in dependence, presumably counselors would still approach patients in the same way, asking them to adopt new behaviors based upon feedback from their environment.

Learning as Motivation

We learn what we like to do by acting in certain ways, experiencing the consequences of our actions, and adjusting our behavior accordingly. In general, it is thought that whereas *drives* primarily initiate behavior, it is *consequences* that determine whether the behavior will be repeated in the future. Feedback from positive and negative reinforcement, as well as punishment, all shape our behavior, and drug-seeking behavior is no exception. In addition, drug use, and even drug dependence and tolerance, can be classically conditioned by contextual factors surrounding drug use.

In the addictions arena, the use of aversion techniques (i.e., pairing drug use with a noxious, painful, or unpleasant stimulus) is an example of the classical conditioning paradigm in action. However, since their heyday in the 1950s, these aversive and punishing regimens have fallen into disuse. More popular in recent years are operant approaches that rearrange the positive and negative incentives for drinking or drug use. For example, some approaches set up negative contingencies for continued use, such as termination from treatment or discontinuation of methadone maintenance. Other approaches use positive incentives such as vouchers to support abstinence among cocaine users (Higgins, Alessi, & Dantona, 2002), or contracting with family members to reward a drinker for abstinence (Meyers & Miller, 2001). Although operant approaches vary widely in the incentives they utilize, their common thread is that they attempt to make sobriety more reinforcing to the client than continued substance use.

Decision Making as Motivation

West (1989) said that the "common sense view of motivation is that people do things because they perceive them as being better in some way than not doing them" (p. 71). From this position it is easy to see motivation as a decision-making process for which a number of models exist. One classic decision-making paradigm is subjective expected utility (SEU; von Winterfeldt & Edwards, 1986). In this "What's in it for me?" approach, people try to anticipate whether a course of action is likely to be useful to them before they act, assessing both the positive and the negative consequences of a behavior. When individuals are confronted with two or more options, they will select the one that, relative to the other options, will provide the most benefit at the least cost. The SEU model is an "as if" model, meaning that individuals do not consciously weigh all the pros and cons of a decision, but they act "as if" they have.

It helped Benjamin Franklin to make difficult decisions by listing his competing motivations in a sort of algebraic equation. After listing the likely pros and cons of an outcome and giving estimated weights to the importance of each item, he added up the two lists and acted accordingly. Two centuries later Janis and Mann (1977) formally proposed the "Decisional Balance Sheet" as a schema for understanding the cognitive, emotional, and motivational aspects of decision making. Within the decisional balance model the perceived gains of undertaking a behavior are contrasted with the costs of that action *and* the costs and benefits of *not* undertaking the behavior. Decisional balance is a comparative model because it is not the total number of gains and losses that influences the decision but the number of gains and losses *in relation to each other.*

Miller and Rollnick (2002) have used a seesaw analogy to illustrate this decision-making dilemma. On each end of the seesaw are possible options, and each option has costs and benefits associated with it. When faced with a new option, individuals weigh the costs and benefits associated with change against the costs and benefits associated with maintaining the status quo, which meta-phorically "tips" the balance from one side to the other. For a drinker consid-ering abstinence, the conflict might be thus: "If I continue to drink, I will con-tinue to enjoy the benefits of being with friends [benefit of status quo]. However, my family relationships and health will continue to deteriorate [costs of status quo]. On the other hand, if I quit drinking, I will feel better physically [benefit of change], but I won't be able to spend the evenings with my friends and will probably feel more stressed [costs of change]."

Decisional balance sheets are now widely used as a therapeutic tool to help frame such a dilemma. One simple way is to draw a line down the middle of a page, label one side "Good Things about My Drug Use" and the other side "Not-So-Good Things about My Drug Use," and have the client com-plete the lists. A slightly more sophisticated version involves listing the pros and cons of both taking action to change and maintaining the status quo in a 2 × 2 matrix (Handmaker & Walters, 2002).

Though popular in practice, some have criticized this simple model of competing assessments as a way to account for behavior change (Frish & Clemen, 1994). First of all, humans are limited in their decision-making capac-ity, and simply cannot gather and process all of the information required to make a fully calculated decision. Simon (1976) coined the term "bounded-ra-tionalists" to describe the way humans make decisions in practice. Because of limited "information-processing capacity," the best that actors can do is to make decisions that seem to be "good enough."

But there are also other problems with the notion of humans as rational actors. As Tversky and Kahneman (1981) have noted, if individuals made deci-sions in a rational manner, we would expect some "consistency" and "coher-ence" in their choices. After all, in making a decision, all individuals weigh rel-evant information and progress through basically the same logical steps. However, in many instances people demonstrate nothing like consistency and coherence in the way they solve problems. Part of the reason for this seeming contradiction may be that it is possible to "frame" a problem in different ways that will preinfluence outcome. Tversky and Kahneman (1981) demonstrated that when two scenarios with identical possible outcomes were presented to subjects, the respondents differed in their stated choices depending on whether the question was framed in terms of possible gains or possible losses. The dif-ference in the way a question was framed caused a significant shift from "risk-aversive" to "risk-taking" styles of decision making, despite the fact that "rationally" the problem was the same.

Thus, the utility model has a second drawback in that it assumes that individuals weigh the pros and cons of behavior in a rational unemotive way. In practice, however, decision making seems to be much more complicated: people may make radically different decisions depending upon the context in which they approach problems, as well as their beliefs about what the outcomes are likely to be. As a compromise, Sutton (1987) introduced a modified form of SEU that incorporated individuals' beliefs in their abilities to succeed in quitting. This has become known as the "value-expectancy" paradigm because it takes into account the perceived importance of the behavior *as well as* the individuals' belief in their ability to achieve the goal. Indeed, when Rollnick, Butler, and Stott (1997) asked smokers in a primary care setting about their readiness to quit smoking, responses tended to be divided into either the *personal value* of change (e.g., its importance to them, or the benefits of changing) or their *ability* to achieve it. Confidence or efficacy in one's ability to master tasks has been demonstrated to be an important psychological component in many other areas (Bandura, 1994), and this modified proposal—that individuals have to *value* the outcome and *expect* that they can achieve it—appears to be a step in the right direction.

Emotion as Motivation

However, this importance/confidence equation still assumes a degree of clear-headedness on the part of the individual. From settings outside the addictions arena, this notion has been challenged. Klar, Nadler, and Malloy (1992) attempted to explain the paradoxical situation in which people pursue outcomes that are very unlikely to happen. They have argued, from analyses of students' attempts to change various aspects, or "domains," of their behavior (e.g., to be more punctual, to stop smoking, to be more sociable), that it is the *desirability* of the outcome that drives behavior much more than the perceived *likelihood of success*. They concluded from the reports of some 200 students, involving more than 25 domains of behavioral change, that individuals may "invest costly resources even when their expectancy to obtain that outcome is meager, or, when their past record with change is poor" (p. 77). In addition, other psychological variables such as low self-worth and a high degree of personal dissatisfaction with life also predicted likelihood of change. For example, the more emotionally "distressed" individuals were, the more likely they were to engage in action.

Cantor and Langston (1989) likewise note that:

> In many cases, individuals give relatively little independent weight to their chance of success and base their decisions and actions on value related information—primarily, how much they would desire a given outcome. The strength of the cos-

metic and fashion industry seems to depend on the fact that people cannot or will not realistically estimate their probability of achieving the sought after goal, but instead base their actions on how much they want the desired outcome. (pp. 217–218)

Similarly, Fitzgibbon and Kirschenbaum (1992) point out that despite a relatively poor track record, the weight loss industry continues to prosper. That is, irrespective of high failure rates, the *appeal* of weight loss keeps people engaging in difficult and costly attempts to diet.

In theory, individuals should make an unbiased choice after taking into account factors such as desirability and likelihood of outcome in a "vigilant" decision-making style. The final decision should be made only after the individual has examined all the information gathered, when he or she can make an informed, "rational" choice. In practice, however, many decisions are made in a less than optimal way. Janis and Mann (1977) discuss four errors that can detract from the quality of an individual's decision:

1. *Unconflicted inertia.* Individuals continue to respond as they are currently doing because they have not systematically evaluated other alternatives.
2. *Unconflicted challenge.* Individuals assume that an alternative must be better than what they are currently experiencing and respond to the alternative option without considering all factors related to the change.
3. *Defense avoidance.* Individuals adopt a particular course of action that may be inappropriate and damaging because they do not see any alternatives as being more favorable.
4. *Hypervigilance.* An individual believes that he or she must act immediately, and so the decision is made without considering the consequences of this option or other alternatives that might be more appropriate.

In employing one or more of these defective coping styles, individuals are more likely to produce a defective balance sheet and consequently make inept decisions. This may be of little consequence to an individual when it comes to minor day-to-day decisions, but the use of these styles may have far-reaching negative implications on major decisions, such as the decision to continue or curtail drug use.

Self-Determination as Motivation

Developed over the last three decades, self determination theory (SDT; Deci & Ryan, 1985; Ryan, 1995; Ryan & Deci, 2000) provides a theoretical framework that solves many of the problems discussed above. In addition, it appears to be particularly promising for application to substance abuse disorders because it (1) takes into account both individual and contextual variables in motivation, and (2) establishes a theoretical basis for explaining the treatment outcomes of brief motivational interventions for substance abuse.

SDT grew out of work by Deci and Ryan (1985) examining the relative contributions of intrinsic and extrinsic motivation on human performance. Research using the SDT framework has found that two factors—the degree of intrinsic motivation and the perceived locus of causality (the extent to which an individual believes that he or she is the active agent in his or her behavior as opposed to being controlled by others)—determine the extent to which an individual will persist in a target behavior. Comparisons between people whose motivation is intrinsic and those who have been externally coerced generally show that those in the former group are more excited and confident about their behavior, which translates into enhanced performance, more creativity, and better overall well-being. Because of the large functional differences between internal and external motivators on behavioral outcome, SDT first asks *what kind* of motivation is operating at any particular time.

According to SDT, human beings are driven to satisfy three basic psychological needs—*autonomy, competence*, and *relatedness*—within contexts that either support or inhibit those needs. Optimal functioning, as well as proper social development and well-being, seem to be produced by these factors. In contrast, behaviors or environments that block any of these needs can result in psychological and behavioral dysfunctions. This conceptualization has been extensively validated outside the field of addiction in a number of experimental and real-world settings, and has recently begun to be applied to addictive behavior as well (Foote et al., 1999; Wild, Newton-Taylor, & Alletto, 1998).

The first basic need, *autonomy*, is focused on having the perception that one is in charge of one's own behavior, that what one does is by one's own choice. Autonomy, or perceived locus of control, in SDT is closely related to concepts such as self-efficacy in other systems (Bandura, 1986). However, whereas "self-efficacy" refers to outcome expectations, "autonomy" is more connected to an individual's perception of him- or herself as the determining agent of an action (Ryan & Connell, 1989). In this theory, threats, deadlines, punitive evaluations, and imposed goals all undermine intrinsic motivation because they promote the perception of an external locus of control. An individual's perception of his or her behavior as freely chosen also affects the way he or she perceives external contingencies. For instance, an alcohol-dependent individual who perceives his or her "recovery" behaviors (e.g., attending support meetings, avoiding alcohol, reducing stress) as freely chosen is more likely to report that he or she engages in those behaviors because they "feel right," rather than for the external rewards they provide (e.g., family support, continued employment, avoiding legal difficulties).

The second basic need is for *competence*, a subjective perception that one is a capable, effective human being who can function adequately in a variety of life contexts. Competence overlaps with the concept of self-efficacy from social learning theory, and is enhanced by positive feedback on effectiveness, "optimal" challenges, and freedom from demeaning evaluations. Individuals who receive feedback like this from their environment are more likely be motivated and persist in a task because they believe that they are good at it.

Finally, SDT postulates a need for *relatedness*, a feeling of belonging and participation in social groups. Because much of behavior is not, strictly speaking, internally motivated, it is also important to understand how autonomy and competence are promoted within the context of *externally* motivated behavior. Because externally motivated behaviors are typically less interesting, one primary reason people engage in them is because the behaviors are modeled or prompted by others to whom they feel attached. Thus, a woman might work two jobs, save her money, or give up drinking because it is meaningful to her sister or because it positively impacts her children. Autonomy is supported in social contexts when people in an individual's environment "take that person's perspective, provide choice, encourage self-initiation, and minimize controls" (Ryan, Sheldon, Kasser, & Deci, 1996, p. 14).

In sum, SDT proposes that those individuals who are intrinsically motivated for behavior change, who feel that they have freely chosen their behaviors, and who are immersed in contexts that support feelings of competence will demonstrate persistently healthy behaviors. These factors also seem to be the key to behavior change. Conversely, for those individuals who are extrinsically motivated, feel that they are not the determining agent in their behavior, and encounter an environment that is controlling, change will be brief, and relapse to old behaviors will occur rapidly once the external contingencies are removed.

SDT has been applied most extensively in the addictions arena to the understanding of motivation to change cigarette smoking. In one early study, Harackiewicz, Sansone, Blair, Epstein, and Manderlink (1987) varied degree of intrinsic versus extrinsic motivation for quitting smoking by assigning subjects to a self-help manual, an intrinsic (self-determined) nicotine gum program, or a physician-directed nicotine gum program without self-help materials. Subjects who chose the intrinsic gum program stopped smoking more rapidly than did those in the other conditions; however, subjects in the self-help group maintained abstinence longer than subjects in either of the other groups.

Curry, Wagner, and Grothaus (1990) also found that intrinsically motivated subjects were more likely to succeed at quitting as compared to subjects whose motivation was more extrinsic. More particularly, smokers who had fully internalized reasons for quitting were more successful at both quitting and in maintaining abstinence. In a second study, Curry, Wagner, and Grothaus (1991) varied the degree of intrinsic versus extrinsic motivation by providing either personalized feedback (intrinsic) or a financial incentive (extrinsic) as adjuncts to a self-help program. Subjects who received the personalized feedback were more likely to quit and abstain than subjects who received a financial incentive. Indeed, in a large survey of former smokers, successful quitting was much more a product of internal motivators such as personal concerns about the health effects of smoking and wanting to set a good example for one's children. In contrast, smokers were more likely to relapse if they had quit for external reasons such as pressure from family and friends and concerns about the costs of smoking (Halpern & Warner, 1993).

In terms of alcohol, Ryan, Plant, and O'Malley (1995) examined client motivations for entering treatment. Using an SDT framework, they developed a questionnaire that rated subjects at entry to an outpatient program on four dimensions: internalized motivation, externalized motivation, help seeking, and confidence. At follow-up, subjects who scored highest on both internal and external motivation scales had the highest treatment retention rates. Compliance with the treatment regimen was associated with both a high degree of internal motivation and a high degree of legal pressure; however, externally motivated subjects had positive treatment outcomes only when they also had concurrently high levels of internal motivation.

In conclusion, SDT shows promise as a theoretical basis for the clinical techniques used in motivational interviewing and other effective brief interventions. In fact, some (e.g., Foote et al., 1999) have already noted that the factors proposed by SDT are remarkably similar to those identified as being commonalities of effective brief interventions for alcohol dependence (Miller & Sanchez, 1994). From the SDT framework, procedures such as personalized feedback and asking clients to identify their own concerns are effective because they increase internal motivation. Emphasizing the responsibility of the client and presenting a menu of options promotes a sense of autonomy. Reinforcing a client's sense of self-efficacy and, when appropriate, giving positive feedback can increase the clients' feelings of competence. Similarly, when it is given, advice should be offered sparingly, so as not to detract from a client's sense of ownership of his or her plan for change. Finally, building a "nest" of empathy between the therapist and the client, as well as involving significant others, can increase motivation during therapy and promote sobriety in the long run.

MOTIVATION AND THE ADDICTIONS FIELD

The controversy over the role of motivation in addiction is nearly as old as addiction treatment itself. There are old debates as to whether addiction is best approached as a genetic defect, a moral shortcoming, a disease-like state, a learned behavior, or any combination of these. One's assumptions have far-reaching implications for understanding the role of motivation in maintenance and quitting.

Alcoholism as a Disease

From a traditional disease model framework, Mindlin (1959) defined *motivation* as the client's willingness to become actively involved in treatment, determination to change, and preparedness to make sacrifices for therapy. Sheehan and Owen (1999) likewise said that "alcoholics" have difficulty initiating abstinence, have an impaired understanding of the severity of their problem, and are likely to exhibit resistance to treatment because of denial of their condition. Based upon these assumptions, Davis (1987) suggested that motivation for change should be inferred by a client's readiness to acknowledge a problem, his or her request for treatment, and his or her cooperation with treatment.

Not surprisingly, after reviewing the literature, Miller (1985) concluded that "motivation is often used as an antonym for terms such as denial and resistance and a synonym for constructs such as acceptance and surrender" (p. 86). For example, when discussing the concept of denial, Wilson (1985) noted that "the alcoholic patient often cannot recognize his disorder and accept the need for treatment because of his own profound denial," and Gitlow (1980) described alcoholism as "the only disease that tells people they don't have it" (p. 94). In one particularly striking example, DiCicco, Unterberger, and Mack (1978) told the story of an employee in "denial" about his drinking problem who was told by the worksite medical director: "Shut up and listen. . . . Alcoholics are liars, so we don't want to hear what you have to say" (p. 599). This commonly held view that problem drug users are untruthful has been reflected in catch-phrases such as "alcoholism is a disease of denial," and the assumption has sometimes been made that without motivation there is nothing the counselor can do for the client.

Fortunately, for problem drug users at least, this traditional view has been challenged, and in some cases superseded, by a more sophisticated model of motivation. Table 11.1 contrasts the theoretical differences between the traditional and the emerging schools of thought and how these are reflected in practice (modified from Miller, 1989, and Stockwell, Gregson, Osbourne, & Bolt, 1989). How these assumptions play out more specifically in the therapy session is the subject of the accompanying chapter by Moyers and Waldorf (see Chapter 12, this volume).

Therapeutic Intervention and Motivational Direction

In the past, the view has often been held that clients need to come to treatment committed to change, and that without this preexisting motivation there is little that can be done for them. However, over the past 20 years it has be-

TABLE 11.1. Perspectives on Motivation and Addictive Behavior

Perspective on . . .	Traditional disease model	Emerging model
Concept of client	Someone who will not face up to the reality of his or her drug use. Confrontation and education required.	Someone who can acknowledge that drug use causes some problems, but who is also aware that drug use provides some very real benefits.
Focus of clinical sessions	To make clients aware of the nature and severity of their drug use.	To elicit and assess the concerns clients may have about drug use and other current drug problems.
Aim of session	To have clients acknowledge their addiction, admit that they cannot control their drug use, and commit themselves to abstinence.	Have clients consider the advantages and disadvantages of continuing, and of stopping, their current drug use and assist them in deciding one way or the other.
Style of session	Therapist-controlled and therapist-directed.	Therapist-led, but client-centered.
Therapist's role	To educate, instruct, advise, confront, and direct clients about the nature of their addiction behavior and tell them how to solve their problems.	To assist clients in making decisions about their future drug use (to continue, to curtail, or to cease) and provide supporting, goal-directed counseling.

come increasingly clear that this is simply not the case. Dozens of descriptive and experimental studies have now shown that there is much that a therapist can do to affect the client's level of motivation and eventual outcome, even within the space of a brief encounter (Dunn et al., 2001; Miller & Wilbourne, 2002).

This change in perspective is in part due to the contribution of Prochaska and DiClemente's theories on behavior change (DiClemente & Prochaska, 1998; Prochaska, DiClemente, & Norcross, 1992). From their work with nicotine users, Prochaska and DiClemente outlined what has become known as the "stages-of-change model," with the idea that drug users go through a decisional and behavioral process that is not unlike that for many other behaviors. As they present to treatment, clients can range from those who are not considering change at all to those who have already made substantial efforts to change. In its simplest form, individuals who have not thought about making a change are described as being in the *precontemplation* stage. For clients in this stage, it is helpful to gently raise their level of awareness of the problems associated with their addictive behavior. When people become aware that their behaviors are causing them problems, they may enter the *contemplation* stage and begin to consider whether they might need to make a change. In this stage, individuals start to weigh the pros and cons of changing versus maintaining the status quo. It is also characteristic for clients at this stage to be ambivalent—literally, feeling two ways—as they evaluate their different options. The task for the counselor at this point is to help clients weigh the pros and cons as they consider whether they would like to make a change. The *preparation* stage is a "window of opportunity" where a client has decided that a change is needed, and is considering how to best approach it. It may be appropriate for the therapist to make suggestions during this phase, or to help the client arrive at an acceptable plan. Next, individuals in the *action* stage have begun to put their plan into action and need support for their efforts. Presumably, it is this group that was traditionally viewed as being motivated, because they came to clinics already wanting to make a change. Finally, in the *maintenance* stage, clients have already developed new behaviors and are in the process of maintaining them. In this stage it is appropriate to give feedback to the client, as well as to explore whether he or she might need to adjust his or her plan. In this model, *relapse* is a normal part of the change process, simply because most people do not succeed in long-term behavior change on their first try. Individuals may have to cycle through the stages of change one or more times before new patterns are reliably maintained.

The importance of this model is, as DiClemente and Prochaska (1998) argue, that different strategies might need to be employed at different stages in the change process. Furthermore, as Tober (1991) has well stated, it is the drug counselor's responsibility to engage effectively with people across the spectrum of change, including precontemplators, and tailor their counseling style to where "the client is at." In fact, from Tober's perspective it can be argued that many of the traits deemed in the past to be hallmark characteristics of problem drug users (e.g., denial, untruthfulness, lack of motivation) were, in fact, natural responses to a mismatched counseling style. That is, clients resisted change because the addiction counselor was locked into strategies that were inconsistent with the client's level of motivation and location in the change process.

In a similar vein, Miller and Rollnick (2002) have argued that "denial" is a product of the interaction between therapist and client and that, rather than being a client-initiated characteristic, denial is in fact a normal reaction to a therapist's aggressive attempts to persuade. Several writers have now explored the therapist styles and qualities thought to be predictive of client outcome. The factor that seems to emerge most consistently is the level of *empathy* exhibited by the therapist during the session (Miller, 2000; Walters, Delaney, & Rodgers, 2001; Wubbolding & Brickell, 1998). In fact, in some studies therapist behavior is a better predictor of outcome than any client characteristic (Project MATCH Research Group, 1998). One early example of this was offered by Patterson and Forgatch (1985) when they experimentally varied the level of confrontation within a single counseling session. They found that the resistance level of clients was driven up or down as counselors switched between empathic and confrontational styles. Along these lines, when Miller, Benefield, and Tonigan (1993) measured drinking outcome in relation to therapist style during a single counseling session, they found that not only was client resistance during the session linked to the level of confrontation the therapist used, but that the client's level of drinking at 1 year was also highly predictable. In short, the more the therapist confronted, the more the client continued to drink.

"Denial" as Cognitive Conflict

Nonetheless, even the most skilled cognitive-behaviorist counselor will encounter clients who seem reluctant to face the nature of their difficulties. While it may be tempting to label this "denial," an alternative perspective is to consider a reluctance to disclose self-damning evidence as a psychological defense induced by cognitive conflict. Orford (1985) has argued that what might be considered the hallmark features of addiction—the ambivalence, the broken promises, the unreliability, the binges, the rationalizations, and even the denial—are in fact the result of an individual being considerably conflicted about a behavior. Orford has written that "what characterizes an 'ism' or a mania, or a strong and troublesome appetite, as distinct from relatively trouble-free, restrained, moderate or normal appetitive behavior, is the upgrading of a state of balance into one of conflict" (p. 233). According to Orford, it is this internal battle between "I want to do this very much, but I know that I really shouldn't" that lies at the heart of compulsive, excessive behavior. As we have long recognized, such conflict is the antithesis to sound decision making. Indeed, Abelson (1963) coined the phrase "hot cognitions" to describe decision making when under emotional duress. As noted earlier, the difficulty with decisions made under such circumstances, as opposed to those reached via "cool cognition," is that they are inherently shortsighted.

Herein, then, lies a possible explanation for the vacillations of problem drug users. Promises to abstain are all too frequently replaced by decisions to use "just once more." While such relapses may look like a lack of motivation, according to Orford, they may in fact mean that the user is acutely troubled by what he or she is doing. Orford (1985) has written that when "subject to opposing motives of great strength it is difficult to know one's own mind, let alone behave with any consistency" (p. 239).

The important paradox in Orford's cognitive conflict model is that a drug user may exhibit all the behavioral features traditionally presumed to be indicative of no motivation, and even denial, at the very time he or she is most conscious of all the dangers and deficits inherent in drug use. The very worst excesses may actually occur when the drug user is most troubled and most conflicted by what he or she is doing. One client recently acknowledged her excessive behavior as being "stupid." But, she pointed out, "There's no point in doing something stupid just a little bit." If it were to be done, it had to be done excessively, and without regard for the consequences. Any reflection on the potential of disaster is too detrimental, too intrusive, to the moment of pleasure. It is also unsettling in the long run, especially when the client is not yet convinced that there is a better way out. And here we arrive full circle at the notion of denial: sometimes, not specific to drug abusers, denial does indeed occur because individuals either don't see a clear way out of their problem or choose not to look. If they did look, they might conclude that a radical change might be in order, and in the stages of change prior to action that is too dreadful a decision to consider.

Motivation and Giving Up Addictive Behaviors

It is relevant to conclude this chapter with reference to the accounts of people who have given up their addictions without formal treatment. Such literature is replete with mystery and ambiguity, but we believe it is not inconsistent with the psychology of motivation we are proposing. As we have seen, our straightforward notions of what things "should" motivate people are often insufficient. Change, when it happens, seems to be the result of a combination of factors—a sort of motivational "alignment"—rather than increased levels of just one factor. Consider Miller and C'de Baca's (2002) account of how one problem drinker resolved his addiction without treatment. While on vacation, he was reading some books on recovery to help an employee who seemed to have a problem with his drinking. A former exercise buff, he had also decided to start running during this vacation time:

> I did a bit of running and I found, God, I couldn't even run a quarter mile. . . . I guess it was that, and some things that were coming out of the reading I had taken along to try and get a handle on how to help the employee [with the drinking problem]. I decided, "I have a problem with alcohol, and the only way to deal with it is to simply put it aside." And all of a sudden, it just dropped away. At that moment I turned into someone who didn't use alcohol. I haven't had a drink since that day two years ago. I can't even remember the last time I had a drink. (p. 36)

The combination of new perspectives and feedback on an important variable, considered at the right time, was enough to motivate this individual to quit drinking.

"Natural" recoveries appear to be the rule rather than the exception (Sobell, Ellingstad, & Sobell, 2000). In fact, only a minority of former alcohol and drug users has been to any formal treatment program at all. The reason that the topic seems to have garnered so little attention may be that clinicians and researchers in the addictions field so seldom come into contact with these people who have recovered on their own. In addition, the emphasis on alcoholism and drug addiction as an "incurable" disease (Dupont, 1993) has often seemed to preclude the many quiet case studies to the contrary. Finally, when therapy does help people to change, it seems to do so by facilitating what is inherently a natural process (DiClemente & Prochaska, 1998).

Motivation and Moving On

Despite the fact that people change every day, accounting for it remains largely a mystery. Nonetheless, the findings as outlined above suggest at least four conclusions:

1. An individual's desire to achieve an outcome, his or her confidence that it can be achieved, and the perception that his or her new behavior is freely chosen seem to be the optimal conditions for behavior change.
2. Often the things that we assume would be motivating to individuals simply aren't. Thus, motivation is a process of finding out what things are reinforcing to a particular individual, as well as what plan will be acceptable for attaining them.
3. Not all moments are created equal. There seem to be "teachable" windows where people are more receptive to feedback from their environment and more interested in trying out new behaviors.
4. In addictions treatment, the qualities of the interaction between therapist and client can have a large impact on client motivation. Radical change sometimes happens as a result of relatively modest efforts.

The many former alcohol and drug users, perhaps the majority, who have made a radical behavior change on their own should be an encouragement to those of us working in the addictions field. People can, and do, get better. When clients present to us who seem "stuck," our task is to nudge them along in this natural process. Once the decision to change has been made, action strategies come into play that will, we hope, sustain the resolution. When they leave our office, it is our hope that external supports, such as family, friends, and job relations, will make this new course of behavior more reinforcing than the old course. Thus, motivation is an ongoing process, involving the initial resolution, action, feedback from external sources, modification of goals, continued resolution, and so on. It is also a process replete with mystery, in which the desire and energy for a goal seems to ebb and flow. All of us, on some days, are more motivated to solve the mystery than on others.

REFERENCES

Abelson, R. (1963). Computer simulation of "hot" cognition. In S. Tomkins & S. Messick (Eds.), *Computer simulation of personality* (pp. 277–298). New York: Wiley.

Bandura, A. (1986). *Social foundations of thought and action.* Englewood Cliffs, NJ: Prentice-Hall.

Bandura, A. (1994). *Self-efficacy: The exercise of control.* New York: Freeman.

Bierut, L. J., Dinwiddie, S. H., Begleiter, H., Crowe, R. R., Hesselbrock, V., Nurnberger, J. I., Jr., Porjesz, B., Schuckit, M. A., & Reich, T. (1998). Familial transmission of substance dependence: Alcohol, marijuana, cocaine, and habitual smoking. A report from the Collaborative Study on the Genetics of Alcoholism. *Archives of General Psychiatry, 55*(11), 982–988.

Cantor, N., & Langston, C. (1989). Ups and downs of life tasks in a life transition. In L. Pervin (Ed.), *Goal concepts in personality and social psychology* (pp. 127–168). Hillsdale, NJ: Erlbaum.

Curry, S., Wagner, E. H., & Grothaus, L. C. (1990). Intrinsic and extrinsic motivation for smoking cessation. *Journal of Consulting and Clinical Psychology, 58,* 310–316.

Curry, S. J., Wagner, E. H., & Grothaus, L. C. (1991). Evaluation of intrinsic and extrinsic motivation interventions with a self-help smoking cessation program. *Journal of Consulting and Clinical Psychology, 59,* 318–324.

Davis, D. (1987). *Alcoholism treatment: An integrative family and individual approach.* New York: Gardner Press.

Deci, E. L., & Ryan, R. M. (1985). *Intrinsic motivation and self-determination in human behavior.* New York: Plenum Press.

DiCicco, L., Unterberger, H., & Mack, J. (1978). Confronting denial: An alcoholism intervention strategy. *Psychiatric Annals, 8,* 596–606.

DiClemente, C. C., Bellino, L. E., & Neavins, T. M. (1999). Motivation for change and alcoholism treatment. *Alcohol Health and Research World, 23*(2), 86–92.

DiClemente, C. C., & Prochaska, J. O. (1998). Toward a comprehensive, transtheoretical model of change: Stages of change and addictive behaviors. In W. R. Miller & N. Heather (Eds.), *Treating addictive behaviors* (2nd ed., pp. 3–24). New York: Plenum Press.

Dunn, C., Deroo, L., & Rivara, F. P. (2001). The use of brief interventions adapted from motivational interviewing across behavioral domains: a systematic review. *Addiction, 96*(12), 1725–1742.

Dupont, R. L. (1993). Forward. In G. R. Ross, *Treating adolescent substance abuse* (pp. xi–xii). Boston: Allyn & Bacon.

Fitzgibbon, M., & Kirschenbaum, D. (1992). Who succeeds in losing weight? In Y. Klar, J. Fisher, J. Chinsky, & A. Nadler (Eds.), *Self change: Social, psychological and clinical perspectives* (pp. 153–178). New York: Springer-Verlag.

Foote, J., DeLuca, A., Magura, S., Warner, A., Grand, A., Rosenblum, A., & Stahl, S. (1999). A group motivational treatment for chemical dependency. *Journal of Substance Abuse Treatment, 17*(3), 181–192.

Frish, D., & Clemen, R. T. (1994). Beyond expected utility: Rethinking behavioral decision research. *Psychological Bulletin, 116*(1), 46–54.

Gitlow, W. (1980). An overview. In S. Gitlow & H. Peyser (Eds.), *Alcoholism: A practical treatment guide* (pp. 1–22). New York: Grune & Stratton.

Halpern, M. T., & Warner, K. E. (1993). Motivations for smoking cessation: A comparison of successful quitters and failures. *Journal of Substance Abuse, 5*(3), 247–256.

Handmaker, N. S., & Walters, S. T. (2002). Motivational enhancement therapy and interviewing. In S. G. Hofman & M. C. Tompson (Eds.), *Handbook of psychological treatments for severe mental disorders* (pp. 215–233). New York: Guilford Press.

Harackiewicz, J. M., Sansone, C., Blair, L. W., Epstein, J. A., & Manderlink, G. (1987). Attributional processes in behavior change and maintenance: Smoking cessation and continued abstinence. *Journal of Consulting and Clinical Psychology, 55*, 372–378.

Higgins, S. T., Alessi, S. M., & Dantona, R. L. (2002). Voucher-based incentives: A substance abuse treatment innovation. *Addictive Behaviors, 27*(6), 887–910.

Janis, I., & Mann, L. (1977). *Decision making: A psychological analysis of conflict, choice and commitment.* New York: Collier Macmillan.

Klar, Y., Nadler, A., & Malloy, T. (1992). Opting to change: Students' informal self-change endeavours. In Y. Klar, J. Fisher, J. Chinsky, & A. Nadler (Eds.), *Self change: Social, psychological and clinical perspectives* (pp. 63–86). New York: Springer-Verlag.

Lemere, F., O'Hollaren, P., & Maxwell, T. (1958). Motivation in the treatment of alcoholism. *Quarterly Journal of Studies on Alcohol, 19*, 428–431.

Meyers, R. J., & Miller, W. R. (2001). *A community reinforcement approach to addiction treatment.* New York: Cambridge University Press.

Miller, W. R. (1985). Motivation for treatment: A review with special emphasis on alcoholism. *Psychological Bulletin, 98*, 84–107.

Miller, W. R. (1989). Increasing motivation for change. In R. K. Hester & W. R. Miller (Eds.), *Handbook of alcoholism treatment approaches: Effective alternatives* (pp. 89–104). Elmsford, NY: Pergamon Press.

Miller, W. R. (2000). Rediscovering fire: Small interventions, large effects. *Psychology of Addictive Behavior, 14*(1), 6–18.

Miller, W. R., Benefield, R. G., & Tonigan, J. S. (1993). Enhancing motivation for change in problem drinking: A controlled comparison of two therapist styles. *Journal of Consulting and Clinical Psychology, 61*, 455–461.

Miller, W. R., & C'de Baca, J. (2002). *Quantum change: When epiphanies and sudden insights transform ordinary lives.* New York: Guilford Press.

Miller, W. R., & Rollnick, S. (2002). *Motivational interviewing (2nd ed.): Preparing people to change.* New York: Guilford Press.

Miller, W. R., & Sanchez, V. C. (1994). Motivating young adults for treatment and lifestyle change. In G. Howard (Ed.), *Issues in alcohol use and misuse by young adults* (pp. 55–82). South Bend, IN: University of Notre Dame Press.

Miller, W. R., & Wilbourne, P. L. (2002). Mesa Grande: a methodological analysis of clinical trials of treatments for alcohol use disorders. *Addiction, 97*(3), 265–277.

Mindlin, D. (1959). The characteristics of alcoholics as related to prediction of therapeutic outcome. *Quarterly Journal of Studies on Alcohol, 20*, 604–619.

Orford, J. (1985). *Excessive appetites: A psychological view of addiction.* Chichester, UK: Wiley.

Patterson, G. R., & Forgatch, M. S. (1985). Therapist behavior as a determinant for client noncompliance: A paradox for the behavior modifier. *Journal of Consulting and Clinical Psychology, 53*, 846–851.

Prochaska, J. 0., DiClemente, C. C., & Norcross, J. C. (1992). In search of how people change: Applications to addictive behaviors. *American Psychologist, 47*, 1102–1114.

Project MATCH Research Group. (1998). Therapist effects in three treatments for alcohol problems. *Psychotherapy Research, 8*(4), 455–474.

Reber, A. (1985). *Dictionary of psychology.* London: Penguin Books.

Robinson, T. E., & Berridge, K. C. (2000). The psychology and neurobiology of addiction: An incentive-sensitization model. *Addiction, 95*(Suppl. 2), S91–S117.

Rollnick, S., Butler, C. C., & Stott, N. (1997). Helping smokers make decisions: The enhancement of brief intervention for general medical practice. *Patient Education and Counseling, 31*(3), 191–203.

Ryan, R. M., & Connell, J. P. (1989). Perceived locus of causality and internalization: Examining reasons for acting in two domains. *Journal of Personality and Social Psychology, 57*, 749–761.

Ryan, R. M., Plant, R., & O'Malley, S. (1995). Initial motivations for alcohol treatment: Relations with patient characteristics, treatment involvement, and dropout. *Addictive Behaviors, 20*, 279–297.

Ryan, R. R. (1995). Psychological needs and the facilitation of integrative processes. *Journal of Personality, 63*, 397–427.

Ryan, R. R., & Deci, E. L. (2000). Self-determination theory and the facilitation of intrinsic motivation, social development and well-being. *American Psychologist, 55*, 68–78.

Ryan, R. R., Sheldon, K. M., Kasser, T., & Deci, E. L. (1996). All goals are not created equal: An organismic perspective on the nature of goals and their regulation. In P. Gollwitzer & J. A. Bargh (Eds.), *The psychology of action: linking cognition and motivation to behavior* (pp. 7–26). New York: Guilford Press.

Schuckit, M. A. (1985). Genetics and the risk for alcoholism. *Journal of the American Medical Association, 254*(18), 2614–2617.

Schuckit, M. A., Tsuang, J. W., Anthenelli, R. M., Tipp, J. E., & Nurnberger J. I. Jr. (1996). Alcohol challenges in young men from alcoholic pedigrees and control families: A report from the COGA Project. *Journal of Studies on Alcohol, 57*(4), 368–377.

Sheehan, T., & Owen, P. (1999). The disease model. In B. S. McCrady & E. E. Epstein (Eds.), *Addictions: A comprehensive guidebook* (pp. 268–286). New York: Oxford University Press.

Simon, H. (1976). *Administrative behavior: A study of decision making processes in administrative organizations.* New York: Free Press.

Sobell, L. C., Ellingstad, T. P., & Sobell, M. B. (2000). Natural recovery from alcohol and drug problems: Methodological review of the research with suggestions for future directions. *Addiction, 95*(5), 749–764.

Sterne, M., & Pittman, D. (1965). The concept of motivation: A source of institutional and professional blockage in the treatment of alcoholics. *Quarterly Journal of Studies on Alcohol, 26*, 41–57.

Stockwell, T., Gregson, A., Osbourne, J., & Bolt, J. (1989, July). *Motivational inter-*

viewing with problem drinkers: A controlled trial of a method for reducing client drop-out*. Paper presented at the Winter School in the Sun Conference, The Alcohol and Drug Foundation, Brisbane, Australia.

Sutton, S. (1987). Social–psychological approaches to understanding addictive behaviours: Attitude–behaviour and decision making models. *British Journal of Addiction, 82*, 355–370.

Tober, G. (1991). Helping the pre-contemplator. In R. Davidson, S. Rollnick, & I. MacEwan (Eds.), *Counselling problem drinkers* (pp. 21–38). London: Tavistock/Routledge.

Tversky, A., & Kahneman, D. (1981). The framing of decisions and the psychology of choice. *Science, 211*, 453–458.

von Winterfeldt, D., & Edwards, W. (1986). *Decision analysis and behavioral research*. Cambridge, UK: Cambridge University Press.

Walters, S. T., Delaney, H. D., & Rodgers, K. L. (2001). Addiction and health: A (not so) new heuristic for change. *Journal of Psychology and Christianity, 20*(3), 240–249.

West, R. (1989). The psychological basis of addiction. *International Review of Psychiatry, 1*, 71–80.

Wild, T. C., Newton-Taylor, B., & Alletto, R. (1998). Perceived coercion among clients entering substance abuse treatment: Structural and psychological determinants. *Addictive Behaviors, 23*(1), 81–95.

Wilson, G. (1985). Intervention by the clinician to motivate the alcoholic. *Australian Alcohol and Drug Review, 4*, 94–100.

Wubbolding, R. E., & Brickell, J. (1998). Qualities of the reality therapist. *International Journal of Reality Therapy, 17*(2), 47–49.

12

Motivational Interviewing
Destination, Direction, and Means

Theresa B. Moyers
V. Ann Waldorf

> I'm here because I got arrested for driving while intoxicated, but it was just a mistake. I did have too much to drink that night, but I'm not an alcoholic.
>
> —*ANDREA B, entering alcohol screening appointment*

Motivational interviewing began as a response to the widespread use of confrontation in the treatment of individuals struggling with alcohol and drug problems, such as the hypothetical client above (Bell & Rollnick, 1995). This confrontational approach was thought necessary to overcome pathological denial and inherent lack of motivation about changing substance use. Miller (1983, 1985), however, conceptualized motivation for changing substance use as generally similar to other difficult behavior change and proposed that the interaction between the client and the provider could be critical in eliciting an appetite for change. Motivational interviewing (Miller & Rollnick, 1991) is a way for providers to maximize their contribution to the change equation. Miller and Rollnick (2002) have defined it as a person-centered, directive method of communication for enhancing intrinsic motivation to change by helping clients to explore and resolve ambivalence.

THE SPIRIT OF MOTIVATIONAL INTERVIEWING

Several important theoretical beliefs underlie the proper use of motivational interviewing and differentiate it from other addictions treatment approaches.

These can be thought of as the theoretical belief system that the practitioner needs in order to use this method well. It has also been called the spirit of motivational interviewing, as differentiated from specific procedures or techniques to be used (Rollnick & Miller, 1995). First, the client must have some intrinsic motivation for change. The practitioner cannot impose a desire for change in the absence of some genuine concern within the client. This is not to say that motivation must be a result of client insight or occur strictly for intrinsic reasons, since change is often prompted by external contingencies. Nevertheless, providers will not be able to use motivational interviewing to elicit an appetite for change in clients who genuinely have no interest or intent to change. Second, using motivational interviewing may mean giving up the worldview of being helpful by educating clients about the urgency of their problems, a cornerstone of many methods. Instead, the provider's style will be quiet and eliciting, meaning that confrontation and vocal cues to persuade will fall away. Third, the relationship between the provider and the client will be one of partnership rather than one of expert–recipient. Although expertise and authority may be helpful for some clients, the motivational interviewer recognizes that they are usually not appropriate for clients who present with ambivalence about complex behavior change. Desire for change is viewed as a product of the partnership, with both the client and the interviewer having some contribution to make to it.

This partnership is similar to a multiplication equation: Client Contribution × Provider Skill = Total Motivation. Clients make an initial contribution of some value. The client contribution, in some circumstances, can be zero since not all clients have concern about a particular behavior, even if it is self-destructive. Nevertheless, for most clients engaging in a maladaptive behavior, there *will* be some amount of concern or intent to change, represented by the first number in the multiplication equation. The skill of the provider, or interviewer, represents the second number in the change equation. Because the equation is multiplicative, not additive, the skills of the provider can significantly enlarge the absolute amount of motivation produced by the change process. For example (using a 0–10 scale to make this point), a client can come to the initial appointment with very little, but at least some, intrinsic motivation to change her drinking behavior after receiving a citation for driving while intoxicated (DWI) or driving under the influence (DUI) (level of 2). The skill of the interviewer now becomes the critical determining variable. A skilled interviewer (with a skill level of 7) will elicit a hypothetical motivational product of 14 whereas a less skilled therapist (with a skill level of 3) will elicit a motivational product of only 6. This metaphor is used to illustrate that providers have a powerful potential to enhance the motivation their clients bring to the change process. They are not likely, however, to elicit much motivation from a client who brings an honest zero to the initial contact.

From the perspective of the transtheoretical model, motivational interviewing is most likely to be useful in the contemplation stage (DiClemente, 2002). It is here that clients weigh the costs and benefits of both the behavior and the possible change. Importantly, motivational interviewing is less likely to be helpful once the client has moved forward into action, and in fact may be counterproductive. The very things that make motivational interviewing useful in coping with ambivalence may be annoying to a client who is ready to implement a change. Of course, if ambivalence recurs, which is not unusual in clinical settings, the practioner should reconsider a motivational interviewing approach.

A Cognitive Map for Motivational Interviewing

How is motivational interviewing done? Like any therapeutic method, the answer is complex. A cognitive map to explain it would contain three elements: the destination, the directions to get to the goal, and the means of getting there.

The Destination: Principles of Motivational Interviewing

The principles of motivational interviewing are the ultimate goal of the provider's actions: they are where the provider wants to "end up." They guide the provider's thinking about all the other behaviors to be employed in the same way that a destination guides a traveler. Because of this, the principles of motivational interviewing are much more important than any specific strategy or skill. Ideally, every strategy or microskill used by the provider attempting motivational interviewing will be in the service of one of these principles. The four principles of motivational interviewing are:

EXPRESS EMPATHY

Studies have repeatedly shown that therapists who are able to employ skillful reflective listening have better outcomes with their substance-using clients than those who do not. This does not imply that the provider must agree with the client, feel sorry for him or her, or have had the same life experiences. This principle is better seen in terms of the therapeutic value of "being understood" first discussed by Rogers (1957). Allowing clients to know that they have been understood, even about something as touchy as ambivalence about changing their substance use, is a powerful therapeutic tool on its own. The provider using motivational interviewing will make many reflections with the goal of letting the client know that he or she has been thoroughly understood. Interestingly, this basic therapeutic skill is often the most difficult to teach to new students of motivational interviewing. A therapist's overlearned habit of relying on questions to elicit information from clients sometimes makes it difficult for therapists to switch gears and allow client information to come in an unfolding fashion. Providers may worry that they will not be able to complete intake forms or will miss a lifesaving bit of information because they have been expressing empathy instead. It is important to have a clear priority in one's interaction with the client. Sometimes a genuine focus on enhancing motivation for change will mean setting aside other goals until momentum has been established. In any case, the best assessment in the world may still leave the provider without the answer to the important question, "How can I help this person change?"

DEVELOP DISCREPANCY

Sometimes substance abuse treatment providers fall into the trap of thinking that their clients glory in self-destructive substance use without any thought to its harmful consequences and cannot be compelled to give it up unless there are severe repercussions. While it may be true that external consequences are helpful in pushing clients toward our doors, it is also usually true that clients have some internal concern if a behavior is genuinely self-destructive. Substance abuse does not remove our clients' ability to experience the discrepancy between what they believe and what they do, and finding that discrepancy and making it explicit can be valuable. Values clarification exercises can be an important part of developing discrepancy and can increase the importance of a contemplated change. An example of this principle is found in a study by Sanchez (2000), who used a values card-sorting exercise in combination with a motivational interview prior to alcohol treatment in a Veterans' Administration (VA) hospital. The intervention focused on identifying core values for participants, as well as the discrepancy between their core values and their levels of alcohol consumption. The group receiving this intervention showed improved drinking outcomes when compared to an attention control group, presumably because exploring values in relation to one's actions highlights a discrepancy between belief and behavior.

ROLL WITH RESISTANCE

There is a natural resistance to giving up something that has both rewards and consequences. The more we are coerced by others to give up something about which we are ambivalent, the more valuable it becomes to us (Brehm & Brehm, 1981). When treating substance abuse, it is not hard to find examples of providers pushing the client hard to change, only to find the client pushing back even harder not to change. This power struggle may actually decrease the chances that clients will change (Miller, Benefield, & Tonigan, 1993), so it is to be explicitly avoided when employing the third principle of motivational interviewing. The provider is fully aware that coercion will not produce change by itself, and the client's option not to change is honored. Even when clients are coerced by external sources (e.g., the legal system, their own health problems), providers cannot assume that this is enough to elicit change. They respond to resistance with strategies designed to keep it as low as possible, so that clients can talk themselves into changing.

SUPPORT SELF-EFFICACY

This principle addresses confidence for making the specific change the client is up against. Often the importance of making a change is low simply because clients do not believe they could change even if they wanted to. Rather, the provider encourages the client to believe that change is possible, drawing on optimism and his or her experience with other clients. Providers who genuinely believe specific changes are possible have better outcomes with clients than those who do not (Leake & King, 1977; Parker, Winstead, & Willi, 1979). Provider optimism can be a client's most important tool.

The destination when using motivational interviewing is to interact with clients in a manner that is deeply empathic, that minimizes resistance, that amplifies natural discrepancy, and that supports optimism. It is as if the therapist assists the client in talking him- or herself into changing. A natural metaphor is that of a boat on a rapidly moving river. The pilot does not try to steer against the force of the water, but moves the boat to take the best advantage of the river's energy.

Direction: How to Get to the Destination

With motivational interviewing, as with most destinations, there is more than one right way to arrive. Once the provider has the goal in mind, how does he or she proceed? Strategies, analogous to turning right and left at certain distances, will give the provider some direction (Miller & Rollnick, 1991; Bell & Rollnick, 1995). The strategies give the provider some ideas about how to maneuver toward the destination.

DECISIONAL BALANCE: THE GOOD AND THE NOT-SO-GOOD
THINGS ABOUT SUBSTANCE USE

The provider asks the client to discuss both sides of the ambivalence equation in order to clarify the nature of the dilemma. He or she starts by asking about the good things associated with the client's substance use and pursues any important benefits that the client mentions. This is followed by asking about the not-so-good things about substance use, in an equally neutral tone. It is important that the provider not assume that the good things will outweigh the bad, and should not use words like "problem" unless the client does. Ideally, a nonjudgmental exploration of the pros and cons of substance abuse will elicit discrepancy in the client.

GIVING FEEDBACK

Many times the provider will have information that is relevant to the client's circumstances, such as assessment results or the content of consults with other professionals or family members. This type of personalized (as opposed to general) information about substance abuse can be extremely valuable in the motivational process because it presents provocative and relevant information gathered from the client's own self-report. When approaching this task from a motivational interviewing perspective, the provider will offer the information and ask permission to provide it. Once received, the provider will give the information in a neutral fashion, avoiding the attitude that it "proves" a diagnosis or a decision the provider wants the client to make. It is the information itself that is confrontational, not the provider. If the client dismisses the information, the provider moves on to another topic without trying to impress the client of its importance.

A special case occurs when the provider feels ethically compelled to give information or advice, even without the client's permission. In this case, the formula of elicit–provide–elicit is recommended (Rollnick, Mason, & Butler, 1999). The provider can minimize resistance by asking the client what he or she already knows about the topic (elicit). Then the provider can give the information in the form of a concern, rather than as a lecture (provide). The feedback is always followed by a request for the client's response (elicit). A common problem of this kind is the pregnant woman who has been engaging in high-risk drinking.

PROVIDER: Anne, tell me what you already know about the effects of drinking during pregnancy.

CLIENT: Everybody knows you are not supposed to drink too much when you are pregnant. It can hurt your baby. I don't want to do that. I'm going to have to live with this baby a long time. I want to drink but keep it at a safe level.

PROVIDER: You of all people have an interest in a healthy baby. I'm worried, though, that we might disagree about what is a safe level. I'm not sure I can agree that there is a safe level of drinking during pregnancy.

CLIENT: Are you saying I shouldn't drink at all?

PROVIDER: That would be my advice, but of course it is your choice in the end. What do you think?

EXPLORING A TYPICAL DAY OR SESSION

Here the provider is trying to get a "snapshot" of the client's relationship with a particular substance by exploring the context. The provider can ask the client to go through a typical day beginning with rising in the morning, and offer prompts for common activities to encourage the client to provide details. If resistance will not be evoked, the provider can ask the client to describe a particular episode where he or she used a substance and again provide prompts for common details as rapport permits. Ideally, reflections will elicit and amplify details about the client's use that can be used to arrive at one of the principles.

VALUES CLARIFICATION EXERCISE

Here the provider makes a detailed exploration about what is important to the client in addition to his or her substance use. With highly verbal clients, this may be accomplished merely by asking them to say what they value. Other clients may require prompts or cues from the provider. For example, "Some veterans say that independence is one of their most important values. They like to be able to live without someone else telling them what to do. Does that fit for you?" Sometimes, as in the veteran study cited above, a formal card sort is used. This strategy involves having the client sort through a stack of 80 cards, each of which is labeled with a particular value (see *http://casaa.unm.edu* for personal values card sort). The client is asked to choose his or her top five values and discuss each one in depth. The provider then gently queries the way substance use fits with each of these important values. Another recent study found that this type of card sort could be successfully modified for use with clients with schizophrenis as part of a highly structured motivational interview (Graeber, Moyers, Griffith, Guajardo, & Tonigan, 2003).

DIRECTIVE REFLECTIONS

By choosing what to reflect and how, the provider can guide the boat in the stream of ambivalence toward one of the principles. From all that a client says, the provider chooses to reflect what will be most useful in moving the client toward a particular goal. For example, if the client describes the embarrassment of an arrest for cocaine possession, the provider might respond by saying, "That was humiliating for you" (simple reflection), thereby conveying understanding and empathy. If a client states that he or she is only in the provider's office to satisfy a legal requirement, the provider might overshoot by saying, "That's the *only* reason you are here"(amplified reflection), thereby inviting the client to step back from the strong statement. When clients express their ambivalence by stating both the consequences and benefits of substance use, the provider can reflect both back by linking the two reflections: "So you see that your drinking is worrying your children and it also helps you to cope with their adolescence" (double-sided reflection). This type of reflection is intended to direct the client to a discrepancy.

MICROSKILLS: THE MEANS OF MOVING

We have already discussed the destination and the directions for getting to it. Now we investigate the means of travel. Just as a traveler might choose an automobile, airplane, or bicycle to move along, so the provider might choose one of the microskills to follow the directions toward the principles of motivational interviewing. Microskills are the basic counseling skills, common to all therapeutic methods, that are essential to building rapport and trust with clients. To continue the travel metaphor, those methods most important to the motivational interviewing approach can be described with the acronym OARS. *Open-ended questions* (O) allow providers to gather information in a manner that facilitates the client exploring his or her own deepest concerns. Asking such questions avoids the question–answer trap in which the therapist asks a series of closed questions and the client learns to respond with a "Yes" or "No." This question–answer trap is the opposite of the motivational interviewing method, in which the therapist helps clients to ask questions of themselves. Within a motivational interviewing approach, open-ended questions are especially useful when they are asked in a manner that evokes concern about a problem, intent to change, or optimism for changing. *Affirming* (A) occurs when providers take something positive about the client and make it explicit. For example, the provider might compliment the client's persistence in coming to the appointment, point out the things he or she has done to be a caring parent, or comment on the positive things still apparent in the person's life. The ability to find the positive and make it explicit is a skill common to helpful providers. *Reflections* (R) form the backbone of the motivational interviewing approach and are used especially to convey empathy and reduce resistance. The ability to form accurate and complex reflections that deftly lead the client where the clinician wishes him or her to go is a critical element of the flow of motivational interviewing; it is one way in which the interviewer "dances" rather than "wrestles" with the client. Finally, the therapist *summarizes* (S) periodically, gathering various important points the client has made and handing them back as a bouquet. As with reflections, summaries can either be simple (a recounting focused on understanding) or complex (designed to move the client's inquiry in another direction). For example, a summary of various examples of how a client has been able to make successful changes when she decided to do so is clearly directional in intent, but it also conveys a clear understanding of what was said. The astute clinician has by now realized that all microskills can be used to supply direction when necessary.

COMBINING THE ELEMENTS: HOW IT MIGHT LOOK

In general, the practitioner will begin by using microskills to help clients tell their stories, with the goal of genuinely understanding the client's point of view about his or her substance use as it fits in the broader picture of his or her life. As the interview progresses, the practitioner might become more directive in structuring the conversation to arrive at empathy, discrepancy, or self-efficacy, or to minimize resistance to change. The practitioner will be helping the client to talk him- or herself into changing, rather than persuading him or her or pushing him or her toward change. As momentum increases, the practitioner will join the client in thinking hypothetically about change, while offering advice sparingly and encouraging a collaborative change plan. Sometimes the practitioner might decide that the appropriate response is to honor the client's determination to avoid change and structure the interaction so as to help the client return to the practioner's door in the future, if his or her circumstances change.

It is important to note that motivational interviewing might look different depending on the setting in which it occurs. For instance, brief negotiation (Rollnick, Mason, & Butler, 1999; Rollnick et al., 2002) is consistent with the methods used in motivational interviewing and is designed for settings where interactions must be short and focused. Motivational interviewing will also look different depending on the style of the therapist. Some therapists will place more emphasis on warmth, some on direction, some on authenticity—all of which will influence the way motivational interviewing is done. Indeed, there are many ways to do it well. However, providers who rely on information gathering as their most important task, who view their job as providing expert advice, who find that confrontation works well for them, or who are extremely uncomfortable when clients remain ambivalent about changing their substance use might have a hard time using motivational interviewing. It is not right for every provider, nor right for every ambivalent client. Let's see an example of how motivational interviewing might work with Andrea, whom we met at the beginning of this chapter.

CASE EXAMPLE: MOTIVATIONAL INTERVIEWING WITH ANDREA B

ANDREA: I'm here because I got arrested for driving while intoxicated, but it was just a mistake. I did have too much to drink that night, but I'm not an alcoholic.

INTERVIEWER: Let me see if I've got this right. You got a DWI and that is why you are here.

ANDREA: Yeah, I had too much to drink and I made a mistake. I admit it. Big deal—everyone drinks and drives at least once. I just got caught.

INTERVIEWER: This seems like a lot of fuss over a little thing. [rolling with resistance]

ANDREA: Well, I know it's not a little thing. I realize that drinking and driving is dangerous. I was lucky I didn't hurt anyone. But I'm not an alcoholic.

INTERVIEWER: You took a chance with your drinking and you also see that your drinking is not serious enough to put you in the category of being alcoholic. [double-sided reflection]

ANDREA: Yeah. Like everyone keeps telling me I am, which I'm not.

INTERVIEWER: Andrea, what if we set aside the idea that we have to find a label for you? I know your evaluation form requires a diagnosis, but it's way too early for me to think about that. I'm more interested in hearing your concerns about your drinking, whatever they might be. [deemphasizing labeling; shifting focus]

ANDREA: What do you mean?

INTERVIEWER: In a situation like this where everyone is telling you there is something wrong with your drinking, it's easy to get sidetracked away from what you might be worried about yourself. It sounds like getting this DWI kind of threw you for a loop. [express empathy]

ANDREA: Well, it was humiliating to get arrested and fingerprinted. Now I find out my name is going to be in the newspaper. This is worse than when I had that blackout thing.

INTERVIEWER: This whole thing has really been embarrassing. [reflection]

ANDREA: My parents don't know yet, but I'm probably going to have to tell them if my name is going to be in the paper.

INTERVIEWER: One of the hardest parts of this whole thing is having everyone know about it. [amplified reflection]

ANDREA: And the money—it's costing a fortune for the lawyer.

INTERVIEWER: So embarrassment and money are two of the worst things about this. What else is bothering you about this whole thing?

ANDREA: Well, if I'm honest, it bothers my conscience. When they arrested me, my blood level was .16, which is, like, twice the legal limit. I was drunker than I thought.

INTERVIEWER: It bothers you that you could be that intoxicated and not really know it. [developing discrepancy]

ANDREA: Yeah, I never saw myself as a drunk driver, but I was really drunk that night. And I did drive.

Several important things have already happened in this brief interview. The provider noticed and responded to the intrinsic concern about her drinking that Andrea brings to this session, rather than attending to her resistance. She did not argue with Andrea about the correctness of her arrest and diagnosis, but shifted focus instead to Andrea's perception of the costs of her drinking. She directed the conversation toward exchanges that elicited change talk from Andrea, even at the expense of gathering information about the enticing subject of blackouts. The interviewer recognized that she could gather this information later, but the chance to increase motivation was too important to pass up with this ambivalent client.

INTERVIEWER: When you think about yourself as the kind of person who would drive intoxicated, it just doesn't fit. [developing discrepancy]

ANDREA: Exactly. My dad was always drinking and driving, and it used to make everyone in my family crazy. He finally sobered up, but I swore I would never get a DWI. I still can't believe I actually did.

INTERVIEWER: It's hard to believe you might be like your dad in this way. [developing discrepancy]

ANDREA: It's disgusting. I need to make sure this doesn't happen again. Believe me, I don't need a treatment program for that.

Rather than arguing for change, the provider has continued to focus on exchanges that "pull" change talk out of Andrea's mouth. When the opportunity was available, the provider commented explicitly on the difference between Andrea's view of herself and her behavior.

INTERVIEWER: Got it. A treatment program is not what you have in mind. How could we be helpful in this situation? [shifting focus]

ANDREA: I need something that will help me in court. They want me to complete this evaluation. You've got the paper right there.

INTERVIEWER: OK, so I could ask you a lot of questions and give you a label. I can see how that would help you with the court, but I'm not sure it will help with the real concern I hear from you. You are worried that your drinking got away from you and you don't really know why. And you don't really think a treatment program is right for you. [reflection]

ANDREA: Yeah, that's true. I wouldn't mind talking with someone about my drinking, but I don't need to quit forever.

INTERVIEWER: You're willing to consider some changes in your drinking, but abstinence is out of the question right now. [amplified reflection]

ANDREA: It's not out of the question if it's temporary. I'm just not willing to say I'm going to quit drinking forever, because I'm not an alcoholic.

INTERVIEWER: I see your point. I wonder if you would be willing to talk with me about your drinking in a little more detail. I'd like to know about both the good things and the not-so-good things about your drinking. [exploring pros and cons]

ANDREA: OK.

INTERVIEWER: Let's start with the good things. What's good about your drinking? What do you like about it?

ANDREA: Well, it's not a problem.

INTERVIEWER: OK, so one of the things you like about it is that it usually doesn't cause a lot of trouble for you. [rolling with resistance] What else is good about your drinking?

Here the interviewer has decided to move in a particular direction, having used microskills to form a working rapport with this client. She is actively attempting to induce discrepancy with a decisional balance, thereby arriving at one of the critical destinations of motivational interviewing. To elicit change talk, the interviewer has chosen to begin with the positives about the client's drinking, knowing that if she is ambivalent she will be likely to bring up the negatives spontaneously.

ANDREA: Oh, I don't know. It's more or less a social thing for me. Believe it or not, I almost never drink by myself. I usually drink with my friends after work. We all work in law offices downtown and we get together a couple of nights after work for happy hour. It helps me to hang out with them and relax—you know, to get rid of stress. I should cut those happy hours back, I guess.

INTERVIEWER: I hear two things: one, it helps you socialize with your friends, and that's important to you. Two, it helps you feel relaxed and let go of some of the stress of your job. I'd like to know more about that job stress.

ANDREA: My job is dull. I mean, really dull. I mostly copy all day long. Plus, the people I work with in that law office treat me like dirt because I don't have a degree.

INTERVIEWER: It's tough to be smart and work in a job where you don't get to use it.

ANDREA: Yeah, and it's my own fault because I dropped out of college. I think about that every day. I should have studied more and partied less, I guess. But I was just a kid.

INTERVIEWER: You might do things differently if you were in college again. [supporting self-efficacy]

ANDREA: You can say that again! Like drink less and hit the damn books.

INTERVIEWER: OK, so we've got visiting with friends and relaxing to help you let go of job stress on the good side here. What else is good about your drinking?

Importantly, the interviewer has not jumped on the first opportunity to shift the topic to the costs of Andrea's drinking. This focus might have been premature and might have elicited resistance. Instead, she has reflected Andrea's internal exploration of what her drinking means and has even taken an opportunity to support some optimism about Andrea's ability to change her life if she chooses. The interviewer continues to probe for the benefits of Andrea's drinking, and will not move to the costs too quickly.

ANDREA: I don't get much else out of it. It's not like I drink every day or anything. I guess it helps when I go out with someone new.

INTERVIEWER: Dating can be stressful, so alcohol helps smooth that out a bit.

ANDREA: Can you imagine going out on a date with someone and not drinking? They'd think I was a loser. I'd never get a second date.

INTERVIEWER: People might not know what to think of you if you didn't drink. Especially on a first date.

ANDREA: They'd think I was an alcoholic.

INTERVIEWER: You don't want to give someone the wrong idea about your drinking.

ANDREA: But I don't want to get drunk either. That's not exactly making the right impression.

INTERVIEWER: It's hard to get it just right. You don't want to drink too much but you don't want to be abstinent either.

ANDREA: I never thought of it that way.

The interviewer might continue in this manner for some time, exploring the meaning of drinking for Andrea within the structure of asking for the positive aspects of it. Eventually, if Andrea was not actively resistant, she would shift to a discussion of the negative aspects of her drinking, preceded by a summary.

INTERVIEWER: So, I'm hearing that the good parts of your drinking are that it helps you socialize, especially on dates and most of all when you're dating someone for the first time. Also, it helps you relax and cope with the fact that you are working at a job that does not challenge you.

ANDREA: Yeah.

INTERVIEWER: So, let's shift focus to the not-so-good things about your drinking. What worries do you have about it?

ANDREA: This DWI is at the top of my list.

INTERVIEWER: Yes, you mentioned that at the beginning. We'll put it at the top in big letters. Anything else?

ANDREA: My family is starting to worry about me. They never really got over my dad's drinking, so they watch how I drink pretty carefully. I drink more than they do, so they think I might be an alcoholic like him.

INTERVIEWER: They don't need to worry about you, but they do.

ANDREA: It's annoying, but I know they care about me.

INTERVIEWER: You might be able to see their point about this a little bit.

The interviewer can move forward with a discussion of the negatives in the same manner as before. She is careful not to push, not to persuade, not to attempt to convince Andrea with logic that she has a problem. Rather, the interviewer is interested in having Andrea express herself how she might benefit from making a change. The interviewer might end the pros and cons exercise with a summary, but one that is heavily weighted in a particular direction.

INTERVIEWER: So, Andrea, I really appreciate you going through this exercise with me. I have a much better picture than before. Let me see if I have it right. What's bothering you the most about all this is that it seems like everyone is trying to convince you that you are an alcoholic, and that just doesn't make sense. You can see some problems with your drinking and you see that it would be good to make a few changes, but you also feel that you use alcohol responsibly most of the time and don't feel it's necessary to give it up completely for the rest of your life. You appreciate the concern of your family and friends, but you know this is something no one else can decide for you. You've been successful at making changes in your life before, and you know that if you put your mind to it, you can make a change in your drinking. But you worry how to socialize without it, and dating would be the biggest challenge. Did I get it right? [summary]

ANDREA: Yeah. Wow, it's strange hearing it all laid out like that.

INTERVIEWER: Strange.

ANDREA: Strange, like I need to do something about this, before it really gets to be a problem in my life. I can see how it could happen.

INTERVIEWER: When you look at it like this, it seems like you might want to make a change of some kind.

Here, the interviewer can begin to discuss hypothetically with the client what changes she might like to make and how those would or would not fit within the structure of the program where the interviewer works. If the client is ready to move forward, the therapist might complete the assessment and treatment plan in the next session or two, taking advantage of the momentum in the interaction.

If the client were to become resistant when discussing specific changes, the therapist might sincerely encourage her to pursue the changes she has endorsed without specific professional help. Interestingly, the interviewer might decide to do little else (Bell & Rollnick, 1995) and encourage her to return if she changes her mind about whether the interviewer can be helpful in the future.

It is important to note that the provider must use an empathic and sincere style to be successful with motivational interviewing. Sarcasm or subtle confrontation will ruin what seem to be perfectly acceptable motivational interviewing interventions, since they convey a contradictory (and clearly discernable) message.

It is worthwhile noting, as well, what this provider has given up by using this method with Andrea. Although research indicates that motivational interviewing-based interventions can be as effective as longer and more intensive interventions (Project MATCH Research Group, 1997; Burke, Arkowitz, & Dunn, 2002), the provider has given up the option of diagnosing quickly, giving strong advice, and presenting an expert prescription for a change plan. In order to achieve the goal of enhancing motivation, the provider has instead invested in a method that is thoughtful, does not always produce the intended result, and relies on the underlying belief that the client will choose what is best for herself. Considering the possibility of using motivational interviewing, like any complex behavior change, involves weighing the gains against the costs.

REFERENCES

Bell, A., & Rollnick, S. (1995). Motivational interviewing in practice: A structured approach. In F. Rotgers, D. S. Keller, & J. Morgenstern (Ed.), *Treating substance abuse: Theory and technique* (pp. 266–285). New York: Guilford Press.
Brehm, S. S., & Brehm, J. W. (1981). *Psychological reactance: A theory of freedom and control.* New York: Academic Press.
Burke, B. L., Arkowitz, H., & Dunn, C. (2002). The efficacy of motivational interviewing and its adaptions: What we know so far. In W. R. Miller & S. Rollnick, *Motivational interviewing* (2nd ed.): *Preparing people for change* (pp. 217–250). New York: Guilford Press.
DiClemente, C. C., & Velasquez, M. M. (1991). Motivational interviewing and the stages of change. In W. R. Miller & S. Rollnick, *Motivational interviewing* (2nd ed.): *Preparing people for change* (pp. 201–216). New York: Guilford Press.
Graeber, D., Moyers, T. B., Griffith, G., Guajardo, E., & Tonigan, J. S. (2003). Comparison of motivational interviewing and an educational intervention in patients with schizophrenia and alcoholism. *Community Mental Health Journal, 39*(3), 189–202.
Leake, G. J., & King, A. S. (1977). Effect of counselor expectations on alcoholic recovery. *Alcohol Health and Research World, 1*(3), 16–22.
Miller, W. R. (1983). Motivational interviewing with problem drinkers. *Behavioural Psychotherapy, 1,* 147–172.
Miller, W. R. (1985). Motivation for treatment: A review with special emphasis on alcoholism. *Psychological Bulletin, 98,* 84–107.

Miller, W. R., Benefield, R. G., & Tonigan, J. S. (1993). Enhancing motivation for change in problem drinking: A controlled study of two therapist styles. *Journal of Consulting and Clinical Psychology, 61,* 455–461.

Miller, W. R., & Rollnick, S. (1991). *Motivational interviewing: Preparing people to change addictive behavior.* New York: Guilford Press.

Miller, W. R., & Rollnick, S. (2002). *Motivational interviewing* (2nd ed.): *Preparing people for change.* New York: Guilford Press.

Parker, M. W., Winstead, D. K., & Willi, F. J. P. (1979). Patient autonomy in alcohol rehabilitation: I. Literature review. *International Journal of the Addictions, 14,* 1015–1022.

Project MATCH Research Group. (1997). Matching alcoholism treatments to client heterogeneity: Project MATCH posttreatment drinking outcomes. *Journal of Studies on Alcohol, 58,* 7–29.

Rogers, C. (1957). The necessary and sufficient conditions for therapeutic personality change. *Journal of Consulting Psychology, 21,* 95–103.

Rollnick, S., Allison, J., Ballasiotes, S., Barth, T., Butler, C., Rose, G., & Rosengren, D. (2002). Variations on a theme: Motivational interviewing and its adaptions. In W. R. Miller & S. Rollnick, *Motivational interviewing* (2nd ed.): *Preparing people to change* (pp. 270–283). New York: Guilford Press.

Rollnick, S., Mason, P., & Butler, C. (1999). *Health behavior change: A guide for practitioners.* New York: Churchill Livingstone.

Rollnick, S., & Miller, W. R. (1995). What is motivational interviewing? *Behavioural and Cognitive Psychotherapy, 23,* 325–334.

Sanchez, F. (2000). *A values-based intervention for alcohol problems.* Doctoral dissertation, University of New Mexico.

13

Integrating Psychotherapy and Pharmacotherapy in Substance Abuse Treatment

Kathleen M. Carroll

Although this book focuses on the theory and technique of psychotherapeutic approaches commonly used in the treatment of substance abuse, medications also play a vital role in the treatment of substance dependence. This chapter (1) describes differences in the roles and functions of psychotherapy and pharmacotherapy in the treatment system; (2) discusses the potential advantages of the two forms of treatment alone and in combination; and (3) concentrates on the treatment of alcohol and opioid dependence (the only classes of substance dependence for which effective pharmacotherapies exist), reviews the major pharmacologic approaches, with emphasis on describing how outcomes from pharmacological treatments can be enhanced and extended through combining them with psychotherapy. It should be noted that, in this chapter, "psychotherapy" is used as a general term for several types of psychosocial treatment, including individual and group counseling, psychotherapy, and behavior therapy.

THE ROLES OF PSYCHOTHERAPY AND PHARMACOTHERAPY

The Roles of Psychotherapy

Most psychotherapies for substance abuse and dependence address several common issues and tasks, despite often wide differences in theory, technique, and strategies. Although different approaches vary in the degree to which emphasis is placed on these common tasks, some attention to these issues is likely to be involved in any successful treatment (Rounsaville & Carroll, 1997).

Moreover, it should be noted that currently available pharmacotherapies for substance dependence would be expected to have little or no effect in following areas commonly addressed by behavioral therapies:

SETTING THE RESOLVE TO STOP

Rare is the substance abuser who seeks treatment without some degree of ambivalence regarding cessation of drug use. Even at the time of treatment seeking, which usually occurs only after substance-related problems have become severe, substance abusers usually can identify many ways in which they want or feel the need for drugs and have difficulty developing a clear picture of what life without drugs might be like (Rounsaville & Carroll, 1997). Moreover, given the substantial external pressures that may precipitate application for treatment, many patients are highly ambivalent about treatment itself. This ambivalence must be addressed if the patient is to experience him- or herself as an active participant in treatment; if the patient perceives treatment as wholly imposed upon him or her by external forces and does not have a clear sense of personal goals for treatment, it is likely that any form of treatment will be of limited usefulness. Treatments based on principles of motivational psychology, such as motivational interviewing (Miller & Rollnick, 2001) or motivation enhancement therapy (Miller, Zweben, DiClemente, & Rychtarik, 1992), concentrate almost exclusively on strategies intended to bolster the patient's own motivational resources. However, most behavioral treatments include some exploration of what the patient stands to lose or gain through continued substance use as a means to enhance motivation for treatment and abstinence.

TEACHING COPING SKILLS

Social learning theory posits that substance abuse may represent a means of coping with difficult situations, positive and negative affects, invitations by peers to use substances, and so on. By the time substance use is severe enough for treatment, use of substances may represent the individual's single, overgeneralized means of coping with a variety of situations, settings, and states. If stable abstinence is to be achieved, treatment must help the patient to recognize the high-risk situations in which he or she is most likely to use substances and to develop other, more effective means of coping with them. Although cognitive-behavioral approaches concentrate almost exclusively on skills training as a means of preventing relapse to substance use (e.g., Carroll, 1998; Marlatt & Gordon, 1985; Monti, Abrams, Kadden, & Cooney, 1989), most treatment approaches touch on the relationship between high-risk situations and substance use to some extent. Another example is the innovative work by Childress and colleagues (Childress, McLellan, & O'Brien, 1984; Childress et al., 1993), on cue exposure and reactivity, which may enhance patients' capacity to cope effectively with craving for substances.

CHANGING REINFORCEMENT CONTINGENCIES

By the time treatment is sought, many substance abusers spend the preponderance of their time involved in acquiring, using, and recovering from substance use to the exclusion of other endeavors and rewards. The abuser may be estranged from family and friends and may have few social contacts who do not use drugs. If the patient is still working, employment often becomes no more than a means of acquiring money to buy drugs; the fulfilling or challenging aspects of work have faded away. Few other activities, such as hobbies, athletics, or involvement with community or church groups can stand up to the demands of substance dependence. Typically, the rewards available in daily life are narrowed progressively to those derived from drug use, and other diversions may be neither available nor perceived as enjoyable. When drug use is stopped, its absence may leave the patient with the need to fill the time that had been spent using drugs and to find rewards that can substitute for those derived from drug use. Thus, most behavioral treatments encourage patients to identify and develop fulfilling alternatives to substance use, as exemplified by the community reinforcement approach (CRA; Azrin, 1976) or contingency management (Budney & Higgins, 1998), both of which stress the development of alternate reinforcers for substance use.

FOSTERING MANAGEMENT OF PAINFUL AFFECT

The most commonly cited reasons for relapse are powerful negative affects (Marlatt & Gordon, 1985). Some clinicians have suggested that failure of affect regulation is a critical dynamic underlying the development of compulsive drug use (Khantzian, 1975; Wurmser, 1978). Moreover, the difficulty many substance abusers have in recognizing and articulating their affect states has been noted in several populations (Keller, Carroll, Nich, & Rounsaville, 1995; Taylor, Parker, & Bagby, 1990). Thus, an important common task in substance abuse treatment is to help patients develop ways of coping with powerful dysphoric affects and to learn to recognize and identify the probable cause of these feelings (Rounsaville & Carroll, 1997). Again, while psychodynamically oriented treatments such as supportive–expressive therapy (Luborsky, 1984) emphasize the role of affect in the treatment of cocaine abuse, virtually all forms of psychotherapy for substance abuse include a variety of techniques for coping with strong affect.

IMPROVING INTERPERSONAL FUNCTIONING AND ENHANCING SOCIAL SUPPORTS

A consistent finding in the literature on relapse to drug abuse is the protective influence of an adequate network of social supports (Longabaugh, Beattie, Noel, Stout, & Malloy, 1993; Marlatt & Gordon, 1985). Typical issues presented by drug abusers are loss of or damage to valued relationships occurring when using drugs was the principal priority, failure to have achieved satisfactory relationships even prior to having initiated drug use, and inability to identify friends or intimates who are not themselves drug users (Rounsaville & Carroll, 1997). Many forms of treatment, including family therapy (McCrady & Epstein, 1995), 12-step approaches (Nowinski, Baker, & Carroll, 1992), interpersonal therapy (Rounsaville, Gawin, & Kleber, 1985), and network therapy (Galanter, 1993), make building and maintaining a network of social supports for abstinence a central focus of treatment.

FOSTERING COMPLIANCE WITH PHARMACOTHERAPY

The difficulties of fostering adequate levels of treatment compliance with substance users is well known (so much so that substance abusers are typically excluded from clinical trials of treatments for other disorders). Thus, when pharmacotherapies are used in the treatment of substance abuse, it is not surprising that high rates of noncompliance are seen. A major role that behavioral treatments plays when pharmacotherapies are used in the treatment of substance use is in fostering compliance: most strategies to improve compliance are inherently psychosocial (Carroll, 1997a). These include, for example, regular monitoring of medication compliance through pill counts or medication serum levels; encouragement of patient self-monitoring of compliance (e.g., through medication logs or diaries); clear communication between patient and staff about the study medication, its expected effects, side effects, and benefits; repeatedly stressing the importance of adherence; contracting with the patients for adherence; directly reinforcing adherence through incentives or rewards; providing telephone or written reminders about appointments or taking medication; preparing and educating patients about the disorder and its treatment; and frequent contact and the provision of extensive support and encouragement to the patient and his or her family (see Meichenbaum & Turk, 1987; Haynes, Taylor, & Sackett, 1979).

It should be noted, however, that some traditional treatment approaches for substance use have a long-standing opposition to pharmacological approaches to the treatment of substance use disorders. While this is changing in that many traditional programs and self-help groups are more accepting of some pharmacotherapies, clinicians may find it helpful to prepare a patient taking medication for the reaction he or she may encounter in such groups, reiterate the rationale and expected benefits of the medication, and point out the difference between drugs of abuse and prescribed pharmacotherapies.

The Roles of Pharmacotherapy

The target symptoms addressed and the roles typically played by pharmacotherapy differ from those of behavioral treatments in their course of action, time to effect, target symptoms, and durability of benefits (Elkin, Pilkonis,

Docherty, & Sotsky, 1988a, 1988b). In general, pharmacotherapies have a much more narrow application than do most behavioral treatments for substance use disorders. That is, most behavioral therapies are applicable across a range of treatment settings (e.g., inpatient, outpatient, residential), modalities (e.g., group, individual, family), and to a wide variety of populations. For example, disease model, behavioral, or motivational approaches have be used, with only minor modifications, regardless of whether the patient is an opiate, alcohol, cocaine, or marijuana user. On the other hand, most available pharmacotherapies are applicable only to a single class of substance use and exert their effects over a narrow band of symptoms. For example, methadone produces cross-tolerance for opioids but has little effect on concurrent cocaine abuse; disulfiram produces nausea after alcohol ingestion but not after ingestion of illicit substances. A notable exception is naltrexone, which is used to treat both opioid and, more recently, alcohol dependence (O'Malley et al., 1992; Volpicelli, Alterman, Hayashida, & O'Brien, 1992).

Common roles and indications for pharmacotherapy in the treatment of substance dependence disorders include the following (Rounsaville & Carroll, 1997):

DETOXIFICATION

For those classes of substances that produce substantial physical withdrawal syndromes (e.g., alcohol, opioids, sedative–hypnotics), medications are often needed to reduce or control the often-dangerous symptoms associated with withdrawal. Benzodiazepenes are often used to manage symptoms of alcohol withdrawal (see Barber & O'Brien, 1999, and Mayo-Smith, 1998, for detailed descriptions). Agents such as methadone, clonidine, naltrexone, and buprenorphine are typically used for the management of opioid withdrawal (see Barber & O'Brien, 1999; O'Connor & Kosten, 1998). Typically, the role of behavioral treatments during detoxification is typically extremely limited due to the level of discomfort, agitation, and confusion the patient may experience. However, recent studies have suggested the effectiveness of behavioral strategies in increasing retention and abstinence in the course of longer term outpatient detoxification protocols (Bickel, Amass, Higgins, Badger, & Esch, 1997).

STABILIZATION AND MAINTENANCE

A widely used example of the use of a medication for long-term stabilization of drug users is methadone maintenance for opioid dependence, a treatment strategy that involves the daily administration of a long-acting opioid (methadone) as a substitute for the illicit use of short-acting opioids (typically heroin). Methadone maintenance permits the patient to function normally without experiencing withdrawal symptoms, craving, or side effects. The large body of research on methadone maintenance confirms its importance in fostering treatment retention, providing the opportunity to evaluate and treat other problems and disorders that often coexist with opioid dependence (e.g., medical, legal, and occupational problems), reducing the risk of HIV infection and other complications through reducing intravenous drug use, and providing a level of stabilization that permits the inception of psychotherapy and other aspects of treatment (see Lowinson, Marion, Joseph,& Dole, 1992; Payte & Zweben, 1998). Another example is nicotine replacement therapies, which effectively provide nicotine while minimizing other harmful aspects of smoking (Hughes, 1995; Schmitz, Henningfield & Jarvik, 1998).

ANTAGONIST AND OTHER BEHAVIORALLY ORIENTED PHARMACOTHERAPIES

A more recently developed pharmacological strategy is the use of *antagonist treatment*, that is, the use of medications that block the effects of specific drugs. An example of this approach is naltrexone, an effective, long-acting opioid antagonist. Naltrexone is nonaddicting, does not have the reinforcing properties of opioids, has few side effects and, most important, effectively blocks the effects of opioids (Barber & O'Brien, 1999; Stine, Meandzija & Kosten, 1998). Therefore, naltrexone treatment represents a potent behavioral strategy: as opioid ingestion will not be reinforced while the patient is taking naltrexone, unreinforced opioid use allows extinction of relationships between conditioned drug cues and drug use. For example, a naltrexone-maintained patient, anticipating that opioid use will not result in desired drug effects, may be more likely to learn to live in a world full of drug cues and high-risk situations without resorting to drug use.

TREATMENT OF COEXISTING DISORDERS

An important role of pharmacotherapy in the treatment of substance use disorders is as a treatment for coexisting psychiatric syndromes that may precede or play a role in the maintenance or complications of drug dependence. The frequent co-occurrence of other mental disorders, particularly affective and anxiety disorders, with substance use disorders is well documented in a variety of populations and settings (Kessler et al., 1994; Regier et al., 1990). Given that psychiatric disorders often precede development of substance use disorders, several researchers and clinicians have hypothesized that individuals with primary psychiatric disorders may be attempting to self-medicate their psychiatric symptoms with drugs and alcohol (Khantzian, 1975; Wurmser, 1978). Thus, effective pharmacological treatment of the underlying psychiatric disorder may improve not only the psychiatric disorder but also the perceived need for and therefore the use of illicit drugs (Rosenthal & Westreich, 1999). Examples of this type of approach include the use of antidepressant treatment for depressed alcohol- (Cornelius et al., 1997; McGrath et al., 1996; Mason, Kocsis,

Rituo, & Cutler, 1996), opioid (Nunes, Quitkin, Brady, & Stewart, 1991), and cocaine-dependent (Margolin, Avants, & Kosten, 1995) individuals. Pharmacological treatment of psychiatric disorders in substance users is not an explicit focus of this chapter; rather, only those medications that target substance use directly are reviewed below.

REVIEW OF SPECIFIC PHARMACOTHERAPIES

As noted above, enormous progress has been made in the development of effective pharmacotherapies for several substance use disorders. Before moving to a review of specific pharmacotherapies, their indications, and how their effectiveness can be enhanced through combining them with behavioral approaches, three major issues regarding pharmacological approaches to treatment substance use disorders should be noted.

First, nonpharmacological, behavioral treatments continue to constitute the bulk of substance abuse treatment in the United States. Numerous uncontrolled studies as well as randomized trials consistently point to the benefits of purely behavioral approaches for many substance use disorders (Hubbard, Craddock, Flynn, Anderson, & Etheridege, 1997; Higgins, 1999; McLellan & McKay, 1998). In most cases, pharmacotherapies (other than those used for detoxification or treatment of comorbid disorders) are typically seen as adjunctive strategies, to be used when behavioral treatment alone has been demonstrated to be insufficient for a particular individual.

Second, for most types of illicit drug use, no effective pharmacotherapies exist. Classes of drug use for which no effective pharmacotherapies have been developed include cocaine, marijuana, hallucinogens, amphetamines, inhalants, phencyclidine, and sedatives/hypnotics/anxiolytics. Although major advances have been made in identifying physiological mechanisms of action for many of these substances, and although in a few cases (such as marijuana) specific receptors have been identified that should accelerate progress in identifying pharmacological treatments, behavioral therapies remain the sole available treatment for these classes of drug dependence (reviewed in O'Brien, 1996).

Third, there is general consensus that even for our most potent pharmacotherapies for drug use, purely pharmacological approaches are insufficient for most substance abusers and best outcomes are seen for combined treatments. Pharmacotherapeutic treatments for substance abusers delivered alone, without psychotherapeutic support, are usually seen as insufficient as a means of promoting stable abstinence in drug abusers. As described above, most pharmacotherapies are comparatively specific and narrow in their actions, and may help to detoxify, stabilize, or treat coexisting disorders, but are rarely considered "complete treatments" in and of themselves. Furthermore, because few patients will persist in or comply with a purely pharmacotherapeutic approach, pharmacotherapies delivered alone, without any supportive or compliance-enhancing elements, are usually not considered feasible.

Even where pharmacotherapy is seen as the primary treatment approach (as in the case of methadone maintenance), some form of psychosocial treatment is used to provide at least a minimal supportive structure within which pharmacotherapeutic treatment can be conducted effectively. Furthermore, it is widely recognized that drug effects can be enhanced or diminished with respect to the context in which the drug is delivered. That is, a drug administered in the context of a supportive clinician–patient relationship, with clear expectations of possible drug benefits and side effects, close monitoring of drug compliance, and encouragement for abstinence, is more likely to enhance its effectiveness than a drug delivered without such elements. Thus, even for primarily pharmacotherapeutic treatments, a psychotherapeutic component is almost always included to foster patients' retention in treatment and compliance with pharmacotherapy and to address the numerous comorbid psychosocial problems that occur so frequently among individuals with substance use disorders (O'Brien, 1996; Rounsaville & Carroll, 1997; Schuckit, 1996).

Pharmacotherapy of Alcohol Dependence

Disulfiram

The most commonly used pharmacological adjunct for the treatment of alcohol dependence and abuse is disulfiram, or Antabuse. Disulfiram interferes with the normal metabolism of alcohol, which results in an accumulation of acetaldhyde; hence drinking following ingestion of disulfiram results in an intense physiological reaction, characterized by flushing, rapid or irregular heartbeat, dizziness, nausea, and headache (Fuller, 1989). Thus, disulfiram treatment is intended to work as a deterrent to drinking.

Despite the sustained popularity and widespread use of disulfiram, empirical support for its effectiveness has been mixed (Garbutt, West, Carey, Lohr, & Crews, 1999).

For example, a large-scale, well-controlled multicenter randomized clinical trial reported that disulfiram was no more effective than inactive doses of disulfiram or no medication in terms of rates of abstinence, time to first drink, unemployment, or social stability (Fuller et al., 1986). However, for subjects who did drink, disulfiram treatment was associated with significantly fewer total drinking days. Moreover, rates of compliance with disulfiram in the study were low (20% of all subjects), although abstinence rates were high (43%) among compliant subjects. This study illustrates several important problems with the use of disulfiram: (1) compliance is a major problem, and (2) many patients are unwilling to take disulfiram, as 62% of those eligible for the study refused to participate. When disulfiram compliance is monitored, data suggesting its effectiveness have been more positive (e.g., Chick et al., 1992).

Thus, several studies have evaluated the effectiveness of psychotherapy as a strategy to improve retention and compliance with disulfiram. One of the most effective strategies may be disulfiram contracts, where the patient's spouse or significant other agrees to observe the patient take disulfiram each day and reward the patient for compliance with disulfiram (O'Farrell & Bayog, 1986). Azrin, Sisson, Meyers, and Godley (1982) reported positive and durable results from a randomized clinical trial comparing unmonitored disulfiram to disulfiram contracts, where disulfiram ingestion was monitored by the patient's spouse or administered as part of a multifaceted behavioral program, the community reinforcement approach (CRA). CRA was developed by Hunt and Azrin (1973) as a broad-spectrum approach (incorporating skills training, behavioral family therapy, and job-finding training) that also includes a disulfiram component. At 6-month follow-up, the traditionally treated group reported over 50% drinking days, while the group that received CRA was almost completely abstinent. The effectiveness of CRA illustrates how psychotherapy can be integrated with pharmacotherapy to produce better outcomes than either treatment alone.

Naltrexone

A major development in the treatment of alcohol dependence was the FDA's recent approval of naltrexone. The application of naltrexone, an opioid antagonist, to the treatment of alcoholism derives from findings that indicate that naltrexone reduces alcohol consumption in animals (Volpicelli, Davis, & Olgin, 1986) and alcohol craving and use in humans (Volpicelli et al., 1990). In randomized clinical trials, naltrexone has been shown to be more effective than placebo in reducing alcohol use and craving, as well as time to first relapse and the severity of relapse when it occurs (O'Malley et al., 1992, 1996; Volpicelli et al., 1992). However, a more recent trial suggested that, as with disulfiram, naltrexone's beneficial effects are limited to the subgroup of patients who are compliant with the daily dosing regimen (Volpicelli et al., 1997). This underscores the importance of delivering naltrexone in conjunction with an effective behavioral approach that addresses compliance.

Thus, it is not surprising that naltrexone's effects have been found to differ somewhat with respect to the nature of the behavioral treatment with which it is delivered; for example, in the O'Malley et al. 1992 study, highest rates of abstinence were found when the patient received naltrexone plus a supportive clinical management psychotherapy condition that encouraged complete abstinence from alcohol and other substances. However, for patients who drank, the combination of a cognitive-behavioral coping skills approach and naltrexone was superior in terms of rates of relapse and drinks per occasion. Anton and colleagues (1999) recently reported high rates of retention (83%), high rates of compliance, and significant effects for naltrexone in a randomized trial comparing naltrexone with placebo among abstinent alcoholics who received cognitive-behavioral therapy, underlining the importance of maximizing naltrexone's effects by delivering it in conjunction with a potent behavioral approach. Evaluation of naltrexone's effectiveness in nontraditional substance abuse treatment settings, such as primary care offices, are ongoing (O'Connor, Farren, Rounsaville, & O'Malley, 1997). A major ongoing multisite trial (Project COMBINE), supported by the National Institute of Alcohol Abuse and Alcoholism is evaluating the most effective level of behavioral therapy for enhancing efficacy of naltrexone and other new alcohol pharmacotherapies.

Acamprosate

Acamprosate, or calcium acetyle homotaurinate, is similar to gamma-aminobutytric acid (GABA) and interacts with the GABAergic system (Litten & Allen, 1998; Schuckit, 1996) and appears to have no abuse potential and a benign side effect profile. The bulk of efficacy data on acamprosate has come from Europe, but several studies, including Project Combine, are ongoing in the United States. While results have been mixed and several studies have had small sample sizes and other methodological problems (Moncrieff & Drummond, 1997), the bulk of the trials suggest acamprosate has some efficacy on drinking frequency and abstinence rates (Garbutt et al., 1999; Litten & Allen, 1998). Moreover, although the mechanism of action of acamprosate is not clear, some data suggests that because acamprosate reduces alcohol withdrawal symptoms (Spanagel, Putzke, Stefferl, Schobitz, & Zieglgansberger, 1996), it may reduce problems associated with protracted withdrawal. Finally, because the bulk of studies in this area have evaluated acamprosate in the context of some psychosocial treatment, but few of these have defined or monitored the psychosocial context, the influence of psychosocial interventions on acamprosate compliance and outcomes has not yet been evaluated.

PHARMACOTHERAPY OF OPIOID DEPENDENCE

Methadone Maintenance

The inception of methadone maintenance treatment revolutionized the treatment of opioid addiction as it displayed the previously unseen ability to keep addicts in treatment and to reduce their illicit opioid use, outcomes with which nonpharmacological treatments had fared comparatively poorly (Brill, 1977; Nyswander, Winick, Bernstein, Brill, & Kaufer, 1958; O'Malley, Anderson, & Lazare, 1972). Beyond its ability to retain opioid addicts in treatment and help control opioid use, methadone maintenance also may reduce risk of HIV infection through reducing intravenous drug use (Sees et al., 2000; Ball, Lange, Myers, & Friedman, 1988), and provides the opportunity to evaluate and treat concurrent disorders, including medical problems, family, and psychiatric problems (Lowinson et al., 1992). The bulk of the large body of literature on the effectiveness of methadone maintenance points to the success of methadone maintenance in retaining opioid addicts in treatment and reducing their illicit opioid use and illegal activity (Ball & Ross, 1991; Sees et al., 2000). However, there is a great deal of variability in the success across different methadone maintenance programs, which is likely to be the result of variability in delivery of adequate dosing of methadone as well as variability in provision and quality of psychosocial services (Ball & Ross, 1991; Corty & Ball, 1987; Strain, Bigelow, Liebson, & Stitzer, 1999). Methadone maintenance treatment, especially when provided at adequate doses and combined with drug counseling, substantially decreases illicit opioid use, injection drug use, criminal activity, and morbidity and mortality risk (O'Brien, 1996).

However, there are several problems with methadone maintenance, including illicit diversion of take-home methadone doses, difficulties with detoxification from methadone maintenance to a drug-free state, and the concurrent use of other substances, particularly alcohol and cocaine, among methadone-maintained subjects (Kosten & McCance, 1996). Thus, a range of psychosocial treatments have been evaluated for their ability to address these drawbacks of methadone maintenance, as well as to enhance and extend the benefits of methadone maintenance. Several types of behavioral approaches have been identified as effective in enhancing and extend the benefits of methadone maintenance treatment. These are summarized below.

Behavioral Treatments in the Context of Maintenance Therapies

Before describing specific approaches that have been demonstrated to be effective in enhancing the effectiveness of opioid maintenance therapies, the context for such approaches should be set by brief review of a study that authoritatively established the importance of psychosocial treatments even in the context of a pharmacotherapy as potent as methadone. McLellan, Arndt, Metzger, Woody, and O'Brien (1993) randomly assigned 92 opiate-dependent individuals to either (1) methadone maintenance alone, without psychosocial services; (2) methadone maintenance with standard services, which included regular meetings with a counselor; and (3) enhanced methadone maintenance, which included regular counseling plus on-site medical/psychiatric, employment, and family therapy, in a 24-week trial. Although some patients did reasonably well in the methadone alone condition, 69% of this group had to be transferred out of this condition within 3 months of the study inception because their substance use did not improve or even worsened, or because they experienced significant medical or psychiatric problems that required a more intensive level of care. In terms of drug use and psychosocial outcomes, best outcomes were seen in the enhanced methadone maintenance condition, with intermediate outcomes for the standard methadone services condition, and poorest outcomes for the methadone alone condition. This study underlines the truths that although methadone maintenance treatment has powerful effects in terms of keeping addicts in treatment and making them available for psychosocial treatments, a purely pharmacological approach will not be sufficient for the large majority of patients and that better outcomes are closely associated with higher levels of psychosocial treatments.

CONTINGENCY MANAGEMENT APPROACHES

Several studies have evaluated the use of contingency management to reduce the use of illicit drugs in addicts who are maintained on methadone. In these studies, a reinforcer is provided to patients who demonstrate specified target behaviors such as providing drug-free urine specimens, accomplishing specific treatment goals, or attending treatment sessions. For example, methadone take-home privileges contingent on reduced drug use is an approach that capitalizes on an inexpensive reinforcer that is potentially available in all methadone maintenance programs. Stitzer and her colleagues (e.g., Stitzer, Iguchi, Kidorf, Bigelow, 1993) have done extensive work in evaluating methadone take-home privileges as a reward for decreased illicit drug use. In a series of well-controlled trials, this group of researchers has demonstrated (1) the relative benefits of positive over negative contingencies (Stitzer, Bickel, Bigelow, & Liebson, 1986); (2) the attractiveness of take-home privileges over other incentives available within methadone maintenance clinics (Stitzer & Bigelow, 1978); (3) the effectiveness of targeting and rewarding drug-free urines over other, more distal behaviors such as group attendance (Iguchi et al., 1996); and (4) the benefits of using take-home privileges contingent on drug-free urines over noncontingent take-home privileges (Stitzer, Iguchi, & Felch, 1992).

Silverman and colleagues (1996), drawing on the compelling work of Steve Higgins and his colleagues (see Budney & Higgins, 1998, and Budney, Sigmon, & Higgins, Chapter 12, this volume), have evaluated a voucher-based contingency management system to address concurrent illicit drug use (typically cocaine) among methadone-maintained opioid addicts. In this approach, urine specimens are required three times weekly in order to systematically detect all episodes of drug use. Abstinence, verified through drug-free urine screens, is reinforced through a voucher system where patients receive points redeemable for items consistent with a drug-free lifestyle that are intended to help the patient develop alternate reinforcers to drug use (e.g., movie tickets, sporting goods). Patients never receive money directly. To encourage longer periods of consecutive abstinence, the value of the points earned by the patients increases with each successive clean urine specimen, and the value of the points is reset when the patient produces a drug-positive urine screen. In a very elegant series of studies, Silverman and his colleagues (Silverman, Higgins, et al., 1996; Silverman, Wong, et al., 1996; Silverman et al., 1998) have demonstrated the efficacy of this approach in reducing illicit opioid and cocaine use and producing a number of treatment benefits among this very-difficult-to-treat population.

There are some drawbacks of this approach: although contingency management procedures appear quite promising in modifying previously intractable problems in methadone maintenance programs, particularly continued illicit drug use among clients, they have rarely been implemented in clinical practice. One major obstacle to the implementation of contingency management voucher approaches in regular clinical settings is their cost (up to $1,200 over 12 weeks). However, a number of investigators are evaluating less expensive contingency management approaches among other populations (Petry & Martin, 2002; Petry, Martin, Cooney, & Kranzler, 2000). Moreover, the positive effects of contingency management procedures diminish over time and drug use increases, sometimes to baseline levels, when the behavioral intervention is terminated (Nolimal & Crowley, 1988; Silverman, Higgins, et al., 1996). This may suggest that in methadone maintenance treatment, specific reinforcers may grow weaker with time and/or be replaced by other reinforcers. Studies evaluating the change in strength or preference of reinforcers over time within methadone maintenance programs are needed. For example, for clients entering a methadone program from the street, contingency payments or dose increases may be highly motivating, whereas for clients who have been stabilized and are working and who may have less free time, other reinforcers, such as take-home doses or permission to omit counseling sessions, may be more attractive later in treatment. While contingency management procedures may prove effective only over short periods of time, they may still be valuable in that they may provide an interruption in illicit drug use (or other undesirable behaviors), and this may serve as an opportunity for other interventions to take effect.

OTHER PSYCHOTHERAPIES

Only a few studies have evaluated other forms of psychotherapy as strategies to enhance outcome from opioid maintenance therapies. The landmark study in this area was done by Woody et al. (1983) and was more recently replicated in community settings by members of this group (Woody, McLellan, Luborsky, & O'Brien, 1995). While the original study is now more than 15 years old, it is reviewed in some detail here because it remains the most impressive demonstration of the benefits and role of psychotherapy in the context of methadone maintenance programs. Moreover, it has generated several substudies that have added greatly to our understanding of the types of patients who benefit from psychotherapy in the context of methadone maintenance programs.

One hundred and ten opiate addicts entering a methadone maintenance program were randomly assigned to one of three treatments: drug counseling alone, drug counseling plus supportive–expressive psychotherapy (SE), or drug counseling plus cognitive psychotherapy (CT). After a 6-month course of treatment, while the SE and CT groups did not differ significantly from each other on most measures of outcome, subjects who received either form of professional psychotherapy evidenced greater improvement in more outcome domains than the subjects who received drug counseling alone (Woody et al., 1983). Furthermore, gains made by the subjects who received professional psychotherapy were sustained over a 12-month follow-up, while subjects receiving drug counseling alone evidenced some attrition of gains (Woody, McLellan, Luborsky, & O'Brien, 1987). This study also demonstrated differential response to psychotherapy as a function of patient characteristics, which may point to the best use of psychotherapy (relative to drug counseling) when resources are scarce: while methadone-maintained opiate addicts with lower levels of psychopathology tended to improve regardless of whether they received professional psychotherapy or drug counseling, those with higher levels of psychopathology tended to improve only if they received psychotherapy. In addition, this study provides indications on differential response to psychotherapy by concurrent psychiatric disorder. For example, depressed addicts improved with psychotherapy, while addicts with antisocial personality disorder tended to show little or no improvement unless they also had a depressive disorder (Woody et al., 1985).

New Maintenance Therapies

In addition, two new maintenance therapies recently developed for opioid dependence also promise to make effective maintenance therapies more broadly available. This is significant because access to methadone treatment is quite limited, and currently fewer than one in five heroin users receives treatment for drug dependence (Regier et al., 1993). Barriers to access to methadone maintenance include limited patient and community acceptance of methadone as well as regulatory restrictions and the lack of availability in many areas of the country (Rounsaville & Kosten, 2000).

Development of alternative maintenance agents, and especially agents that can be more readily administered with reduced clinic attendance and outside of traditional methadone maintenance settings, may address some of the problems associated with limited access to treatment. LAAM (L-alpha-acetylmethadol) has recently gained U.S. Food and Drug Administration (FDA) approval as the first alternative to methadone as a maintenance treatment for opioid dependence. Although similar to methadone in terms of the level of physical dependence it produces (Fraser & Isbell, 1952), LAAM is much longer acting than methadone, and can suppress symptoms of opiate withdrawal for more than 72 hours (Fraser & Isbell, 1952; Jaffe, Schuster, Smith, & Blachley, 1970). Like methadone, LAAM acts as a pure agonist at the mu receptor, and its pharmacological profile suggests that many of the same problems (such as the potential for overdose and the difficulty of withdrawal from maintenance treatment) will occur with its use as with methadone (Greenstein, Fudula, O'Brien, 1992). One important advantage of LAAM over methadone is its efficacy when administered on a thrice-weekly dosing schedule, which permits reduced clinic attendance, obviates the need for take-home bottles, and reduces dispensing costs. Because it is administered on a thrice-weekly schedule, LAAM is potentially suitable for use outside of traditional maintenance clinics, but current regulations severely restrict implementation of LAAM maintenance. Despite FDA approval for its use in opioid agonist maintenance treatment, LAAM has not been widely used in most programs that provide maintenance treatment. Possible reasons for its limited use include somewhat reduced efficacy for reducing illicit opioid use and greater attrition, compared to methadone, as well as patient preference (Stine et al., 1998).

Buprenorphine, a partial mu agonist and kappa antagonist, represents a promising alternative to either methadone or LAAM (Blaine, 1992). Because of its unique pharmacological properties, there may be a number of advantages to its use, compared to either methadone or LAAM, as a maintenance agent for the treatment of opioid dependence settings. Ceiling effects at higher buprenorphine doses result in a lower risk of overdose, compared with methadone (Walsh, Preston, Bigelow, & Stitzer, 1995; Walsh, Preston, Stitzer, Cone, & Bigelow, 1994), and buprenorphine may also have a reduced abuse liability in opiate-dependent individuals (and thus less likelihood for diversion) because its use may precipitate withdrawal symptoms (Strain, Preston, Liebson, & Bigelow, 1995; Walsh, June, et al., 1995). Withdrawal symptoms following abrupt discontinuation of buprenorphine are also usually relatively mild (Fudala, Jaffe, Dax, & Johnson, 1990; Negus & Woods, 1995; Amass, Bickel, Higgins, & Hughes, 1994). Results of random assignment, double-blind clinical trials generally support the safety and dose-dependent efficacy of daily sublingual buprenorphine (Kosten, Schottenfeld, Ziedonis, & Falcioni, 1993; Ling, Wesson, Charavastra, & Klett, 1996; Schottenfeld, Pakes, Oliveto, Ziedonis, & Kosten, 1997). The lower abuse liability of buprenorphine suggests that, once approved, buprenorphine may not be governed by the same stringent regulatory requirements that apply to methadone and LAAM.

Because LAAM and buprenorphine have been made available only recently, very few studies have been done on identifying the minimal and optimal intensity of behavioral treatment to be administered in conjunction with these maintenance agents. However, it is likely that the same principles regarding use of behavioral therapies to enhance outcome with these agents as have with the methadone literature will emerge over time.

Naltrexone/Agonist Treatment

Opioid antagonist treatment (naltrexone) offers many advantages over methadone maintenance, including that is nonaddicting and can be prescribed without concerns about diversion, has a benign side effect profile, and may be less costly, in terms of demands on professional time and of patient time, than the daily or near-daily clinic visits required for methadone maintenance (Rounsaville, 1995). Most important are behavioral aspects of the treatment, as unreinforced opiate use allows extinction of relationships between cues and drug use. While naltrexone treatment is likely to be attractive only to a minority of opioid addicts (Greenstein, Arndt, McLellan, O'Brien, & Evans, 1984), naltrexone's unique properties make it an important alternative to methadone maintenance.

However, naltrexone has not, despite its many advantages, fulfilled its promise. Naltrexone treatment programs remain comparatively rare and underutilized with respect to methadone maintenance programs (Rounsaville, 1995). This is in large part due to problems with retention, particularly during the induction phase, where on average 40% of patients drop out during the first month of treatment and 60% drop out by 3 months (Greenstein et al., 1992). Naltrexone treatment has other disadvantages compared with methadone, including (1) discomfort associated with detoxification and protracted withdrawal symptoms, (2) lack of negative consequences for abrupt discontinuation, and (3) no reinforcement for ingestion, all of which may lead to inconsistent compliance with naltrexone treatment and high rates of attrition.

Preliminary evaluations of behavioral interventions targeted to address naltrexone's weaknesses were encouraging. Several investigators (Grabowski et al., 1979; Meyer, Mirin, Altman, & McNamee, 1976) reported success using contingency payments as reinforcements for naltrexone consumption. Family therapy and counseling have also been used to enhance retention in naltrexone programs. For example, in a nonrandomized study of multiple family therapy, Anton, Hogan, Jalali, Riordan, and Kleber (1981) reported that during the first month of naltrexone therapy, addicts in family therapy had a much lower dropout rate compared to those not in family therapy (92% vs. 62%).

More recently, some of the most promising data regarding strategies to enhance retention and outcome in naltrexone treatment has come from investigators evaluating contingency management approaches. Preston and colleagues (1999) found improved retention and naltrexone compliance for an approach that provided vouchers for naltrexone compliance versus an approach that provided noncontingent or no vouchers. However, possibly because drug use was not targeted by the incentives, significant differences in drug use were not seen. Moreover, it is not clear to what extent these procedures can be implemented outside of research settings, nor how durable they are after the termination of the incentive program.

PHARMACOTHERAPY OF COCAINE DEPENDENCE

To date, an effective pharmacotherapy for cocaine dependence has not been identified (O'Brien, 1997). Common targets for cocaine pharmacotherapies have been similar to those of other abused substances: agonists, antagonists, anticraving agents, and agents directed toward underlying or co-occurring conditions. More than 30 medications have been evaluated in clinical trials, and although a large number of agents have shown promise in open-label or pilot studies, none have consistently been demonstrated to be more effective than placebo or behavioral treatment alone when evaluated in rigorous randomized, double-blind evaluations. These include antidepressant agents such as desipramine (Arndt, Dorozynsky, Woody, McLellan, & O'Brien, 1992) and fluoxetine (Batki, Washburn, Delucchi, & Jones, 1996; Petrakis et al., 1998), anticonvulsant agents such as carbamazepine (Halikas, Crosby, Pearson, & Graves, 1997), and other agents including amantadine (Kampman et al., 1996), ritanserin (Johnson et al., 1997), gepirone (Jenkins et al., 1992), mazindol (Margolin et al., 1995), and many more. Gorelick (1998), Kosten and McCance (1996), and O'Brien (1997) have provided excellent reviews of the pharmacotherapy literature.

Although no medication has been found to be effective for general populations of cocaine users, it is important to note that some medications do have a place in the treatment of cocaine dependence, particularly medications for treating co-occurring psychiatric or substance use disorders. These agents are often useful because many of the comorbid disorders that accompany cocaine dependence may play a role in perpetuating cocaine dependence (as in the case of individuals who are self-medicating psychiatric symptoms with cocaine) and even impede treatment progress if left unmonitored and treated. Thus, even though there are currently no effective pharmacotherapies for cocaine dependence, there are a number of effective pharmacotherapies for the many psychiatric disorders that frequently accompany cocaine dependence, and these may also benefit cocaine abusers with these comorbid disorders. These include antidepressants in the case of individuals with comorbid depressive disorders (Margolin et al., 1995; Nunes et al., 1991) and agents such as methylphenidate for cocaine abusers with residual attention deficit disorders (Levin, Evans, McDowell, & Kleber, 1998).

A similar strategy involves the use of pharmacotherapies to target substance use disorders that frequently co-occur with cocaine dependence. For example, several investigators have noted high rates of comorbid alcohol dependence among clinical populations of cocaine-dependent individuals (Brady, Sonne, Randall, Adinoff, & Malcolm, 1995; Carroll, Rounsaville, & Bryant, 1993). Thus, targeting alcohol use in this population via suitable pharmacotherapies may be effective for several reasons. First, one benefit of these treatments is that they may reduce patients' exposure to alcohol, which, by virtue of being frequently paired with cocaine use, acts as a powerful conditioned cue for cocaine use for many patients. Second, this strategy may be helpful in reducing alcohol-related disinhibition and impairment of judgment that are common antecedents of cocaine use. Finally, reduction or elimination of alcohol use through alcohol pharmacotherapies may also reduce cocaethylene effects, making cocaine potentially less reinforcing and reducing toxicity resulting from the combined use of cocaine and alcohol (Jatlow et al., 1991).

The Yale group has recently completed one randomized clinical trial with 122 individuals with co-occurring cocaine and alcohol dependence, which suggested that disulfiram was associated with significantly better retention, longer periods of abstinence from cocaine and alcohol, and significantly fewer cocaine-positive urine specimens (Carroll, Nich, Ball, McCance, & Rounsaville, 1998; Carroll et al., 2000). Two subsequent pilot studies also have suggested that disulfiram may be a promising approach for treating cocaine dependence without co-occurring alcohol use (George et al., 2000; Petrakis et al., 2000), but these results should be replicated before disulfiram is more widely used as treatment for cocaine dependence in individuals who do not abuse alcohol.

Compared with the results of trials evaluating pharmacological treatment of cocaine dependence, evaluations of behavioral therapies, and particularly contingency management and cognitive-behavioral, and manualized disease-model approaches have been much more promising (Higgins, Budney, Bickel, & Hughes, 1993; Higgins et al., 1994; Maude-Griffin et al., 1998; McKay et al., 1997; Carroll, Nich, Ball, McCance, & Rounsaville, 1998). Because of the lack of an effective pharmacological platform for cocaine dependence (analogous to methadone maintenance for the treatment of opioid dependence), behavioral therapies for cocaine-dependent individuals have had to focus on key outcomes such as retention and the inception and maintenance of abstinence, rather than placing initial emphasis on secondary psychosocial problems (e.g., family, psychological, legal problems).

CONCLUSIONS

Even for those classes of substance abuse for which there are powerful and effective pharmacotherapies, the availability of methadone, naltrexone, and antabuse have by no means cured substance abuse. These very powerful agents tend to work primarily on the symptoms of substance abuse that are time-limited and autonomous, but have little impact on the enduring behavioral characteristics of substance use. Moreover, pharmacotherapies work only if substance abusers see the value of stopping substance use, but substance abusers have consistently found ways to circumvent these pharmacological interventions. It is unlikely that we will develop a pharmacological intervention that gives addicts the motivation to stop using drugs, helps them see the value in renouncing substance use, improves their ability to cope with the day-to-day frustrations in living, or provides alternatives to the reinforcements drugs and the drug-using lifestyle provide. The bulk of the evidence suggests that pharmacotherapies can be very effective treatment adjuncts, but in most cases the effects of pharmacotherapies can be broadened, enhanced, and extended by the addition of psychotherapy (Carroll & Rounsaville, 1993).

Psychotherapy and pharmacotherapies work through different mechanisms, and address different problems. Neither is completely effective by itself. As the bulk of the evidence in the treatment of substance abuse suggest that the two forms of treatment tend to work better together than apart, integrated treatments, carefully matching the particular needs of particular patients, may provide our best hope for helping patients whose lives have been devastated by substance abuse (Carroll, 1997b).

ACKNOWLEDGMENT

Support was provided by NIDA Grant Nos P50-DA09241, K02-DA00248, and U10-DA13038.

REFERENCES

Amass, L., Bickel, W. K., Higgins, S. T., & Hughes, J. R. (1994). A preliminary investigation of outcome following gradual or rapid buprenorphine detoxification. *Journal of Addictive Disease, 13,* 33–45.

Anton, R. F., Hogan, I., Jalali, B., Riordan, C. E., & Kleber, H. D. (1981). Multiple family therapy and naltrexone in the treatment of opiate dependence. *Drug and Alcohol Dependence, 8,* 157–168.

Anton, R. F., Moak, D. H., Waid, L. R., Latham, P. K., Malcolm, R. J., & Dias, J. K. (1999). Naltrexone and cognitive behavioral therapy for the treatment of outpatient alcoholics: Results of a placebo-controlled trial. *American Journal of Psychiatry, 156,* 1758–1764.

Arndt, I. O., Dorozynsky, L., Woody, G. E., McLellan, A. T., & O'Brien, C. P. (1992). Despramine treatment of cocaine dependence in methadone maintained patients. *Archives of General Psychiatry, 49,* 888–893.

Azrin, N. H. (1976). Improvements in the community-reinforcement approach to alcoholism. *Behaviour Research and Therapy, 14,* 39–348.

Azrin, N. H., Sisson, R. W., Meyers, R., & Godley, M. (1982). Alcoholism treatment by disulfiram and community reinforcement therapy. *Journal of Behavior Therapy and Experimental Psychiatry, 13*, 105–112.

Ball, J. C, Lange, W. R., Myers, C. P., & Friedman, S. R. (1988). Reducing the risk of AIDS through methadone maintenance treatment. *Journal of Health and Social Behavior, 29*, 214–216.

Ball, J. C., & Ross, A. (1991) *The effectiveness of methadone maintenance treatment.* New York: Springer-Verlag.

Barber, W. S., & O'Brien, C. P. (1999). Pharmacotherapies. In B. S. McCrady & E. E. Epstein (Eds.), *Addictions: A comprehensive guidebook* (pp. 347–369). New York: Oxford University Press.

Batki, S. L., Washburn, A. M., Delucchi, K., & Jones, R. T. (1996). A controlled trial of fluoxetine in crack cocaine dependence. *Drug Alcohol Dependence, 41*, 137–142.

Bickel, W. K., Amass, L., Higgins, S. T., Badger, G. J., & Esch, R. A. (1997). Effects of adding behavioral treatment to opioid detoxification with buprenorphine. *Journal of Consulting and Clinical Psychology, 65*, 803–810.

Blaine, J. D. (Ed.). (1992). *Buprenorphine: An alternative treatment for opioid dependence* (National Institute on Drug Abuse Research Monograph Series No. 121). Rockville, MD: National Institute on Drug Abuse.

Brady, K. T., Sonne, E., Randall, C. L., Adinoff, B., & Malcolm, R. (1995). Features of cocaine dependence with concurrent alcohol use. *Drug and Alcohol Dependence, 39*, 69–71.

Brill, L. (1977). The treatment of drug abuse: Evolution of a perspective. *American Journal of Psychiatry, 134*, 157–160.

Budney, A. J., & Higgins, S. T. (1998). *A community reinforcement plus vouchers approach: Treating cocaine addiction.* Rockville, MD: National Institute on Drug Abuse.

Carroll, K. M. (1993). Psychotherapeutic treatment of cocaine abuse: Models for its evaluation alone and in combination with pharmacotherapy. In F. M. Tims & C. G. Leukefeld (Eds.), *Cocaine treatment: Research and clinical perspectives* (National Institute on Drug Abuse Research Monograph Series No. 135, pp. 116–132). Rockville, MD: National Institute on Drug Abuse.

Carroll, K. M. (1997a). Manual guided psychosocial treatment: A new virtual requirement for pharmacotherapy trials? *Archives of General Psychiatry, 54*, 923–928.

Carroll, K. M. (1997b). Integrating psychotherapy and pharmacotherapy to improve drug abuse outcomes. *Journal of Addictive Behaviors, 22*, 233–245.

Carroll, K. M. (1998). *A cognitive-behavioral approach: Treating cocaine addiction* (NIH Publication No. 98-4308). Rockville, MD: National Institute on Drug Abuse.

Carroll, K. M., Nich, C., Ball, S. A., McCance, E., & Rounsaville, B. J. (1998). Treatment of cocaine and alcohol dependence with psychotherapy and disulfiram. *Addiction, 93*, 713–728.

Carroll, K. M., Nich, C., Ball, S. A., McCance-Katz, E. F., Frankforter, T., & Rounsaville, B. J. (2000). One year follow-up of disulfiram and psychotherapy for cocaine-alcohol abusers: Sustained effects of treatment. *Addiction, 95*, 1335–1349.

Carroll, K. M., & Rounsaville, B. J. (1993). Implications of recent research on psychotherapy for drug abuse. In G. Edwards, J. Strang, & J. H. Jaffe (Eds.), *Drugs, alcohol, and tobacco: Making the science and policy connections* (pp. 211–221). New York: Oxford University Press.

Carroll, K. M., Rounsaville, B. J., & Bryant, K. J. (1993). Alcoholism in treatment seeking cocaine abusers: Clinical and prognostic significance. *Journal of Studies on Alcohol, 54*, 199–208.

Chick, J., Gough, K., Falkowski, W., Kersahw, P., Hore, B., Mehta, B., Ritson, B., Ropner, R., & Torley, D. (1992). Disulfiram treatment of alcoholism. *British Journal of Psychiatry, 161*, 84–89.

Childress, A. R., Hole, A. V., Ehrman, R. N., Robbins, S. J., McLellan, A. T., & O'Brien, C. P. (1993). Cue reactivity and cue reactivity interventions in drug dependence. In L. S. Onken, J. D. Blaine, & J. J. Boren (Eds.), *Behavioral treatments for drug abuse and dependence* (National Institute on Drug Abuse Research Monograph Series No. 137, pp. 73–95). Rockville, MD: National Institute on Drug Abuse.

Childress, A. R., McLellan, A. T., & O'Brien, C. P. (1984). Assessment and extinction of conditioned withdrawal-like responses in an integrated treatment for opiate dependence. In L. S. Harris (Ed.), *Problems of drug dependence, 1984* (National Institute on Drug Abuse Research Monograph Series No. 55, pp. 202–210). Rockville, MD: National Institute on Drug Abuse.

Cornelius, J. R., Salloum, I. M., Ehler, J. G., Jarrett, P. J., Cornelius, M. D., Perel, J. M., Thase, M. E., & Black, A. (1997). Fluoxetine in depressed alcoholics: A double-blind, placebo-controlled trial. *Archives of General Psychiatry, 54*, 700–705.

Corty, E., & Ball, J. C. (1987). Admissions to methadone maintenance: Comparisons between programs and implications for treatment. *Journal of Substance Abuse Treatment, 4*, 181–187.

Elkin, I., Pilkonis, P. A., Docherty, J. P., & Sotsky, S. M. (1988a). Conceptual and methodological issues in comparative studies of psychotherapy and pharmacotherapy, I: Active ingredients and mechanisms of change. *American Journal of Psychiatry, 145*, 909–917.

Elkin, I., Pilkonis, P. A., Docherty, J. P., & Sotsky, S. M. (1988b). Conceptual and methodological issues in comparative studies of psychotherapy and pharmacotherapy, II: Nature and timing of treatment effects. *American Journal of Psychiatry, 145*, 1070–1076.

Fraser, H. F., & Isbell, H. (1952). Actions and addiction liabilities of alpha acetylmethadols in man. *Journal of Pharmacology and Experimental Therapeutics, 105*, 458–465.

Fudala, P. J., Jaffe, J. H., Dax, E. M., & Johnson, R. E. (1990). Use of buprenorphine in the treatment of opioid addiction, II: Physiologic and behavioral effects of daily and alternate-day administration and abrupt withdrawal. *Clinical Pharmacology Therapeutics, 47*, 525–534.

Fuller, R. K. (1989). Antidipsotropic medications. In W. R. Miller & R. K. Hester (Eds.), *Handbook of alcoholism treatment approaches: Effective alternatives* (pp. 117–127). New York: Pergamon Press.

Fuller, R. K., Branchey, L., Brightwell, D. R., Derman, R. M., Emrick, C. D., Iber, F.

L., James, K. E., Lacoursiere, R. B., Lee, K. K., & Lowenstein I. (1986). Disulfiram treatment for alcoholism: A Veterans Administration cooperative study. *Journal of the American Medical Association, 256,* 1449–1455.

Galanter, M. (1993). *Network therapy for alcohol and drug abuse: A new approach in practice.* New York: Basic Books.

Garbutt, J. C., West, S. L., Carey, T. S., Lohr, K. N., & Crews, F. T. (1999). Pharmacological treatment of alcohol dependence: A review of the evidence. *Journal of the American Medican Association, 281,* 1318–1325.

George, T. P., Pakes, J., Chawarski, M. C., Carroll, K. M., Kosten, T. R., & Schottenfeld, R. S. (2000). Disulfiram versus placebo for cocaine abuse in buprenorphine-maintained subjects: A preliminary trial. *Biological Psychiatry, 47,* 1080–1086.

Gorelick, D. A. (1998). Pharmacologic therapies for cocaine and other stimulant addiction. In A. W. Graham & T. K. Schultz (Eds.), *Principles of addiction medicine* (2nd ed., pp. 531–544). Chevy Chase, MD: American Society of Addiction Medicine.

Grabowski, J., O'Brien, C. P., Greenstein, R., Ternes, T., Long, M., & Steinberg-Donato, S. (1979). Effects of contingency payment on compliance with a naltrexone regimen. *American Journal of Drug and Alcohol Abuse, 6,* 355–365.

Greenstein, R. A., Arndt, I. C., McLellan, A. T., O'Brien, C. P., & Evans, B. (1984). Naltrexone: A clinical perspective. *Journal of Clinical Psychiatry, 45,* 25–28.

Greenstein, R. A., Fudala, P. J., & O'Brien, C. P. (1992). Alternative pharmacotherapies for opiate addiction. In J. H. Lowinsohn, P. Ruiz, & R. B. Millman (Eds.), *Comprehensive textbook of substance abuse* (2nd ed., pp. 562–573). New York: Williams & Wilkins.

Halikas, J. A., Crosby, R. D., Pearson, V. L., & Graves, N. M. (1997). A randomized double-blind study of carbamazepine in the treatment of cocaine abuse. *Clinical Pharmacology and Therapeutics, 62,* 89–105.

Haynes, R. B., Taylor, D. W., & Sackett, D. L. Eds.). (1979). *Compliance in health care.* Baltimore: Johns Hopkins University Press

Higgins, S. T. (1999). We've come a long way: Comments on cocaine treatment outcome research. *Archives of General Psychiatry, 56,* 516–518.

Higgins, S. T., & Budney, A. J. (1993). Treatment of cocaine dependence through the principles of behavior analysis and behavioral pharmacology. In L. S. Onken, J. D. Blaine, & J. J. Boren (Eds.), *Behavioral treatments for drug and alcohol dependence* (National Institute on Drug Abuse Research Monograph Series, No. 137, pp. 97–121). Rockville, MD: National Institute on Drug Abuse.

Higgins, S. T., Budney, A. J., Bickel, W. K., Foerg, F. E., Donham, R., & Badger, G. J. (1994). Incentives improve outcome in outpatient behavioral treatment of cocaine dependence. *Archives of General Psychiatry, 51,* 568–576.

Higgins, S. T., Budney, A. J., Bickel, W. K., & Hughes, J. R. (1993). Achieving cocaine abstinence with a behavioral approach. *American Journal of Psychiatry, 150,* 763–769.

Higgins, S. T., Delaney, D. D., Budney, A. J., Bickel, W. K., Hughes, J. R., Foerg, F., & Fenwick, J. W. (1991). A behavioral approach to achieving initial cocaine abstinence. *American Journal of Psychiatry, 148,* 1218–1224.

Hubbard, R. L., Craddock, S. G., Flynn, P. M., Anderson, J., & Etheridge, R. M.

(1997). Overview of 1-year follow-up outcomes in the Drug Abuse Treatment Outcome Study (DATOS). *Psychology of Addictive Behaviors, 11,* 261–278.

Hughes, J. R. (1995). Combining behavioral therapy and pharmacotherapy for smoking cessation: An update. In L. S. Onken & J. D. Blaine (Eds.), *Integrating psychosocial therapies with pharmacotherapies in the treatment of drug dependence* (National Institute on Drug Abuse, Research Monograph No. 105, pp. 92–109). Rockville, Maryland: National Institute on Drug Abuse.

Hunt, G. M., & Azrin, N. H. (1973). A community-reinforcement approach to alcoholism. *Behavior Research and Therapy, 11,* 91–104.

Iguchi, M. Y., Lamb, R. J., Belding, M. A., Platt, J. J., Husband, S. D., & Morral, A. R. (1996). Contingent reinforcement of group participation versus abstinence in a methadone maintenance program. *Experimental and Clinical Psychopharmacology, 4,* 1–7.

Jaffe, J. H., Schuster, C. R., Smith, B. B., & Blachley, P. H. (1970). Comparison of acetylmethadol and methadone in the treatment of long-term heroin users: A pilot study. *Journal of the American Medical Association, 211,* 1834–1836.

Jatlow, P., Ellsworth, J. D., Bradberry, C. W., Winger, G., Taylor, R., & Roth, R. K. (1991). Cocaethylene: A neuropharmacologically active metabolite associated with concurrent cocaine-ethanol ingestion. *Life Sciences, 48,* 1787–1794.

Jenkins, S. W., Warfield, N. A., Blaine, J. D., Cornish, J., Ling, W., Rosen, M. I., Urshel, H., Wesson, D., & Ziedonis, D. (1992). A pilot trial of gepirone vs. placebo in the treatment of cocaine dependency. *Psychopharmacology Bulletin, 28,* 21–26.

Johnson, B. A., Chen, Y. R., Swann, A. C., Schmitz, J., Lesser, J., Ruiz, P., Johnson, P., & Clyde, C. (1997). Ritanserin in the treatment of cocaine dependence. *Biological Psychiatry, 15,* 932–940.

Kampman, K., Volpicelli, J. R., Alterman, A., Cornish, J., Weinrieb, R., Epperson, L., Sparkman, T., & O'Brien, C. P. (1996). Amantadine in the early treatment of cocaine dependence: A double-blind, placebo-controlled trial. *Drug and Alcohol Dependence, 41,* 25–33.

Keller, D. S., Carroll, K. M., Nich, C., & Rounsaville, B. J. (1995). Differential treatment response in alexithymic cocaine abusers: Findings from a randomized clinical trial of psychotherapy and pharmacotherapy. *American Journal on Addictions, 4,* 234–244.

Kessler, R. C., McGonagle, K. A., Zhao, S., Nelson, C. B., Hughes, M., Eshlemen, S., Wittchen, H., & Kendler, K. S. (1994). Lifetime and 12-month prevalence of DSM-III-R psychiatric disorders in the United States: Results from the National Comorbidity Survey. *Archives of General Psychiatry, 51,* 8–19.

Khantzian, E. J. (1975). Self-selection and progression in drug dependence. *Psychiatry Digest, 10,* 19–22.

Kosten, T. R., & McCance, E. F. (1996). A review of pharmacotherapies for substance abuse. *American Journal on Addictions, 5,* 58–64.

Kosten, T. R., Schottenfeld, R., Ziedonis, D., & Falcioni, J. (1993). Buprenorphine versus methadone maintenance for opioid dependence. *Journal of Nervous and Mental Disease, 181,* 358–364.

Levin, F. R., Evans, S. M., McDowell, D. M., & Kleber, H. D. (1998). Methylphenidate treatment for cocaine abusers with adult attention-deficit/hyperactivity disorder: A pilot study. *Journal of Clinical Psychiatry, 59*, 300–305.

Ling, W., Wesson, D. R., Charavastra, C., & Klett, C. J. (1996). A controlled trial comparing buprenorphine and methadone maintenance in opioid dependence. *Archives of General Psychiatry, 53*, 401–407.

Litten, R. Z., & Allen, J. P. (1998). Advances in development of medications for alcoholism treatment. *Psychopharmacology, 139*, 20–33.

Longabaugh, R., Beattie, M., Noel, R., Stout, R., & Malloy, P. (1993). The effect of social support on treatment outcome. *Journal of Studies on Alcohol, 54*, 465–478.

Lowinson, J. H., Marion, I. J., Joseph, H., & Dole, V. P. (1992). Methadone maintenance. In J. H. Lowinsohn, P. Ruiz, & R. B. Millman (Eds.), *Comprehensive textbook of substance abuse* (2nd ed., pp. 550–561). New York: Williams & Wilkins.

Luborsky, L. (1984). *Principles of psychoanalytic psychotherapy: A manual for supportive-expressive treatment.* New York: Basic Books.

Margolin, A., Avants, S. K., & Kosten, T. R. (1995). Mazindol for relapse prevention to cocaine abuse in methadone-maintained patients. *American Journal of Drug and Alcohol Abuse, 21*, 469–481.

Marlatt, G. A., & Gordon, J. R., (Eds.). (1985). *Relapse prevention: Maintenance strategies in the treatment of addictive behaviors.* New York: Guilford Press.

Mason, B. J., Kocsis, J. H., Ritvo, E. C., & Cutler, R. B. (1996). A double-blind, placebo-controlled trial of desipramine for primary alcohol dependence stratified on the presence or absence of major depression. *Journal of the American Medical Association, 275*, 761–767.

Maude-Griffin, P. M., Hohenstein, J. M., Humfleet, G. L., Reilly, P. M., Tusel, D. J., & Hall, S. M. (1998). Superior efficacy of cognitive-behavioral therapy for crack cocaine abusers: Main and matching effects. *Journal of Consulting and Clinical Psychology, 66*, 832–837.

Mayo-Smith, M. (1998). Management of alcohol intoxication and withdrawal. In A. W. Graham & T. K. Schultz (Eds.), *Principles of addiction medicine* (2nd ed., pp. 431–441). Chevy Chase, MD: American Society of Addiction Medicine.

McCrady, B. S., & Epstein, E. E. (1995). Marital therapy in the treatment of alcohol problems. In N. S. Jacobson & A. S Gurman (Eds.), *Clinical handbook of couple therapy* (pp. 369–393). New York: Guilford Press.

McGrath, P. J., Nunes, E. V., Stewart, J. W., Goldman, D., Agosti, V., Ocepek-Welikson, K., & Quitkin, F. M. (1996). Imipramine treatment of alcoholics with primary depression: A placebo controlled clinical trial. *Archives of General Psychiatry, 53*, 232–240.

McKay, J. R., Alterman, A. I., Cacciola, J. S., Rutherford, M. J., O'Brien, C. P., & Koppenhaver, J. (1997). Group counseling versus individualized relapse prevention aftercare following intensive outpatient treatment for cocaine dependence. *Journal of Consulting and Clinical Psychology, 65*, 778–788.

McLellan, A. T., Arndt, I. O., Metzger, D. S., Woody, G. E., & O'Brien, C. P. (1993). The effects of psychosocial services in substance abuse treatment. *Journal of the American Medical Association, 269*, 1953–1959.

McLellan, A. T., & McKay, J. R. (1998). The treatment of addiction: What can research offer practice? In S. Lamb, M. R. Greenlick, & D. McCarty (Eds.), *Bridging the gap between practice and research: Forging partnerships with community based drug and alcohol treatment* (pp. 147–185). Washington, DC: National Academy Press.

Meichenbaum, D., & Turk, D. C. (1987). *Facilitating treatment adherence.* New York: Plenum Press.

Meyer, R. E., Mirin, S. M., Altman, J. L., & McNamee, B. (1976). A behavioral paradigm for the evaluation of narcotic antagonists. *Archives of General Psychiatry, 33,* 371–377.

Miller, W. R., & Rollnick, S. (2001). *Motivational interviewing* (2nd ed.): *Preparing people for change.* New York: Guilford Press.

Miller, W. R., Zweben, A., DiClemente, C. C., & Rychtarik, R. G. (1992). *Motivational enhancement therapy manual: A clinical research guide for therapists treating individuals with alcohol abuse and dependence.* National Institute on Alcohol Abuse and Alcoholism Project MATCH Monograph Series Vol. 2, DHHS Publication No. [ADM] 92-1894). Rockville, MD: National Institute on Alcohol Abuse and Alcoholism.

Moncrieff, J., & Drummond, D. C. (1997). New drug treatments for alcohol problems: A critical appraisal. *Addiction, 92,* 939–947.

Monti, P. M., Abrams, D. B., Kadden, R. M., & Cooney, N. L. (1989). *Treating alcohol dependence: A coping skills training guide in the treatment of alcoholism.* New York: Guilford Press.

Negus, S. S., & Woods, J. H. (1995). Reinforcing effects, discriminative stimulus effects, and physical dependence liability of buprenorphine. In A. Cowan & J. W. Lewis (Eds.), *Buprenorphine: Combating drug abuse with a unique opioid* (pp.71–101). New York: Wiley-Liss.

Nolimal, D., & Crowley, T. (1988). Difficulties in a clinical application of methadone dose contigency contracting. In L. S. Harris (Ed.), *Problems of drug dependence, 1988* (National Institute on Drug Abuse Research Monograph Series No. 90, p. 69). Rockville, MD: National Institute on Drug Abuse.

Nowinski, J., Baker, S., & Carroll, K. M. (1992). *Twelve-step facilitation therapy manual: A clinical research guide for therapists treating individuals with alcohol abuse and dependence* (National Institute on Alcohol Abuse and Alcoholism Project MATCH Monograph Series Vol. 1, DHHS Publication No. [ADM] 92-1893). Rockville, MD: National Institute on Alcohol Abuse and Alcoholism.

Nunes, E. V., Quitkin, F. M., Brady, R., & Stewart, J. W. (1991). Imipramine treatment of methadone maintenance patients with affective disorder and illicit drug use. *American Journal of Psychiatry, 148,* 667–669.

Nyswander, M., Winick, C., Bernstein, A., Brill, I., & Kaufer, G. (1958). The treatment of drug addicts as voluntary outpatients: A progress report. *American Journal of Orthopsychiatry, 28,* 714–727.

O'Brien, C. P. (1996). Recent developments in the pharmacotherapy of substance abuse. *Journal of Consulting and Clinical Psychology, 64,* 677–686.

O'Brien, C. P. (1997). A range of research-based pharmacotherapies for addiction. *Science, 278,* 66–70.

O'Connor, P. G., Farren, C. K., Rounsaville, B. J., & O'Malley, S. S. (1997). A preliminary investigation of the management of alcohol dependence with naltrexone by primary care providers. *American Journal of Medicine, 103,* 477–482.

O'Connor, P. G., & Kosten, T. R. (1998). Management of opioid intoxication and withdrawal. In A. W. Graham & T. K. Schultz (Eds.), *Principles of addiction medicine* (2nd ed., pp. 457–464). Chevy Chase, MD: American Society of Addiction Medicine.

O'Farrell, T. J., & Bayog, R. D. (1986). Antabuse contracts for married alcoholics and their spouses: A method to insure Antabuse taking and decrease conflict about alcohol. *Journal of Substance Abuse Treatment, 3,* 1–8.

O'Malley, J. E., Anderson, W. H., & Lazare, A. (1972). Failure of outpatient treatment of drug abuse, I: Heroin. *American Journal of Psychiatry, 128,* 865–868.

O'Malley, S. S., Jaffe, A. J., Chang, G., Rode, S., Schottenfeld, R., Meyer, R. E., & Rounsaville, B. J. (1996). Six month follow-up of naltrexone and psychotherapy for alcohol dependence. *Archives of General Psychiatry, 53,* 217–224.

O'Malley, S. S., Jaffe, A. J., Chang, G., Schottenfeld, R. S., Meyer, R. E., & Rounsaville, B. J. (1992). Naltrexone and coping skills therapy for alcohol dependence: A controlled study. *Archives of General Psychiatry, 49,* 881–887.

Payte, J. T., & Zweben, J. E. (1998). Opioid maintenance therapies. In A. W. Graham & T. K. Schultz (Eds.), *Principles of addiction medicine* (2nd ed., pp. 557–570). Chevy Chase, MD: American Society of Addiction Medicine.

Petrakis, I., Carroll, K. M., Gordon, L., Nich, C., Kosten, T. R., & Rounsaville, B. J. (1998). Fluoxetine treatment of depressive disorders in methadone maintained opioid addicts. *Drug and Alcohol Dependence, 50,* 221–226.

Petrakis, I. L., Carroll, K. M., Gordon, L., Nich, C., McCance, E., Katz, E. F., Frankforter, T., & Rounsaville, B. J. (2000). Disulfiram treatment for cocaine dependence in methadone maintained opioid addicts. *Addiction, 95,* 219–228.

Petry, N. M., & Martin, B. (2002). Low-cost contingency management for treating cocaine and opioid abusing methadone patients. *Journal of Consulting and Clinical Psychology, 70,* 398–405.

Petry, N. M., Martin, B., Cooney, J. L., & Kranzler, H. R. (2000). Give them prizes and they will come: Lower-cost contingency management treatment of alcohol dependence. *Journal of Consulting and Clinical Psychology, 68,* 250–257.

Preston, K. L., Silverman, K., Umbricht, A., DeJusus, A., Montoya, I. D., & Schuster, C. R. (1999). Improvement in naltrexone treatment compliance with contingency management. *Drug and Alcohol Dependence, 54,* 127–135.

Regier, D. A., Farmer, M. E., Rae, D. S., Locke, B. Z., Keith, S. J., Judd, L. L., & Goodwin, F. K. (1990). Comorbidity of mental disorders with alcohol and other drug use. *Journal of the American Medical Association, 264,* 2511–2518.

Regier, D. A., Narrow, W. E., Rae, D. S., Manderscheid, R. W., Locke, B. Z., & Goodwin, F. K. (1993). The de facto US mental and addictive disorders service system: Epidemiologic catchment area prospective 1-year prevalence rates of disorders and services. *Archives of General Psychiatry, 50,* 85–94.

Rosenthal, R. N., & Westreich, L. (1999). Treatment of persons with dual diagnoses of substance use disorder and other psychological therapies. In B. S. McCrady & E. E. Epstein (Eds), *Addictions: A comprehensive textbook* (pp. 439–476). New York: Oxford University Press.

Rounsaville, B. J. (1995). Can psychotherapy rescue naltrexone treatment of opioid addiction? In L. S. Onken & J. D. Blaine (Eds.), *Potentiating the efficacy of medications: Integrating psychosocial therapies with pharmacotherapies in the treatment of drug dependence* (National Institute on Drug Abuse Research Monograph Series No. 105, pp. 37–52, NIH Publication No. 95–3899). Rockville, MD: National Institute on Drug Abuse.

Rounsaville, B. J., & Carroll, K. M. (1997). Individual psychotherapy for drug abusers. In J. H. Lowinsohn, P. Ruiz, & R. B. Millman (Eds.), *Comprehensive textbook of substance abuse* (3rd ed., pp. 430–439). New York: Williams & Wilkins.

Rounsaville, B. J., Gawin, F. H., & Kleber, H. D. (1985). Interpersonal psychotherapy adpated for ambulatory cocaine abusers. *American Journal of Drug and Alcohol Abuse, 11*, 171–191.

Rounsaville, B. J., & Kosten, T. R. (2000). Treatment for opioid dependence: Quality and access. *Journal of the American Medical Association, 283*, 1337–1339.

Schmitz, J. M., Henningfield, J. E., & Jarvik, M. E. (1998). Pharmacologic therapies for nicotine dependence. In A. W.Graham & T. K. Schultz (Eds.), *Principles of addiction medicine* (2nd ed., pp. 571–582). Chevy Chase, MD: American Society of Addiction Medicine.

Schottenfeld, R. S., Pakes, J. R., Oliveto, A., Ziedonis, D., & Kosten, T. R. (1997). Buprenorphine vs. methadone maintenance treatment for concurrent opioid dependence and cocaine abuse. *Archives of General Psychiatry, 54*, 713–720.

Schuckit, M. A. (1996). Recent developments in the pharmacotherapy of alcohol dependence. *Journal of Consulting and Clinical Psychology, 64*, 669–676.

Sees, K. L., Delucchi, K. L., Masson, C., Rosen, A., Clark, H. W., Robillard, H., Banys, P., & Hall, S. M. (2000). Methadone maintenance vs. 180-day psychosocially enriched detoxification for treatment of opioid dependence: A randomized controlled trial. *Journal of the American Medical Association, 283*, 1303–1310.

Silverman, K., Higgins, S. T., Brooner, R. K., Montoya, I. D., Cone, E. J., Schuster, C. R., & Preston, K. L. (1996). Sustained cocaine abstinence in methadone maintenance patients through voucher-based reinforcement therapy. *Archives of General Psychiatry, 53*, 409–415.

Silverman K., Wong, C. J., Higgins, S. T., et al. (1996). Increasing opiate abstinence through voucer-based reinforcement therapy. *Drug and Alcohol Dependence, 41*, 157–165.

Silverman, K., Wong, C. J., Umbricht-Schneiter, A., Montoya, I. D., Schuster, C. R., & Preston, K. L. (1998). Broad beneficial effects of cocaine abstinence reinforcement among methadone patients. *Journal of Consulting and Clinical Psychology, 66*, 811–824.

Spanagel, R., Putzke, J., Stefferl, A., schobitz, B., Zieglgansberger, & W. (1996). Acamprosate and alcohol, II: Effects on alcohol withdrawal in the rat. *European Journal of Pharmacology, 305*, 45–50.

Stine, S. M., Meandzija, B., & Kosten, T. R. (1998). Pharmacologic therapies for opioid addiction. In A. W. Graham & T. K. Schultz (Eds.), *Principles of addiction medicine* (2nd ed., pp. 545–555). Chevy Chase, MD: American Society of Addiction Medicine.

Stitzer, M. L., Bickel, W. K., Bigelow, G. E., & Liebson, I. A. (1986). Effect of methadone dose contingencies on urinalysis test results of polydrug-abusing methadone maintenance patients. *Drug and Alcohol Dependence, 18*, 341–348.

Stitzer, M. L., & Bigelow, G. E. (1978). Contingency management in a methadone maintenance program: Availability of reinforcers. *International Journal of the Addictions, 13*, 737–746.

Stitzer, M. L., Iguchi, M. Y., & Felch, L. J. (1992). Contingent take-home incentive: Effects on drug use of methadone maintenance patients. *Journal of Consulting and Clinical Psychology, 60*, 927–934.

Stitzer, M. L., Iguchi, M. Y., Kidorf, M., & Bigelow, G. E. (1993). Contingency management in methadone treatment: The case for positive incentives. In L. S. Onken, J. D. Blaine, & J. J. Boren (Eds.), *Behavioral treatments for drug abuse and dependence* (National Institute on Drug Abuse Research Monograph Series No. 137, pp. 19–36). Rockville, MD: National Institute on Drug Abuse.

Strain, E. C., Bigelow, G. E., Liebson, I. A., & Stitzer, M. L. (1999). Moderate vs. high dose methadone in the treatment of opioid dependence. *Journal of the American Medical Association, 281*, 1000–1005.

Strain, E. C., Preston, K. L., Liebson, I. A., & Bigelow, G. E. (1995). Buprenorphine effects in methadone-maintained volunteers: Effects at two hours after methadone. *Journal of Pharmacology Experimental Therapeutics, 272*, 628–638.

Taylor, G. J., Parker, J. D., & Bagby, R. M. (1990). A preliminary investigation of alexithymia in men with psychoactive substance dependence. *American Journal of Psychiatry, 147*, 1228–1230.

Volpicelli, J. R., Alterman, A. I., Hayashida, M., & O'Brien, C. P. (1992). Naltrexone and the treatment of alcohol dependence. *Archives of General Psychiatry, 49*, 876–880.

Volpicelli, J. R., Davis, M. A., & Olgin, J. E. (1986). Naltrexone blocks the post-shock increase of ethanol consumption. *Life Sciences, 38*, 841–847.

Volpicelli, J. R., O'Brien, C. P., Alterman, A. I., et al. (1990). Naltrexone and the treatment of alcohol dependence. In L. D. Reid (Ed.), *Opioids, bulimia, and alcohol abuse and alcoholism*. New York: Springer-Verlag.

Volpicelli, J. R., Rhines, K. C., Rhines, J. S., Volpicelli, L. A., Alterman, A. I., & O'Brien, C. P. (1997). Naltrexone and alcohol dependence: Role of subject compliance. *Archives of General Psychiatry, 54*, 737–742.

Walsh, S. L., June, H. L., Schuh, K. J.., Preston, K. L., Bigelow, G. E., & Stitzer, M. L. (1995). Effects of buprenorphine and methadone in methadone-maintained subjects. *Psychopharmacology, 119*, 268–276.

Walsh, S. L., Preston, K. L., Bigelow, G. E., & Stitzer, M. L. (1995). Acute administration of buprenorphine in humans: Partial agonist and blockade effects. *Journal of Pharmacology Experimental Therapy, 274*, 361–372.

Walsh, S. L., Preston, K. L., Stitzer, M. L., Cone, E. J., & Bigelow, G. E. (1994). Clinical pharmacology of buprenorphine: Ceiling effects at high doses. *Clinical Pharmacology and Therapeutics, 55*, 569–580.

Woody, G. E., Luborsky, L., McLellan, A. T., O'Brien, C. P., Beck, A. T., Blaine, J., Herman, I., & Hole, A. (1983). Psychotherapy for opiate addicts: Does it help? *Archives of General Psychiatry, 40*, 639–645.

Woody, G. E., McLellan, A. T., Luborsky, L., & O'Brien, C. P. (1985). Sociopathy and psychotherapy outcome. *Archives of General Psychiatry, 42,* 1081–1086.

Woody, G. E., McLellan, A. T., Luborsky, L., & O'Brien, C. P. (1987). Twelve-month follow-up of psychotherapy for opiate dependence. *American Journal of Psychiatry, 144,* 590–596.

Woody, G. E., McLellan, A. T., Luborsky, L., & O'Brien, C. P. (1995). Psychotherapy in community methadone programs: A validation study. *American Journal of Psychiatry, 152,* 1302–1308.

Wurmser, L. (1978). *The hidden dimension.* New York: Aronson.

14

Integration of Theory, Research, and Practice
A Clinician's Perspective

Edward Rubin

Research over the past 15–20 years has made significant contributions to the advancement of knowledge in the field of alcohol and drug use disorders and treatment efficacy. "Treatment professionals are now in the fortunate position of being able to look to this literature and to make informed treatment decisions based on findings derived from this body of work" (Read, Kahler, & Stevenson, 2001, p. 232). Despite this proliferation of information, a considerable gap has been observed to exist between what science has shown to be effective and what is often practiced by the majority of clinicians in the substance abuse treatment field (Read et al., 2001). This present volume is replete with compilations and reviews of current findings in the field therefore is an important resource for practitioners and others who choose to avail themselves of the current knowledge and research.

This chapter illustrates how current research and a variety of treatment approaches can be integrated into a coherent approach to clinical practice. The challenge addressed here is to bring the thinking, clinical understanding, and decision making of the psychologist directly into the clinical situation. In an attempt to meet this challenge, information from firsthand experience is shared with readers in an expository, informal style. The author's approach in writing this chapter is to reveal his thinking and philosophy throughout his work with patients. In that manner, there may be a clearer example of how treatment research has influenced the thinking of a particular clinician, and how it has been incorporated into the treatment philosophy and approaches he uses.

GETTING STARTED

It is important to understand that my treatment approach is, at least in part, determined by my understanding that *therapist* effects have a profound impact on treatment outcome. I believe that what I bring into the therapy session can significantly influence treatment outcome. In my approach to treating addictions, I do not engage in what has traditionally been called "confrontation," although I do think that the way material is elicited and reflected back to the client can be confrontive in nature. By that I mean that it can aid clients in reflecting on themselves or their behavior (Yahne & Miller, 1999). You may also note that nowhere in this chapter do I refer to the "disease" of alcoholism or drug addiction. Frankly, it doesn't really matter to me *what* it is. In the context of treatment, it is much more important how the person seeking services conceptualizes the problem he or she is having. I am willing to accept whatever way he or she has found to explain his or her problem to him- or herself. I have not found it helpful to insist that a client label him- or herself in any certain way to be able to recover, so if someone wants to talk about his or her disease, I can accept and use that concept in our treatment together. If someone else thinks about his or her problem as a bad habit, I can also accept and work with that notion of the problem. In that sense, as well as in my general therapeutic stance, I have been described by other treatment professionals as "nontraditional" in my treatment approach (Washburne, 2001).

For me, treatment begins long before I see the client. In my practice, I make my own appointments most of the time. Therefore, I have an opportunity to speak to the person seeking my services before we meet in person. This provides the initial occasion for me to offer a therapeutic intervention, begin to establish rapport with this person, and provide the caller with a "taste" of my style and approach (Carroll, 1997). Quite a bit can happen in what most often is only a 5- to 10-minute phone interaction.

Most often, this conversation begins with me asking the person on the phone how I can help and how he or she got my name. Many of my referrals originate in managed care organizations or with other professionals, and this can be important for me to know. Obviously, these first questions allow the individual an opportunity to reveal a bit of the reason why he or she is calling. It is important to understand that he or she may be revealing the crux of the issue or very little of it. However, it does give me a chance to respond to him or her, which is the most important part of the exchange in terms of my engagement of this individual in the treatment process. During this brief exchange, my goal is to listen carefully to what the individual is saying, to reflect accurately and with empathy what I hear, and to begin to communicate my belief that change is possible. I also try to communicate my conviction that it lies within the power of this individual to positively effect any changes that he or she may choose to make in his or her (Miller & Rollnick, 2002). I take this initial approach almost without exception with clients seeking services with me.

I specialize in the treatment of addictions, so many of the referrals that I get are people who have had previous experiences with substance abuse treatment services. They are seeking help because they are struggling again with their addictive behavior. As a clinician whose treatment includes a variety of treatment interventions, I believe that there is "more than one way to skin a cat," and I often convey this message at the initial phone contact, if it seems indicated. This is my attempt to convey a sense of hope and positive expectation about the treatment experience that the individual may have with me. If people have had previous contact with a therapist, this also allows them to get some brief sense of my style to compare with their last treatment experience. This initial conversation ends with my asking if this individual still wants to schedule an appointment with me, and with an additional opportunity for the individual on the phone to ask me any immediate questions or express any concerns. I also provide directions to my office, discuss parking, and address insurance coverage briefly. I have found it helpful to inquire about insurance at this early juncture to make sure that we both know whether I am part of the insurance provider panel, should the individual have some sort of managed mental health and substance abuse coverage. This saves time and trouble if we discover that my services will not be covered, but it can also alert the caller if he or she needs to contact his or her insurance company prior to an initial visit to get a first session preauthorized. If we find that I am not going to be covered by the individual's behavioral health coverage, we discuss other payment options. If that is not acceptable, I always offer to recommend someone who is on their panel, if they are willing to share the provider list with me. When I am able to engage in this process, I find that 85–90% of clients will come for their initial appointment with me.

INITIAL ASSESSMENT

My practice takes place in two settings. Most of my time is spent as a psychologist in the Outpatient Behavioral Health Service at Aurora Sinai Medical Center, located in the central part of the city of Milwaukee, Wisconsin, where I am the clinical coordinator of dual diagnosis services. I also work in a private practice, located close to downtown Milwaukee, in the near northeastern suburbs of the city. Although these settings draw different clientele with very diverse experiences and backgrounds, it is obvious that much of the information that needs to be gathered about people seeking service is the same in both settings. The information that needs to be collected is determined in part by the various state and national licensing regulations under which outpatient clinics and hospitals operate in Wisconsin (Joint Commission on Accreditation of

Healthcare Organizations, 2002; Wisconsin Administration Code ss. HFS 75, 2001). Various professional codes of ethics (American Psychological Association, 1992) also mandate that enough data is gathered about the person seeking services so that clinical decisions can be made with confidence, and so that the practitioner can know that he or she is practicing within his or her range of expertise.

Data gathering obviously will take the form of a clinical interview, but it also may include information from collateral sources, as well as the use of psychological screening or assessment instruments (Allen & Columbus, 1995; Center for Substance Abuse Treatment [CSAT], 1999; Rubin, 1999). The decision about the use of assessment instruments depends upon the reason for the referral, one's usual practice patterns, and reimbursement considerations. Assessment instruments also may be used later in the process to aid in increasing motivation to change (CSAT, 1999). Most clinicians have developed their own outline of the information that they want to collect in the course of initial sessions with clients. There are also references that offer suggestions for information to be collected (Zuckerman, 2000). As part of my own process, however, I get some particular information that I may want to use later as part of engagement and motivational strategies (Miller, Zweben, DiClemente, & Rychtarik, 1992).

If one of the issues to be addressed is an addiction problem, it is important for me to inquire about periods of abstinence, sobriety, or moderation in the client's experience. This inquiry often leads to information about what has worked for the individual in the past to contribute to abstinence or control. This provides something positive to build on in the early stages of treatment and allows further expression of self-efficacy and hope.

Testing can also provide useful individualized information and feedback to the individual seeking treatment for his or her alcohol or drug addiction. I have found several instruments helpful in this regard, although I do not routinely administer them to everyone. They include the DrInC/InDuC (Drinkers Inventory of Consequences/Inventory of Drug Use Consequences); Audit (Alcohol Use Disorders Identification Test); CAGE Questions; and the RTC (Readiness to Change Questionnaire) (Rubin, 1999; Allen & Columbus, 1995). These all provide additional opportunities for more feedback to the client about his or her drug use and how it has affected him or her. The State of Wisconsin has also developed a tool to help determine any particular client's severity of need and the level of care that is suggested by that need. Called the Wisconsin Uniform Placement Criteria (WI-UPC), it or some acceptable, state-approved equivalent tool such as the ASAM-PPC (Gartner & Mee-Lee, 1995) is now mandated by administrative rule (Wisconsin Administrative Code ss. HFS 75, 2001) to be used statewide by all certified clinics providing substance use treatment for anyone seeking substance use treatment services. It was developed by workgroups of stakeholders (e.g., payers, providers, administrators, etc.) and is to be used not only to help determine initial need and level of care, but to determine any change in the level of care as well as to determine discharge from treatment services. Information about this tool can be obtained at the website for the Bureau of Substance Abuse Services, State of Wisconsin Department of Health and Family Services (*www.dhfs.state.wi.us/substabuse/index.htm*).

Challenge, confrontation, or "breaking through denial" are not part of my therapeutic approach at all. I utilize a strong motivation enhancement approach (Miller & Rollnick, 1991), and conceptualize therapeutic movement through the transtheoretical stages of change model (Prochaska, Norcross, & DiClemente, 1994). From this position, I do not find it helpful or therapeutic to "argue" with the client about whether or not he or she is an addict or alcoholic. In addition, I have found no value in having someone accept a particular label that he or she is an addict (Hester & Miller, 1995). I have realized that if the client and I engage in a power struggle, I will ultimately and always lose. It enhances engagement with the client to accept his or her view or philosophy or explanation of his or her problems, and to use that as a starting point for our treatment together.

SHAPING THE RELATIONSHIP

Often I find that the client is already being quite critical of him- or herself, especially if he or she has had treatment experiences in the past. These past treatments are often interpreted as failures now that the individual is again seeking help for the same problem. I frequently try to reframe the client's experience with stopping an addiction as being like learning to ride a bicycle. It is rare that someone learning this new behavior gets it right the first, the second, or even the third time he or she tries. Often, learning entails stopping or falling off the bicycle until the individual finally learns *all* the new behaviors needed to get this complex behavior correct. It is similar in working on changing addictive behavior too. It is sometimes hard to learn all of the new things that must be incorporated and synthesized to be able to do this. So, to succeed, the client must continue to work at it over and over until he or she gets it "right." This image seems to take some of the sting out of thoughts about previous unsuccessful efforts, and also proves useful during relapses.

One of my goals, not only during the "intake" or assessment phase of treatment, but throughout, is to shape my relationship with this individual such that it is different than any other that he or she has encountered in life. I do not want our relationship to "replicate" that with a parent, sibling, boss, lover, child, neighbor, or anybody else; rather, I want this therapeutic relationship to be unique. It is not that I deny the possibility of transference (or countertransference), but I recognize that there are likely already many people in this person's life who have criticized him or her and told him or her what, when, where, and how to do things. Our relationship needs to be different: it needs to be uncritical and empathic so that motivation to change can be increased (Miller, 2000).

As part of the assessment process, I gather both quantity and frequency data about drinking or drug use from the individual. As part of the individual feedback that I provide, I almost always try to estimate an annualized dollar amount that the individual has been spending on alcohol or other drugs. Obviously, this can add up to thousands or even tens of thousands of dollars, depending upon the drug of choice. After I calculate this figure and share it with the client, I almost invariably will hear that he or she "never thought about it like that before." I follow up this "revelation" by asking what else he or she might have done with that money. This begins to create some discrepancy between the client's reality of drug use or drinking and what he or she might have as goals or plans for his or her future. In addition, at least where alcohol is concerned, I provide information about how the client's quantity of consumption compares to general U.S. norms for drinking (Alcohol Research Group, 1995). I also may provide information about the caloric intake the client's drinking has entailed, and then translate that into weight gained. Another extremely helpful piece of data can be an estimate of BAC (blood alcohol concentration). This can be obtained from several World Wide Web sites (*www. ou.edu/oupd/bac.htm*; Markham & Miller, 1991). These pieces of information provide specific and individualized feedback that is unique to the particular person, and can be highly motivating as he or she considers changing addictive behavior. As part of this process, I inquire about the client's reaction to the individual pieces of information that I have provided. This gives me an opportunity to heighten discrepancies between what the client believes about his or her substance use and what the data is suggesting about it, further increasing client motivation to change.

AGREEING ON A PLAN OF ACTION

After an initial assessment period of gathering data (in whatever form that may take), it is useful to establish a treatment plan. Often, this is required by state certification and licensing authorities as well as by third-party payers, but it is a very powerful tool for establishing rapport and engagement with the client as well as providing direction for the treatment. After providing some feedback from the intake procedure, I ask the client what he or she would like to work on. It is important to note that I do not *tell* the client what I think the problem is (at least not right away), or what I think he or she should emphasize during the treatment. By asking what the *client* wants to focus on, I create an opportunity to model a collaborative relationship and support the idea that the ultimate responsibility for any changes that take place rests with the client (Hester & Miller, 1995). None of this precludes my sharing with the client my opinion about these matters—it is just that I find the timing for that interaction is very important.

I always hope that the client is going to establish at least one goal that has something to do with his or her use of alcohol or other drugs, but I must admit that there are times when I am surprised by the goals that some people want to set for themselves. It is not uncommon that the person sitting across from me has no intention of identifying substance use as an issue, at least at this time. Rather, a variety of other problems may be mentioned (e.g., marital difficulties, job problems, financial problems, stress, etc.). I know it may sound trite, but my work with clients leads me to really attempt to begin "where the client is at." In my experience as a consultant and supervisor, I have often found that this approach is paid lip service, but not practiced. To continue the engagement process, I find it is important to have that approach, so that the person with whom I am talking feels understood.

A number of years ago, Milwaukee County (1990) funded a study to examine the dropout of clients from publicly funded substance abuse treatment. This study concluded that there were two variables that contributed most to treatment dropout in this population. One factor had to do with access and ease of service delivery. More important for this discussion, the other factor was the perception on the part of those clients referred into or seeking substance abuse services that the therapist or counselor was not listening to what the client had to say. The clinician was perceived as having his or her own agenda to pursue, and therefore did not seem to value the issues the clients were sharing or said were important to them. Others (Center for Substance Abuse Treatment, 1999) have discussed the value of building a trustworthy working relationship with the client. Taking the client's agenda suggests that abstinence may not be the goal articulated by the client. A goal of moderation or controlled drinking or drug use may need to be seriously considered and, at least initially, become part of the treatment. In my experience, this is not uncommon. Often this goal may include a desire to stop using one drug (e.g., cocaine), but not another (e.g., marijuana). If the treating clinician cannot incorporate this harm-reduction approach (Marlatt, 1998; Volpicelli & Szalavitz, 2000) into his or her treatment philosophy, he or she should have a frank discussion with the client, and then make a referral to a clinician who can pursue harm reduction as a legitimate goal of treatment.

That is not to say that the therapist has to blindly agree that moderation or controlled use is the only, best, or safest treatment goal. However, if the agenda of the therapist (e.g., only and always abstinence) is not a goal that the client is willing to acknowledge and work toward achieving, the chances are great that either the client will terminate treatment prematurely because he or she feels that his or her issues are not being adequately addressed, or that he or she will continue to sit in the therapist's office, but to be passively unengaged in treatment. In either case, there is a reduced probability that the therapy experience with be of any help to the client. At this point, early in the treatment process, a decision will need to be made on the part of the therapist about whether he or she is willing to work on a non-substance-abuse goal or take a harm–reduction or moderation approach (Kishline, 1996) with this client. This willingness to work with articulated client goals reflects a number of the six elements used in brief motivational counseling approaches associated with positive change in behavior (Miller & Sanchez, 1994). The acronym FRAMES describes them:

FEEDBACK about personal risk or impairment
Emphasis on personal RESPONSIBILITY for change
Clear ADVICE to change
A MENU of alternative change options
Therapist EMPATHY
Facilitation of client SELF–EFFICACY or optimism

It is important to note that the giving of advice is clearly an integral part of this treatment approach. If the therapist finds him- or herself in a situation in which the client goal(s) is one with which he or she disagrees, the therapist can certainly let that be known at some point, but the therapist should not simply dismiss these goals out-of-hand because of that disagreement. It is also noteworthy that Miller and Hester (1995) have suggested that there are multiple treatment approaches that can be effective and incorporated into treatment systems. When an individual client is involved in selecting his or her own treatment goals and approach, his or her motivation and energy to stay engaged and commit to the change behavior is enhanced, and therefore treatment outcome is more likely to improve and treatment dropout is reduced.

My style and the therapeutic interventions described here are designed to match a client early in the change process – in either the precontemplation or contemplation stage of change (Prochaska et al., 1994). Various other therapeutic tasks and interventions are more appropriate for clients in the later stages of change (Miller & Rollnick, 2002). In terms of the transtheoretical stages of change model (Prochaska, DiClemente, & Norcross, 1992), when a client has moved into the preparation phase where he or she has decided that there is a problem that now must be addressed, my therapeutic stance shifts a little. Although continuing to utilize some of the techniques listed above, I generally move toward a more cognitive–behavioral approach (Monti, Abrams, Kadden, & Cooney, 1989).

Establishing goals for treatment begs the question about how the goals can be accomplished. This, too, is a question that should be addressed to the client. This change model suggests that if someone moves *too quickly* into the action of making changes, without adequate planning for that change, there can be a higher risk for relapse or recurrence of the problem behavior. Information as well as suggestions and advice may be offered by the therapist, if desired by the client, but the client does the work of change, and so the primary options and alternatives should come from the client him- or herself. This style also further reinforces the collaborative and respectful nature of the therapeutic relationship.

It is at this juncture that I generally present a menu of choices or treatment options to the client. I have not done this earlier in the treatment process because the client has not been ready to even consider change until now. Discussing ways to go about making changes before this stage would have been premature, and therefore it is quite likely that the client would have been unwilling or unable to follow through on any therapist suggestions or options. Options discussed now may be in response to interventions or treatment modalities about which the client has expressed some earlier interest, may be something he or she has tried in the past with some success in changing other behaviors, or may be the result of my question to the client about whether he or she would like to know what treatments are available.

Treatment options selected by the client are more likely to be carried through than those initially suggested, recommended, or insisted upon by the therapist. Choices may include the obvious alternatives; individual or group therapy, couple or family therapy, and services with a variety of intensities, such as a partial hospitalization program, an intensive outpatient program, or a level of involvement that is at the lowest intensity, which might include weekly individual, group, couple, or family sessions.

Outpatient detoxification is also discussed at this juncture, if warranted, and the use of other medications for the treatment of addictions (e.g., Antabuse, ReVia, Depade)might also be offered (McCrady & Epstein, 1999; Volpicelli & Szalavitz, 2000). In my case, as the result of an affiliation between the Aurora Sinai Medical Center and the Center for Addiction and Behavioral Health Research at the University of Wisconsin–Milwaukee, various medication and substance abuse treatment research trials may be going on, and I might offer these as alternatives for my client to consider. For example, in the recent past, there has been research on the effectiveness of the medication acamprosate, not yet available in the United States, as an adjunct treatment for alcohol dependence. In addition, this is one of the research sites for Project COMBINE (a follow-up to Project MATCH). The presence of this research unit at the medical center adjacent to the Behavioral Health Clinic presents a variety of additional treatment opportunities and client choices that otherwise might not be available.

After discussion about the choices available to the client and whatever preferences he or she may have, I often ask if I may offer some advice or suggestions. At this time, I may suggest a particular service or intensity of treatment to the client based on the information that the client has already presented to me and based on my experience in working with others with similar problems. I do not insist that the client accept the form of treatment that I recommend, as I do not want to get into a power struggle with the client (which I can only lose). I only offer my recommendations based on my observations of the person. However, as part of the stage of preparation for change, no matter what the client's choices may be, it is always worth asking how the client thinks that he or she will go about following through on those choices. If the client decides that part of his or her program will include attendance at some form of community-based self-help meeting, I almost invariably will inquire about the frequency with which he or she thinks he or she will attend. In fact, I may also challenge him or her a bit, asking if he or she thinks that that frequency is enough, too much, and so on. I ask about which particular meetings he or she thinks that he or she will attend as a way to help focus on issues of geography, time, and travel. Also, we talk about the start time of the intended meetings. This allows for a conversation about other things that might conceivably interfere with the client's good intentions. I ask the client when he or she thinks he or she might actually begin attending the meetings. All of this is designed to help the client think through how meeting attendance will impact on the rest of his or her life so that he or she can decide if there are things that need to be changed or rearranged to allow him or her to follow through. Finally, I often ask what he or she can foresee that might interfere with meeting attendance. This is designed to allow anticipation of any problems and to permit some problem solving ahead of time. That way, any "bumps in the road" are less likely to destroy positive plans for behavior change. This discussion is also a model for how I approach other involvements in which the client may be willing to participate as part of his or her treatment. We discuss therapy times, schedules, frequency, and anticipated interference in the same way that we discuss meeting attendance.

BEGINNING TREATMENT

Whether or not the client accepts my particular suggestions, we proceed to make the necessary arrangements to begin that treatment to which he or she agrees. This is when the client moves into the action stage of change. As part of this stage, almost invariably I will accept the level of care in which the individual is willing to participate. Although I may disagree, accepting the client's own sense about the level of care that he or she needs is much more likely to encourage the client to continue to participate in some form of treatment. I find that this approach also reinforces the idea that the client is always the final arbiter of his or her own fate, and so places in a very real way the responsibility for change upon the client. In addition it acknowledges that he or she knows him- or herself better than I do or ever can. Therefore, it is the client who is in a better position to know what would or would not be helpful for him or her. I have too often had the experience of an individual dropping out of treatment prematurely as a result of a mismatch between what I thought he or she needed (and referred him or her to), and what the client was willing to accept. If someone leaves treatment prematurely, I have no hope of being able to help him or her change their problem behaviors. If the client is willing to engage in *some* form of treatment experience, I can engage, motivate, and encourage change at the level the client is willing to accept and perhaps help that client eventually accept a different level of treatment if the original choice is inadequate.

Although I have already mentioned harm reduction, it is worthy of another discussion. That is because it is at this juncture that the client and I may be faced with a decision about the goals of treatment. Some clients are willing to consider the goal of abstinence for themselves, some want to work on moderating their substance use, and yet others want to quit using one drug or another, but continue using something else that they see as nonproblematic. From my perspective, all of these are goals may be reasonable and worthy of consideration. From the point of view of engagement and treatment adherence, it is important to recognize and accept the goals of the individual seeking our services rather than to impose our agenda on him or her. Of course, these original goals may not be our ultimate treatment goals. In addition, even though I may identify a substance abuse problem and a suitable goal at the outset of treatment, the client may not. I am willing to engage with the client in working on the issues that he or she has identified as meaningful and important. Although I feel free to offer my opinion about additional issues or goals that I may think are worth considering, I do not insist that someone work on goals that I have identified. It is the client's agenda that needs to be recognized and acknowledged as important, not mine. If I can acknowledge and begin with issues that the client has already identified as important (after all, that is what brought him or her in to see me in the first place), later I can often bring up the relationship between these problems that the client is willing to discuss and any addictive behaviors in which the client might also be engaging. Conversely, I also feel free to comment on whether or not it appears that we are making progress in treatment. If we seem to be foundering, I am not unwilling to point this out to the client. Hopefully, this will encourage a discussion of the current treatment goals and what we each see may be interfering with treatment. This will allow me to discuss the role that substance use may play. Ultimately, I am free to continue or not continue working in therapy with someone. If we do not seem to be able to make any treatment progress, I can end treatment and make an appropriate referral.

When creating a menu of options and choices for treatment services, a variety of treatment modalities are available. These range from services that are most intensive (e.g., inpatient detoxification) through decreasing levels of care and intensity. The system for which I work provides outpatient detoxification, residential care, partial hospitalization, and intensive outpatient treatment, as well as usual outpatient treatment. Modalities can include individual, group, family, or couple therapy.

SUPPORT GROUPS AND TREATMENT

There is an array of community-based self-help groups available. Although there are primarily 12-step programs (Alcoholics Anonymous, 1976) in Milwaukee, there are also a few Women for Sobriety (1993) and Secular Organizations for Sobriety (undated) groups available. I am hopeful that soon S.M.A.R.T. Recovery (1996) groups will also begin meeting, perhaps right at the medical center.

A discussion of the value of community-based self-help groups is always part of my work with clients. Over time, my enthusiasm for these programs has waxed and waned. Initially, during my first employment at a center for the treatment for substance use disorders, I worked at a traditional, 12-step-based treatment facility. This was, and I think continues to be, the treatment approach of the overwhelming majority of treatment centers available in the United States. At that time, virtually every clinician had, at the core of his or her clinical armamentarium, a 12-step-based philosophy as part of his or her treatment approach. Virtually every clinician also had *his or her own* 12-step experiences as part of *his or her own* recovery to draw on and share with the clients. At that time, I saw how the 12 steps were integrated into the universal, standard treatment program for alcohol and other drug abuse. Every patient at this facility was expected to attend 12-step meetings and everyone was expected to complete a certain number of steps prior to successful discharge. This included "doing" a fourth and fifth step (Alcoholics Anonymous, 1976). If this was not completed as expected, patients could be "unsatisfactorily" discharged from the program. As I gained experience, however, I began to see how this approach did not fit everyone. In the context of this setting, however, I found this a thorny issue to raise. I think now that I have come to a more balanced view of the role of self-help groups. Both anecdotally and in reviewing the findings of the Project MATCH Research Group (1997), I see that there are certain people for whom this is a great fit and for whom it can be of great use. I also understand the value of community or social connections as factors that can mitigate the risk of relapse to addiction. So, 12-step groups have become part of a more general discussion of community connections that I have with clients. This might also include a mention of other community support groups available, for example, involvement in a religious group, social activities, classes, and so on. The importance of these options varies depending upon each individual client, and what he or she brings into the treatment.

Choosing Specific Modalities

At Aurora Sinai Medical Center, there is not *a* substance abuse treatment "program" that everyone gets if they have the *proper* diagnosis. I present the array of services to the client, and then a negotiation takes place as to what seems to be indicated by the clinical aspects of the case and what the client is willing to do. Part of the initial assessment for substance abuse problems that I helped develop for Aurora Sinai specifically asks, "What does the client think will be helpful?" Often, in accepting the client's choice about treatment options, I will suggest that if what he or she has decided does not achieve the desired results, I will want to revisit the decision in the future, when I may suggest other treatment options. In addition, I want to point out that not achieving treatment goals at one level of care does not automatically result in a referral to a higher, more intensive, level of care. In fact, sometimes it is just the opposite. One of the assumptions that I make—and that I have helped integrate into the thinking and philosophy of other substance abuse treatment providers at the medical center—is that if one does not achieve his or her stated treatment goals at one treatment level, it may be because there has been a mismatch between what the client wants or is willing to do and what the treatment expected or provided. Therefore, at times this can result in a referral to a *less* intensive level of care (corresponding to an earlier stage of change).

With this in mind, one of the treatment experiences that clients are often willing to enter when they are unwilling to do something else is a group that I facilitate based on the transtheoretical stages of change and using a motivational enhancement treatment approach. Called the "Decision Group," it does not require abstinence prior to or even during participation; participants do not have to label themselves with any particular diagnosis, and no random urine drug screens are performed. The only requirements, as explained to the participants, is that they agree to attend, not to be intoxicated, and be willing to discuss the role of addiction in their lives. I have found the book by Velasquez, Maurer, Crouch, and DiClemente (2001) on group treatment very helpful in this regard. This group has become a resource as a "least restrictive" treatment option available to clients who do not seem to be ready for more intensive or demanding services. It provides an additional referral so that people do not have to be discharged from services as "unmotivated" or "in denial" (Hester & Miller, 1995, p. 68). Clients who have had previous treatment experiences elsewhere are often dumbfounded by this particular group. It is non-confrontational, encouraging, and positive about client participation. There are no overriding group goals or agendas except to enhance motivation for change, and no "hot seat." Rather, individual participants are able to set their own goals with regard to their addictive behavior. Therefore, it is not unusual to have some group members exploring the possibility of abstinence from some drug, others working on moderating their use, and yet others working on abstaining from one drug while moderating another. Most interesting to me is that the group members seem to have little problem dealing with these different and varying treatment goals. It seems that just as I am able to model acceptance of a variety of goals as reasonable and am also willing to engage with the client in trying to really achieve those goals, the group members are able to do the same.

The reactions of the substance abuse treatment staff to the Decision Group, however, have been a very different experience for me. When I began this group, the staff and former medical director accused me of being "an enabler." I was told that what I was proposing to do was unethical since I would be encouraging and permitting people to use drugs or drink. Also, by not taking a strong, confrontive, negative (or "anti-") stance, I would be exposing the medical center and myself to liability if something untoward were to occur. Over time, staff and administrative attitudes have changed significantly. Through training, consultation, ongoing seminars, and exposure to current literature (as well as some staff turnover), this treatment group, and the attitude and philosophy behind it, have become an accepted methodology and treatment modality at our facility and throughout the Aurora Behavioral Health substance abuse treatment services.

As mentioned previously, discussion takes place with the client about possible future renegotiations of treatment, depending upon the outcome of the current plan at the current level of intensity. That is, if an agreement is reached that the current goal of treatment is moderation of drinking, we also agree on a time frame in which we will work together on this goal. I then work *actively* with the client to teach behavioral ways to moderate his or her drinking or drug use. At the end of that time, as part of the review of the treatment plan, a new goal may be established. Often what occurs is that if the moderation goal is not achieved after the agreed-upon time, the goal of abstinence might then be reconsidered as more reasonable. Even when moderation is ultimately achieved, it is not unusual for the individual to decide that abstinence is really the outcome he or she seeks. Frequently, the client realizes while working on moderation that this particular goal requires significant work and concentration. It necessitates, for example, that the individual decide if he or she wishes to drink on any particular day. If he or she does, on that day he or she must then count his or her drinks, watch the passage of time, alternate alcoholic with nonalcoholic drinks, and so on. Individuals often reach the conclusion that it is simply easier to quit using altogether than to go through a rather elaborate formula each time they decide to drink. Nonetheless, from the perspective of engagement and motivation, it is much more powerful and respectful to work on the client's stated goal rather than to impose my own goal on the client. In addition, I know that it is possible for some people to moderate, since I have seen it done a number of times. Because of my willingness to acknowledge and respect the client's goals, and engage with each client in working on those goals, I find that my clients are more likely to continue to work with me even if their goals are not accomplished, and so dropout is reduced. Also, they are more likely to consider abstinence at this later point in the treatment process, even though they may have been reluctant to do so earlier.

INVOLVING OTHERS

Another service I frequently offer clients with substance abuse problems is meeting with a significant other. This is not "marriage counseling," although that may also be needed. The substance abuse treatment field recognizes that there is tremendous power in a collateral person to either positively or negatively influence behavior change, and that there is "evidence of reciprocal relationships between marital-family interactions and abusive drinking" (O'Farrell, 1995, p. 195). Thus, the value of meeting with a significant other in an attempt to engage her or him in supporting and contributing to the behavior change of the client can be quite potent in enhancing motivation and commitment to change (O'Farrell & Fals-Stewart, 2000). Such a meeting affords the spouse or partner a chance to relate to the substance abuser how his or her drinking or drug-using behavior has affected the couple and their relationship. It also provides an opportunity for the spouse or significant other to gain a clearer understanding of the problem, and to have input into the development of treatment goals.

One of my goals in involving others is to change "ineffective alcohol-related interactional patterns such as nagging about past drinking and drug use but ignoring current sober behavior" (O'Farrell & Fals-Stewart, 1999, p. 295) Positive interactions that can enhance and support the behavior change of the client can be identified and reinforced. Identification of interactions that interfere with or impede the treatment goals can also occur, and then be modified. Fletcher (2001) includes a chapter in her book on the role family members can play in supporting or hindering the recovery of a loved one, written from the perspective of the addicts themselves. All this can serve to increase marital or relationship satisfaction, which further enhances motivation to change the problem behavior.

THE PROCESS OF CHANGE

It is rewarding and fulfilling for me to see someone proceed through the stages of change from precontemplation to action. Although this process can take some time, it can also proceed relatively quickly. I have seen clients pass through two or three stages within one or two therapy sessions. Nonetheless, early in treatment, I may not meet weekly with an individual. He or she may not be ready for even that level of intensity of service. Of course, levels of intensity of treatment can be modified as the client moves through the stages. It is rare, however, for me to see someone through to the maintenance stage. Obviously, this takes place much later in his or her process of recovery. It may be as many as 6–9 months after the action of recovery begins that someone reaches the maintenance stage. Because of the time frame and the vicissitudes of behavioral health reimbursement, people who are doing this well in sustaining the changes that they have made seldom remain in treatment this long. My hope, assumption, and experience are, however, that if they run into trouble, they will feel that they can recontact me for additional help, if they need it.

Things seldom go smoothly. Changing problematic substance use is difficult, and there is no reason to expect that the client will "get it right" the first, the second, or even the third time that he or she tries, although I want to be encouraging and support his or her repeated attempts. This means that another stage that both the client and I frequently face is that of relapse, or recurrence. Often this occurs when change efforts have broken down, and the person has returned to drinking or drug use. It is important for the client to understand that I see this is a normal part of the change process for many people. My usual manner of dealing with this is to be supportive and encouraging. Even my language can contribute to conveying my attitude about this. As do others in the field, I often speak about "slips" or "lapses" rather than use the word "relapse." The latter, I teach, is a full return not only to drinking or drug use, but to the entire way of life engendered by that behavior. The other words ("slip," "lapse") I define as being much shorter in duration, with many fewer consequences. I am encouraging and supportive about the client's willingness to return to talk to me about the slip rather than dropping out of therapy.

I am positive about the experience of slips or lapses (e.g., the client stopped drinking or using drugs after a very short time, the client came in right away to discuss it, etc.), and focus instead on helping the client to see that somehow he or she managed *this* use differently than previously in his or her addiction experience. I also remind the person that this is a normal part of changing almost any behavior or habit, and then refocus the client's attention on how it happened. I try to reframe the client's perspective on the return to drinking or drug use as a learning experience. I wonder with the client about what he or she learned from this lapse and ask how he or she might do things differently in the future to avoid this happening in the same way again. There are similarities between some discussions that take place during this stage and those that took place during the preparation stage of change. We need to understand how the return to drinking took place and identify what the high-risk situation was or what the thinking or feelings were prior to the drinking or drug use that triggered the lapse or relapse. All this I hope to do without the client becoming so demoralized that he or she returns to and becomes stuck in earlier stages of change. Rather, I hope to encourage the client to keep moving on the earlier stages back to action again.

THE ROLE OF MEDICATION IN TREATMENT

It is important to discuss the role of medication in the treatment process—at least as I see it. My perspective is that the hard work of recovery rests with the individual who I am seeing. Ultimately, he or she is the one who must make the cognitive and behavioral changes that will result in the reduction of his or her drinking/drug use or his or her abstinence. Nonetheless, I also think that medication can play an adjunctive role in this process. I am not speaking to the important role of medication in the treatment of withdrawal, detoxification, or some of the medical consequences of withdrawal (i.e., DT's). Neither am I addressing the role that medication can play in the treatment of co-occurring psychiatric disorders, although much of my work has been with people suffering from multiple psychological problems in addition to addictions. Rather, I particularly address the role that I see medication can play in helping an individual maintain abstinence from alcohol (Antabuse), the reduction in urges or craving for cocaine (Seroquel) or in the reduction of urges or cravings, as well as the ultimate effect, of alcohol (ReVia, Depade, Neurontin, Topamax). These medications become part of the menu of options that I discuss with my client during the initial phases of treatment.

Often, I have found that patients are not initially interested in medication. They see its use as a "crutch," suggesting that they are not strong enough to do this on their own. Although not necessarily accepting their characterization of the use of medication, I will go with their treatment preference, reminding them that if things don't go as planned, they always have these additional options available at another time to reconsider, if they would like. In the course of my practice, I have found that there is little awareness of naltrexone and its apparent value in reducing the urges, craving, and effect of alcohol in some people. Once explained, however, I have found that there is more interest in that medication than in Antabuse. Volpicelli et al.'s work (1992) has convinced me that naltrexone should be an integral part of the menu of options offered for alcohol treatment. In any case, medication is most often seen by my clients primarily as a secondary option in their recovery. I am pleased to see that these options are available, and am anxiously awaiting the results of Project COMBINE to see if the medication acamprosate will also be useful in this phase of treatment. The more options and choices available to someone who is trying to recover, the more likely he or she will be able to find an approach, or combination of approaches, that will be successful for him or her. I always like to be in the position of telling a client that if something doesn't work for him or her, there are always more things that can be tried.

I should also mention that I am not at all opposed to working with people who may be taking methadone as part of a treatment program for opiate addiction or for chronic pain. I have found a certain prejudice among substance abuse treatment professionals and programs against those who may be using methadone as part of their recovery. My understanding of the research (Gerstein & Harwood, 1991) leads me to conclude that methadone maintenance is one of the most successful treatment approaches for opiate addiction. I found that I had to examine this prejudice against people taking methadone, where the primary treatment goal for the treatment I am working on with a client is abstinence from some other drug. I have been told by some counselors that the person using methadone is "stoned," "high," or intoxicated, and therefore is unable to fully utilize any therapy. In addition, others have said that they are "still using drugs," having only substituted one opiate for another. In my view, this latter perspective is a gross oversimplification, and I have not found the former view to be true. I will work toward *sobriety and abstinence* with them, as well as whatever other recovery issues may arise.

If the client is taking medication as prescribed, and is not using any other drugs, I have no difficulty describing this as "abstinence," or in seeing methadone as the harm-reduction technique that it is. There have also been times in my clinical experience where I have challenged a client's motivation by suggesting that he or she may not yet be ready for abstinence, or that it might be too difficult a goal for him or her to obtain at this time. At that time, I have suggested methadone maintenance as a viable alternative. Although generally not accepted by the client, it has allowed for a good discussion of the role of methadone in treatment as well as an examination of the client's current motivation and goals. There have also been times when the client thought about the suggestion, and returned wanting to pursue it. At those times, I have been more than willing to provide a referral to a local methadone maintenance program. Continuing to maintain my therapeutic relationship with that client becomes more difficult in that circumstance, however. This is because the methadone maintenance programs in this area take over the entirety of treatment once the client becomes involved with them. More methadone options will be available soon, however, as private physicians, with some additional training and education, will be able to prescribe methadone for maintenance programs in their own practices. It seems to me that closer collaboration in treatment will then be available among the client, the prescribing physician, and me.

CONCLUDING THOUGHTS

This chapter provides a brief sense of my style and approach to the treatment of addictions. Growing into this approach has been an evolution for me. When I first entered this field, over 25 years ago, treatment seemed simple: we knew what everyone's problem was, and everyone got exactly the same treatment (28 days of inpatient hospital stay). The longer I have been in the field, the more complex it has seemed to become. The field has certainly grown more sophisticated in its understanding of addictive behavior and behavior change. The people entering the addictions treatment field have changed over time and the clinicians have grown more sophisticated and open to advances in the field. We have rightly become more concerned with the integration of research and technology into the practice of our profession and see the value of applied research in our chosen area. We are also able to see more of the individual differences among those with addiction problems rather than seeing addictions, and addicts, as identical. The field has undergone a revolution during my time as a psychologist and addiction specialist. My practice has certainly undergone radical changes over time as addiction science has influenced myth and ritual, and I have moved from being seen as a pariah, enabler, and unethical practioner to a respected "mind healer." I want to stick around a while longer to see what else we learn.

REFERENCES

Alcohol Research Group. (1996). *1995 National Alcohol Survey of 10,000 households.* Berkeley, CA: Author.

Alcoholics Anonymous. (1976). *Alcoholics anonymous: The story of how many thousands of men and women have recovered from alcoholism* (3rd ed.). New York: Alcoholics Anonymous World Services.

Allen, J. P., & Columbus, M. (Eds.). (1995). *Assessing alcohol problems: A guide for clinicians and researchers.* (National Institute on Alcohol Abuse and Alcoholism Treatment Handbook Series 4, NIH Publication No. 95-3745). Bethesda, MD: U.S. Government Printing Office.

American Psychological Association. (1992). Ethical principles of psychologists and code of conduct. *American Psychologist, 47,* 1597–1611.

Beck, A. T., Wright, F. D., Newman, C. F., & Liese, B. S. (1993). *Cognitive therapy of substance abuse.* New York: Guilford Press.

Carroll, K. M. (1997). *Improving compliance with alcoholism treatment* (National Institute on Alcohol Abuse and Alcoholism Project MATCH Monograph Series Vol. 6, NIH Publication No. 97-4143). Bethesda, MD: National Institute on Alcohol Abuse and Alcoholism.

Center for Substance Abuse Treatment. (1999). *Enhancing motivation for change in substance abuse treatment* (Treatment Improvement Protocol Series No. 34, DHHS Publication No. [SMA] 99-3354). Washington, DC: U.S. Government Printing Office.

Fletcher, A. M. (2001). *Sober for good.* Boston: Houghton Mifflin.

Gartner, L., & Mee-Lee, D. (1995). *The role and current status of patient placement criteria in the treatment of substance use disorders* (Treatment Improvement Protocol Series No. 13). Rockville, MD: Center for Substance Abuse Treatment.

Gerstein, D. R., & Harwood, H. J. (Eds.). (1991). *Treating drug problems* (Vol. 1). Washington, DC: National Academy Press.

Hester, R. K., & Miller, W. R. (Eds.). (1995). *Handbook of alcoholism treatment approaches: Effective alternatives* (2nd ed.). Boston: Allyn & Bacon.

Joint Commission on Accreditation of Healthcare Organizations. (2002). *www.jcaho.org*

Kishline, A. (1996). *Moderate drinking: The moderation management guide for people who want to reduce their drinking.* New York: Crown.

Markham, M. R., & Miller, W. R. (1991). BACCuS: Blood alcohol concentration calculation system. (Version 2.01a) [Computer Software]. Albuquerque: University of New Mexico.

Marlatt, G. A. (Ed.). (1998). *Harm reduction: Pragmatic strategies for managing high-risk behaviors.* New York: Guilford Press.

McCrady, B. S., & Epstein, E. E. (Eds.). (1999). *Addictions: A comprehensive guidebook.* New York: Oxford University Press.

Miller, W. R. (2000). Rediscovering fire: Small interventions, large effects. *Psychology of Addictive Behaviors, 14*(1), 6–18.

Miller, W. R., & Rollnick, S. (2002). *Motivational interviewing* (2nd ed.): *Preparing people for change.* New York: Guilford Press.

Miller, W. R., & Sanchez, V. C. (1994). Motivating young adults for treatment and lifestyle change. In G. Howard & P. E. Nathan (Eds.), *Alcohol use and misuse by young adults* (pp. 55–81). South Bend, IN: University of Notre Dame Press.

Miller, W. R., Zweben, A., DiClemente, C. C., & Rychtarik, R. G. (1992). *Motivational enhancement therapy manual: A clinical research guide for therapists treating individuals with alcohol abuse and dependence* (National Institute on Alcohol Abuse and Alcoholism Project MATCH Monograph Series Vol. 2, DHHS Publication No. [ADM] 92-1894). Rockville, MD: National Institute on Alcohol Abuse and Alcoholism.

Milwaukee County. (1990). [Treatment of publicly funded substance abuse clients in Milwaukee County]. Unpublished raw data.

Monti, P., Abrams, D. B., Kadden, R. M., & Cooney, N. L. (1989). *Treating alcohol dependence: A coping skills training guide in the treatment of alcoholism.* New York: Guilford Press.

O'Farrell, T. O. (1995). Marital and family therapy. In R. K. Hester & W. R. Miller (Eds.), *Handbook of alcoholism treatment approaches: Effective alternatives* (2nd ed., pp. 195–220). Boston: Allyn & Bacon.

O'Farrell, T. J., & Fals-Stewart, W. (1999). Treatment models and methods: Family models. In B. S. McCrady & E. E. Epstein (Eds.), *Addictions: A comprehensive guidebook* (pp. 287–305). New York: Oxford University Press.

O'Farrell, T. J., & Fals-Stewart, W. (2000). Behavioral couples therapy for alcoholism and drug abuse. *Journal of Substance Abuse Treatment, 18,* 51–54.

Prochaska, J. O., DiClemente, C. C., & Norcross, J. C. (1992). In search of how people change: Applications to addictive behaviors. *American Psychologist, 47*(9), 1102–1114.

Prochaska, J. O., Norcross, J. C., & DiClemente, C. C. (1994). *Changing for good: The revolutionary program that explains the six stages of change and teaches you how to free yourself from bad habits.* New York: Morrow.

Project MATCH Research Group. (1997). Matching alcoholism treatment to client heterogeneity: Project MATCH posttreatment drinking outcomes. *Journal of Studies on Alcohol, 58,* 7–29.

Read, J. P., Kahler, C. W., & Stevenson, J. F. (2001). Bridging the gap between alcoholism treatment research and practice: Identifying what works and why. *Professional Psychology: Research and Practice, 32*(3), 227–238.

Rubin, E. M. (1999). Essentials of substance abuse assessment. In M. J. Ackerman (Ed.), *Essentials of forensic psychological assessment* (pp. 208–233). New York: Wiley.

Secular Organizations for Sobriety. (undated). *Secular Organizations for Sobriety: A self-empowerment approach to recovery.* Buffalo, NY: Author.

S.M.A.R.T. Recovery. (1996). *S.M.A.R.T. Recovery: Self-management and recovery training. Member's manual.* Beachwood, OH: S.M.A.R.T. Recovery Self-Help Network.

Velasquez, M. M., Maurer, G. G., Crouch, C., & DiClemente, C. C. (2001). *Group treatment for substance abuse: A stages-of-change therapy manual.* New York: Guilford Press.

Volpicelli, J. R., Alterman, A. I., Hayashida, M., & O'Brien, C. P. (1992). Naltrexone in the treatment of alcohol dependence. *Archives of General Psychiatry, 49,* 876–880.

Volpicelli, J., & Szalavitz, M. (2000). *Recovery options: The complete guide.* New York: Wiley.

Washburne, C. K. (2001, February). Mind healers. *Milwaukee Magazine,* pp. 43–53.

Wisconsin Administrative Code ss. HFS 75. (2001).

Women for Sobriety. (1993). *Welcome to WFS and the new life program.* Quakertown, PA: Author.

Yahne, C. E., & Miller, W. R. (1999). Enhancing motivation for treatment and change. In B. S. McCrady & E. E. Epstein (Eds.), *Addictions: A comprehensive guidebook* (pp. 235–249). New York: Oxford University Press.

Zuckerman, E. L. (2000). *Clinician's thesaurus* (5th ed.). New York: Guilford Press.

Index